FORENSIC MEDICINE AND TOXICOLOGY

VOLUME 1: BRIDGING SCIENCE, LAW, AND THE HUMAN BODY

Mohamed Amine Kerdoun

ALLIED HEALTH PRESS

Forensic Medicine and Toxicology

Volume 1: Bridging Science, Law, and the Human Body

Author: **Mohamed Amine Kerdoun**

Allied Health Press
4164 Lakeshore Road
Burlington ON L7L 1A4
Canada
www.alliedhealthpress.com
Email: orders@arclereducation.com

ISBN: 978-1-77956-842-7

ABOUT THE AUTHOR

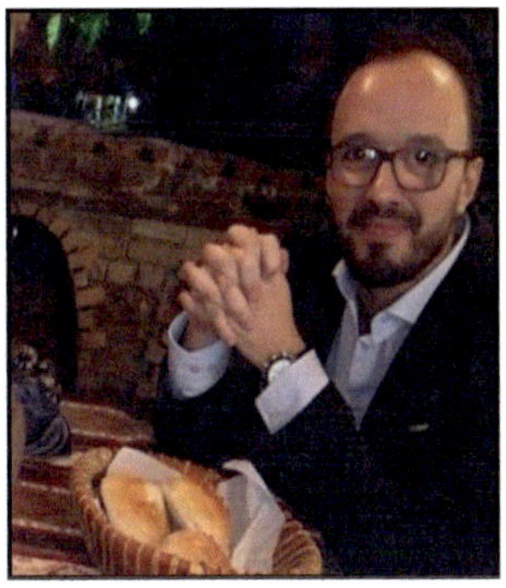

Amine Kerdoun, PharmD, PhD, is an associate professor of Toxicology at the Faculty of Medicine, Kasdi Merbah University in Ouargla, Algeria. A specialist in medical and environmental toxicology, he brings over a decade of academic, clinical, and regulatory experience to his work. Dr. Kerdoun holds a Doctorate in Medical Sciences with a focus on toxicology, along with degrees in pharmacy and specialized medical studies from leading Algerian institutions. His research focuses on chemical risk assessment, heavy metals, endocrine disruptors, and cosmetic safety, with numerous peer-reviewed publications in international journals. A respected educator and scientific communicator, Dr. Kerdoun combines rigorous toxicological expertise with a commitment to public health protection and regulatory excellence across global frameworks.

Brief Table of Contents

Getting Started with This Book

Chapter Openers

A list of Chapter Outline is presented providing a brief Introduction to what will be covered in the chapter.

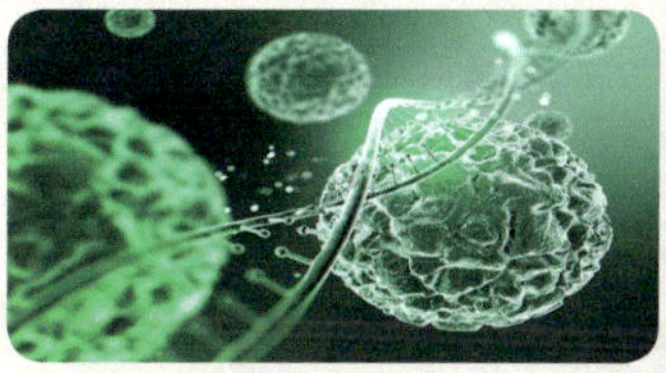

LEARNING OBJECTIVES

After studying this chapter, you will be able to:

1. Discuss the scientific method in biology;
2. Explain the cell theory;
3. Discuss the genetics and heredity;
4. Evolution and natural selection;
5. Focus on ecology and ecosystems;
6. Learn about human biology;
7. Evaluate the plant biology;
8. Explain the microbiology;
9. Focus on current trends in biology.

Introduction

Often referred to as the science of life, biology is a broad field of study aimed at comprehending the several kinds of life on Earth, from tiny creatures to sophisticated multicellular entities. Comprising several subfields, including molecular biology, ecology, and evolutionary biology, each of which advances our knowledge of living systems, this field clarifies the mechanisms controlling life events, including development, reproduction, and interaction with the surroundings, which is the central goal of biology. Moreover, biology fills in the void between the natural sciences and medicine by offering a necessary understanding of health, illness, and the interactions between organisms and their environments. Dealing with urgent global issues such as climate change, biodiversity loss, and new diseases depends on an awareness of these complex biological interactions, therefore highlighting the critical part biology plays in modern civilization. Fundamentally, biology explores and tests ideas about the living world using the scientific method. Through methodical observation and experimentation,

1.1. The Scientific Method in Biology

Learning Outcome

1. Describe the steps of the scientific method;
2. Focus on hypothesis formation;
3. Learn about experimental design.

Learning Outcomes

The beginning of each section of every chapter contains a set of Learning Outcomes that inform students of concepts they should understand. These outcomes help students understand what they should be able to do if they have mastered the material in that section.

Test Your Knowledge

Throughout each chapter, Test Your Knowledge cues you to note which topics have been covered and to self-test your understanding of the material presented.

Test Your Knowledge

1. Explain why correlation does not imply causation in scientific experiments.
2. How does the scientific method help reduce the influence of personal opinions in research?

Chapter Summary

The Summary Section appear at the end of each chapter and summarize main concepts covered throughout the chapter. These points provide key concepts in an engaging and meaningful way.

Summary

The investigation of biological principles highlights the importance of a comprehensive view of life by reflecting the intricate interactions that occur within living systems. The complexity of biology goes beyond individual species or systems, as this essay highlights; it also includes the interactions that mold ecosystems and affect biodiversity. Researchers can conduct in-depth analyses of metabolomic data using sophisticated technologies like MetaboAnalyst, which offer insights into the molecular mechanisms underlying these interactions. As demonstrated by the developments in MetaboAnalyst, for example, the integration of diverse omics data promotes a thorough understanding of metabolic pathways and helps identify important biological markers necessary for research on development and disease (Chong et al., 2018). Additionally, the phenomenon of ecological invasions is a key component of biological research and a vital field of study. The introduction of non-native species into unfamiliar habitats has significant ramifications and calls for multidisciplinary management strategies. Examining the origins and effects of these biological incursions, invasion science has become a crucial field that highlights the need to comprehend ecological dynamics and community interactions. As interest in biological invasions increases, new findings are emerging that put conventional ecological theories and practices to the test. The importance of incorporating various scientific viewpoints is shown by this developing discipline, which also highlights how invasive species shape ecosystems and advances our knowledge of ecological resilience (David et al., 2013). When taken as a whole, these discoveries from invasion science and metabolomics highlight the value of multidisciplinary biology research. Fostering cross-disciplinary collaboration and utilizing technological breakthroughs to improve our comprehension of intricate biological interactions are crucial as we look to the future of biological research. In addition to deepening our understanding of the complexities of life, this method lays the groundwork for tackling urgent environmental issues. Future studies can ensure the continued relevance of biology in a world that is constantly changing by acknowledging the interconnection of biological systems and opening the door to creative solutions that support sustainability and biodiversity conservation. We might imagine a thorough comprehension of life that serves both academia and society at large through ongoing investigation and integration of scientific knowledge.

Knowledge Assessment

The chapter includes material designed to review and reinforce each content. It includes Critical Thinking Questions to help test of your understanding of information presented in the chapter and Short answer Questions to review your understanding of the key concepts presented in the chapter.

Critical Thinking Questions

1. **Who is known as the "Father of Modern Biology"?**
   a. Aristotle
   b. Charles Darwin
   c. Gregor Mendel
   d. Louis Pasteur
2. **What is the basic unit of life?**
   a. Atom
   b. Molecule
   c. Cell
   d. Organism
3. **Which branch of biology studies the interaction of organisms with their environment?**
   a. Genetics
   b. Ecology
   c. Physiology
   d. Botany
4. **Which macromolecule is the main source of energy for living organisms?**
   a. Proteins
   b. Lipids
   c. Carbohydrates
   d. Nucleic acids
5. **DNA is primarily responsible for which function in living organisms?**
   a. Energy production
   b. Protein synthesis
   c. Storing genetic information
   d. Regulating body temperature

Short Answer Questions

1. What is biology, and why is it important to study biology?
2. What are the three main domains of life, and how are they different from one another?
3. Define homeostasis and give an example of how it works in living organisms.
4. What is the cell theory, and why is it fundamental to biology?
5. How do autotrophs and heterotrophs differ in the way they obtain energy?
6. What is the scientific method, and how is it applied in biological research?
7. Discuss how biology helps address global challenges such as climate change, disease, and food security.
8. Explain the levels of biological organization from the smallest unit to the largest. Provide examples at each level.
9. Describe the relationship between structure and function in biology, giving specific examples from cells or organs.
10. How has the discovery of genetics shaped our understanding of inheritance and variation among organisms?

Supplementary Materials

Key Terms: A list of key terms is given for quick reference

KEY TERMS FROM THIS CHAPTER

Annotation enrichment analysis	Biological structure	Cell
Cell theory	Cellular structure	Ecology
Ecosystems	Genetics	Human biology
Microbiology	Natural selection	Organism
Plant biology		

Further Resources: Recommendations for additional readings, websites, and multimedia resources.

References

1. Argelaguet, R., Velten, B., Arnol, D., Dietrich, S., Zenz, T., Marioni, J. C., Buettner, F., et al. (2018). Multi-omics factor analysis—A framework for unsupervised integration of multi-omics data sets. *Molecular Systems Biology, 14*. https://doi.org/10.15252/msb.20178124.
2. Bacher, S., Blackburn, T. M., Essl, F., & Genovesi, P. (2017). *Socio-Economic Impact Classification of Alien Taxa (SEICAT)*. https://core.ac.uk/download/286567949.pdf (accessed on 8th March 2025).
3. Barnett, R., Brace, S., Cucchi, T., & Dobney, K. (2013). *Divergent Evolutionary Processes Associated with Colonization of Offshore Islands*. https://core.ac.uk/download/20664364.pdf (accessed on 8th March 2025).

Detailed Table of Contents

CHAPTER 3

Identification in Forensic Medicine and Toxicology 65

CHAPTER 4

CHAPTER 5

Postmortem Changes 119

CHAPTER 6

Medico-Legal Autopsy 153

CHAPTER 8

Mechanical Injuries 211

CHAPTER 9

Firearm Injuries 241

LIST OF FIGURES

PREFACE

Forensic medicine and toxicology are important at the meeting point of medicine, science and law. Clinical knowledge, laboratory work and investigative methods are used in this field to respond to questions that occur in legal cases. To find the time of death, the cause and any toxins, forensic scientists rely on anatomy, pathology, chemistry and pharmacology. Being skilled in these areas helps collect, analyze and present evidence scientifically which supports strong decisions made by the courts.

Toxicology helps us spot and measure substances that may change how people behave, make them unable to function or cause death. They use advanced tools such as gas chromatography–mass spectrometry and immunoassays, to look for poisons, drugs of abuse and environmental contaminants. When experts know about dose–response relationships, metabolic pathways and how chemicals are absorbed and excreted, they can determine the role of chemicals in various injuries or deaths. Because new types of drugs and chemicals are always being discovered, knowing the latest in toxicology is essential for handling all types of cases.

Forensic Medicine and Toxicology introduces the main ideas and methods used in medico-legal investigations. The book is written to be used as a textbook and a reference manual and it merges theory with practical examples. Strong focus is given to modern approaches, standard practices and what is expected of practitioners in terms of ethics. The book includes pictures and examples to link the findings in the lab with what doctors observe and what is needed in court. The book is set up so that the reader can follow a logical sequence of topics.

Chapters 1–3 explain the terms used, describe important events in history and review the laws that oversee expert testimony. Chapter 1 outlines the main areas of forensic medicine, explains important ideas and explains how a medical expert fits into the process. The second chapter looks at the rules for conducting trials which evidence is allowed and how medical reports are involved in court decisions. Chapter 3 covers how to identify individuals by fingerprinting, dental records and using molecular methods and it explains the proper handling of samples in toxicology.

The focus of chapters 4–7 is on the legal side of death. Chapter 4 explains that death can be natural, accidental, suicidal, homicidal or undetermined and it looks at how evidence at the scene and a person's medical history help reach a conclusion. In Chapter 5, the sequence of changes after death such as rigor mortis, livor mortis and putrefaction, is described, along with the things that can alter the speed of decomposition. Chapter 6 explains how to perform an autopsy by covering the external check, internal examination, organ sampling and documenting the results. The chapter explains the process of finding the cause, manner and mode of death by using differential diagnosis and combining autopsy findings with toxicology and histology.

In these chapters (8–12), the book explores the different ways injuries occur and how to interpret them. Chapter 8 discusses mechanical injuries, including abrasions, lacerations, contusions and fractures and looks at the way wounds form and the biomechanical forces involved.

Chapter 9 deals with firearm wounds by looking at ballistics, entrance and exit traits and how to reconstruct the events. Chapter 10 discusses transportation incidents, paying attention to the way vehicles crash, the movements of victims and the pattern of injuries. Chapter 11 examines thermal injuries which include burns and asphyxia from fire, by discussing how to classify them, measure their depth and tell the difference between pre- and postmortem scorching. Chapter 12 discusses deaths caused by asphyxia such as strangulation, suffocation and drowning and explains the signs found in the body that agree with what witnesses and experiments show.

The book is written for medical students, postgraduate trainees, forensic pathologists, toxicologists, legal professionals and allied experts who are involved in medicolegal investigations. Clear explanations, lists of steps to follow and examples of cases are included to show how things are done in both normal and challenging situations. It can be used as a primary learning tool or a desk reference and this book Forensic Medicine and Toxicology aids in making practitioners knowledgeable, skilled and dedicated to scientific accuracy and justice.

INTRODUCTION TO FORENSIC MEDICINE

1

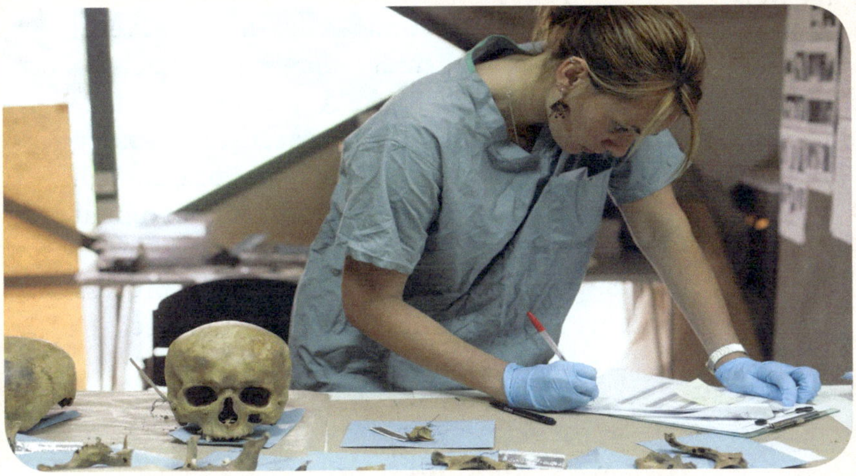

LEARNING OBJECTIVES

After studying this chapter, you will be able to:

1. Understand the role of forensic pathology;
2. Explain forensic toxicology;
3. Focus on forensic anthropology;
4. Describe forensic psychology.

Introduction

Medicine and law sometimes meet in ways that lead to surprising arguments and this is becoming more noticeable lately. With our society becoming more complicated, forensic medicine appears as a helpful link between medical information and court decisions which also raises ethical issues. Handling ethical problems that arise when health laws are questioned is as important as solving crimes in the field. Look at how technology is shaking things up, for instance, 3D printing has flipped the script on making patient-specific body models, giving surgeons a better chance to plan and execute surgeries with greater care and precision (Aimar et al., 2019). Then there's image segmentation driven by deep learning, which is increasingly stepping in to sort evidence and even piece together crime scenes in ways we haven't seen before (Aggarwal et al., 2021). Generally, following these changes is important for knowing how forensic medicine is improving and what it could mean for future cases.

Definition of Forensic Medicine

There are times when medicine and law come together and it's especially interesting when medical knowledge helps solve tough legal issues. Forensic medicine helps connect the knowledge from hospitals to the legal world and it often introduces a new point of view to legal arguments. It deals with the specifics, checking injuries, figuring out how someone died and analyzing biological evidence which are usually important in criminal and civil cases. As well as assembling the facts of a case, this area can also influence legal rules that could help avoid similar crimes in the future. Understanding the significance of these forensic hints can make sure that verdicts are based on real science which helps keep the public safe. And then, breakthroughs like using biodegradable polymers in gathering evidence show that this area is always evolving—pushing for creative, innovative methods (Bairoch, 2018; Samir et al., 2022).

Historical Background

Medicine and law have been linked for a long time which has influenced the development of forensic science in messy ways. With time, the use of blood and hair analysis in criminal cases has grown to be very important. Hair toxicology, for example, popped up as a way to spot long-term drug use, even though its reliability hinges on the natural texture of hair and the risk of outside contamination, things you need to get a handle on (Hubbard, 2025). Also, alcohol influence charts are interesting; for example, the DuBowski table. It was first introduced way back in 1957 and has been tweaked over the years to break down how alcohol affects someone based on blood-alcohol levels, while also factoring in personal differences that can throw off breath tests and stir up legal issues (Jones, 2024). In short, these changes prove that forensic medicine is always evolving and sometimes mixes old methods with new ones.

Importance in the Legal System

Many courtroom decisions are influenced by scientific analysis and this is especially clear when forensic medicine and the law intersect. Forensic specialists connect the evidence from a medical report to the legal questions and occasionally they help fill in gaps that nobody expected.

Take toxicology tests, for instance—they're pretty much key to figuring out the circumstances around a death, as several studies have repeatedly shown (Candiaet al., 2022). Modern tools, like AI platforms such as ChatGPT, are now helping speed up research and smooth out legal document work, though there are still some nagging concerns about ethics and accuracy (Sallam, 2023). Basically, joining forensic science with the legal process improves justice and points out the need to update methods to follow today's laws.

Role of Forensic Medicine in Criminal Investigations

Investigating crimes can be messy and you often need to use information from various areas. Forensic medicine comes in with its science and expert opinions which often have a big impact on the outcome of a case. Mass graves are often examined at international tribunals and the process of looking at the remains can link specific evidence to a bigger legal case in surprising ways. In many situations, the careful process of collecting and making sense of forensic details builds what some call a dependable "forensic truth" that's strong enough to face tough courtroom challenges (Klinkner et al., 2008). Generally speaking, the confidence in these findings comes from solid methods like cross-checking details and even presenting different expert views (Klinkner et al., 2009). All in all, forensic medicine is essential to the stability of our justice system.

Interdisciplinary Nature of Forensic Medicine

Forensic medicine encounters many tough problems that require specialists from many areas. Knowledge of law, psychology, biology and sociology adds to the understanding of both criminal acts and what happens around them. Sexual crimes are a good example – the combination of physical signs and social factors adds complexity that is usually very important in court and in investigations. Criminal sexology has, in most cases, underlined the need to look at things from several angles when dealing with debates around consent and even the subtle dynamics of violence, as noted in recent changes in criminal law (Volobuyeva, 2024). At the same time, forensic science appearing in movies and news demonstrates that it involves serious research as well as things we see in daily life. All in all, cooperating with different experts allows forensic medicine to adapt to the changes in society.

Overview of Forensic Medicine Subfields

Many branches of forensic medicine work together to make the field rich and varied. Forensic pathologists often do autopsies to determine the cause of death which often reveals important facts for homicide investigators. At the same time, forensic toxicology examines bodily fluids to find drugs or toxins which is very important in both criminal and civil matters. If soft tissues are missing, forensic anthropology takes over to find and identify bones, using its skills. Lately, new technology has led to digital forensics—a branch that uses artificial intelligence and data analysis to unravel intricate digital evidence (Adel, 2023). Generally speaking, as techniques keep evolving these areas are leaning on ideas from one another, slowly reshaping the whole investigative process (Vodanović et al., 2023).

Ethical Considerations in Forensic Medicine

Forensic medicine calls for a new approach to the ethical principles it follows. Those in this profession often have to balance seeking justice with the duty to protect the rights of the people involved, mainly when the individuals are vulnerable. In many cases, the picture gets even murkier when new tech like AI is thrown into the mix in healthcare; it might bring impressive perks yet also stir up risks such as hidden bias and murky transparency, as noted in 58/60 records flagging clinical ethics concerns (Sallam, 2023). When crises hit—think the SARSCoV2 pandemic—the rapid whirlwind of information makes it clear that contact tracing needs some solid ethical guardrails to protect privacy while still addressing widespread health challenges (Ferretti et al., 2020). Maintaining trust and the integrity of forensic work depends mainly on having a solid ethical framework in place.

Current Trends and Developments

Because of modern approaches to education and data management, forensic medicine is going through unexpected changes. During the COVID-19 period, for example, med students experienced a move to online classes that, in most cases, saved them time and proved effective—even though they still bumped into tech glitches and sometimes found the way content was delivered a bit off (Khalil et al., 2020). At the same moment, changing methods for handling data are pushing forensic pathology ahead, mainly because many systems are still stuck using paper which slows down information access and leads to confusing reports. This lag can end up blocking deeper research and stop tailored public health studies in forensic contexts, as noted in recent findings (Prahladh et al., 2020). In short, embracing digital advances helps with learning and also leads to better data handling and better outcomes in forensic medicine.

1.1. The Role of Forensic Pathology

Learning Outcome

1. Understand the definition and scope of forensic pathology;
2. Explain autopsy procedures and techniques;
3. Know the determining cause and manner of death;
4. Discuss the identification of decomposed bodies;
5. Describe the role in homicide investigations;
6. Focus on forensic pathology in civil cases;
7. Identify challenges faced by forensic pathologists;
8. Explain future directions in forensic pathology.

Forensic pathology is very important in solving legal cases—it is a key part of finding justice. This area isn't limited to using checklists; it involves examining a body closely and using tests to find out the cause of death which can greatly influence a criminal case. Experts here use both practical tests and lab methods, sometimes finding evidence that changes or supports the main story presented in court. What forensic scientists discover helps law enforcement solve crimes and also guides how the legal process is carried out, making sure justice is done fairly. And as forensic science keeps evolving, new tools like next-generation sequencing (NGS) are increasingly stepping into the picture—boosting both the clarity and precision of these tests and underscoring the lasting impact of forensic pathology in the broader realm of forensic medicine (Sane et al., 2023; Satam et al., 2023).

1.1.1. Definition and Scope of Forensic Pathology

Forensic pathologists have to use their medical skills and understanding of the law to solve puzzling cases about death. It is located where healthcare and the justice system meet – autopsies and postmortem exams help solve cases in court. Forensic pathologists go into great detail examining injuries, laboratory findings and diseases to ensure all reasons for death are clear in the legal documents. Most of the time, they do not limit their role to naming the crime; they also collect evidence needed for criminal investigations and trials. With cases getting trickier, especially amid new health challenges, there's a growing push to mix in modern tools like machine learning for sharper diagnostic accuracy, as pointed out in several healthcare studies (Qayyum et al., 2020). Ultimately, the wide-ranging nature of forensic pathology truly mirrors its key role in linking scientific insight with the demands of societal justice (Lechien et al., 2020) (Figure 1.1).

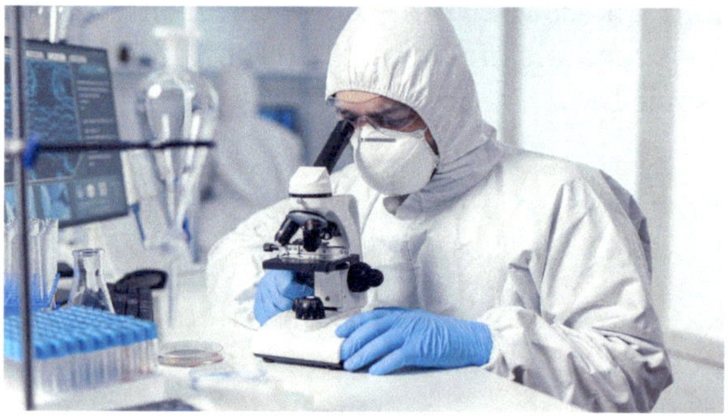

Figure 1.1. Forensic pathology.

Source: https://medlifemastery.com/wp-content/uploads/2023/09/Best-Medical-Schools-for-Forensic-Pathology.jpg.

1.1.2. Autopsy Procedures and Techniques

Forensic science has developed a lot, bringing new imaging technology into the autopsy process. Nowadays you see methods like post-mortem computed tomography (PMCT)—which quickly reveals a body's internal layout—and post-mortem computed tomographic angiography (PMCTA) that, in many cases, spots lesions more effectively; this combination often beats the old-school approach when it comes to flagging key anatomical irregularities. In most studies, research even shows that PMCTA picks up around 96.1% of skeletal lesions compared to roughly 65.4% using traditional autopsy methods (Grabherr et al., 2018). Meanwhile, although PMCT is valued for its rapid peek at internal structures, advances such as three-dimensional surface scanning can enhance external assessments, thereby broadening what forensic investigators have at their disposal (Grabherr et al., 2017). To summarize, merging modern imaging with time-tested practices seems to not only refine post-mortem investigations but also nudge diagnostic accuracy in forensic medicine just a bit higher (Figure 1.2).

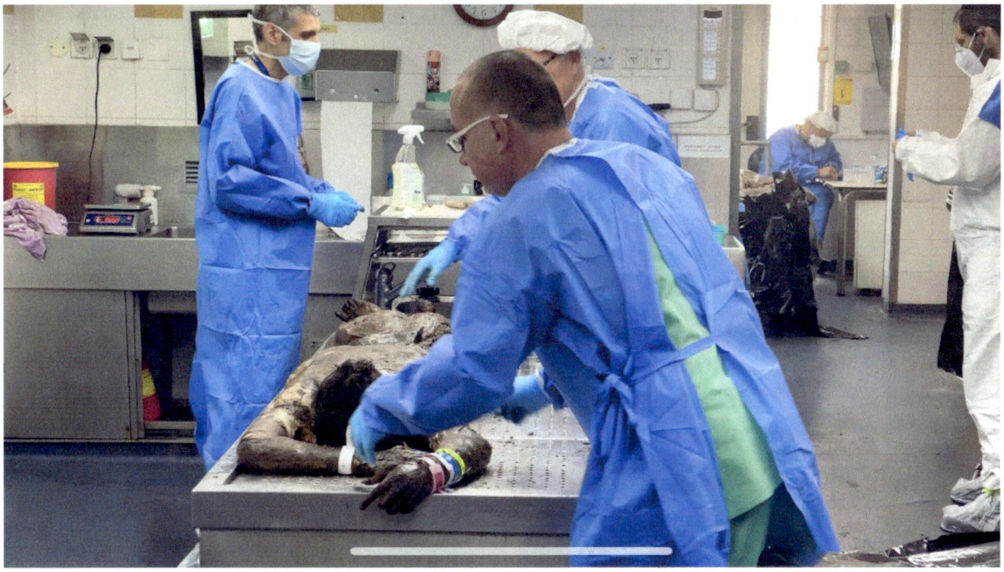

Figure 1.2. Autopsy procedures.

Source: https://themedialine.org/wp-content/uploads/2023/10/IMG_2899-e1697755199710.jpg.

1.1.3. Determining Cause and Manner of Death

Such exams are not only about identifying the deceased—they also try to figure out the cause of death. In a lot of cases, medicolegal autopsies examine both obvious changes and the less noticeable signs in the body to determine how and why someone died, especially if the death was sudden or had no clear reason. One recent study even pointed out using bladder wash samples for toxicology, hinting that these less common specimens could come in handy when the usual ones aren't up to the task (Rodda et al., 2025). Generally, this argument is moving forensic pathologists to consider new possibilities which is quietly changing how forensic science is practiced. Evaluating deaths from accidents, poisonings, and other unnatural causes also shows why it's so important to keep a thorough, systematic eye on how these patterns emerge, all of which feeds into public health strategies (Ranjan et al., 2024). To summarize, figuring out not just the cause but also the manner of death remains a cornerstone of forensic work, steering legal processes and preventive action alike (Figure 1.3).

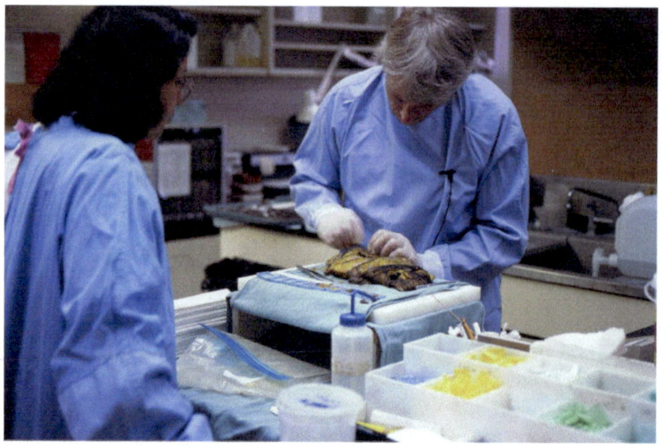

Figure 1.3. Determining cause and manner of death.

Source: https://s.hdnux.com/photos/01/40/01/46/25172370/3/ratio3x2_1920.jpg.

1.1.4. Identification of Decomposed Bodies

When a body is very decomposed, forensic investigators must use exhumation to find out what happened. The process is started when a judicial magistrate gives permission which may be affected by legal, cultural or social factors. According to one study involving 258 forensic exhumations, the decomposition of internal organs makes it very hard to determine the exact cause of death.

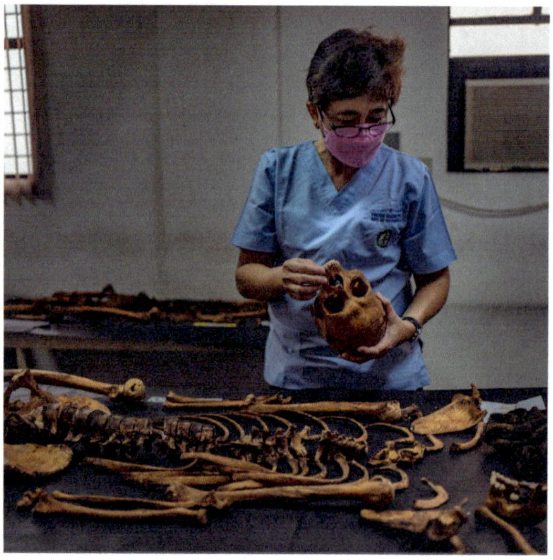

Figure 1.4. Exhumation is vital for forensic investigators trying to figure out what happened in a death—especially when a body is so decomposed that little remains intact.

Source: https://static01.nyt.com/images/2022/06/03/world/03philippines-pathologist-profile-01/03philippines-pathologist-profile-01-mediumSquareAt3X.jpg.

How long a body's been buried, the local environmental conditions, and the type of injuries all play their part, frequently resulting in findings that aren't clear-cut because soft tissue markers may no longer be present (Awan et al., 2023). With rising legal disputes about death causes, there's, in most cases, a growing push for better, more efficient protocols—highlighting the urgent need for procedures that are both careful and thorough (Samir et al., 2022) (Figure 1.4).

1.1.5. Role in Homicide Investigations

Many people might not realize that entomology is important, but even tiny insects found at crime scenes can give important details about the timing of the death. Forensic medicine dives into these details, piecing together nature's own hints—as Lutz et al. (2021) point out, bug traces on remains, thanks to species that follow almost clockwork life cycles under certain environmental conditions, can sketch out a rough timeline. It is especially important to be this precise, mainly when determining when a person died which is a key issue in legal cases. At the same time, looking at a suspect's behavior—for instance, noticing signs of psychopathy—can offer extra insights into motives and possible dangers; Sanz-García et al. (2021) even stress that these psychological angles can gently steer interrogation methods and help ward off future crimes. In a lot of situations, the combination of natural signs and clues from the suspect's actions helps investigators understand what happened. All in all, forensic medicine helps protect our communities as well as help solve crimes.

1.1.6. Forensic Pathology in Civil Cases

Civil cases often rely on forensic pathologists when we need to understand the cause of sudden deaths or injuries.

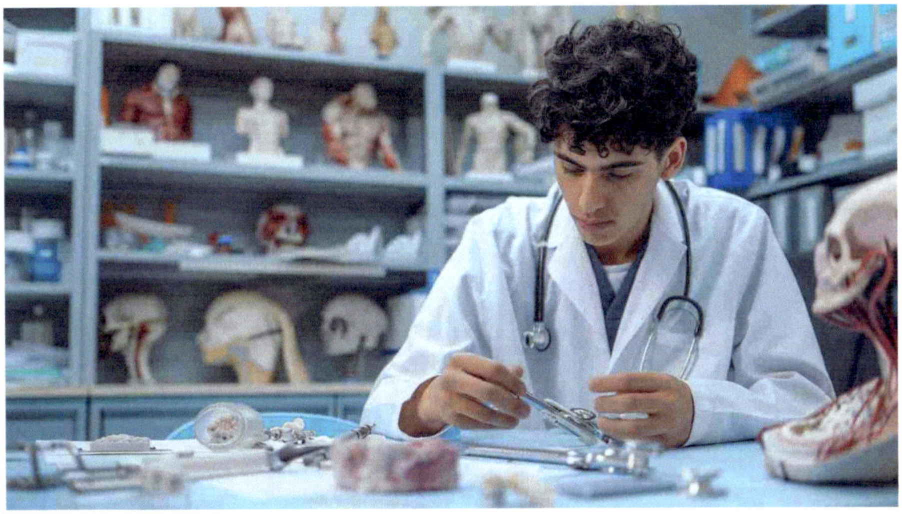

Figure 1.5. Forensic pathologists are a key part of civil cases—especially when sudden deaths or injuries leave us with unanswered questions.

Source: https://www.apoia.com.br/_next/image/?url=https%3A%2F%2Fapoia-images-production.s3.amazonaws.com%2Fb1aa9ccd-df6d-405c-b7ba-977d3f1bf5ba.png&w=3840&q=15.

They are involved in many cases, not only criminal, by helping to decide who is liable, what insurance covers and how much compensation should be given. Today, civil litigation relies heavily on scientific research, so these experts change complex events into accounts that ordinary people and legal staff can understand. Sometimes they join forces with forensic anthropologists and forensic odontologists, who both help find and study the remains of victims. For instance, recent progress in forensic anthropology has proven pretty crucial for disaster victim identification—a strong hint that messy, complex cases benefit from a mixed-method approach (de Boer et al., 2018). Also, forensic odontology has grown into a trusted tool, making a noticeable impact in civil cases, particularly those involving mass disasters (Prajapati et al., 2018) (Figure 1.5).

1.1.7. Challenges Faced by Forensic Pathologists

Discovering the real identity of a person after they die is not easy and forensic pathologists run into many difficulties at the outset. Since these experts are essential to our justice system, they must deal with moral questions about unidentified bodies which are found in huge numbers worldwide and often remain unclaimed for many reasons. Disasters and humanitarian crises add more confusion; research from lower-income regions has been revealing a growing number of unknown remains which makes things even harder. Then, the COVID-19 outbreak threw a wrench in things by forcing universities to close and putting body donation programs on hold—both of which are key to practical forensic education and hands-on training (Brassett et al., 2020). With fewer resources and a shortage of skilled professionals, the push for detailed forensic analysis and the pursuit of justice becomes all the more uphill (Suwalowska et al., 2023). To summarize, it's becoming increasingly clear that setting up clear, well-coordinated strategies and embracing cross-disciplinary teamwork is absolutely essential if we're to tackle these pressing challenges (Figure 1.6).

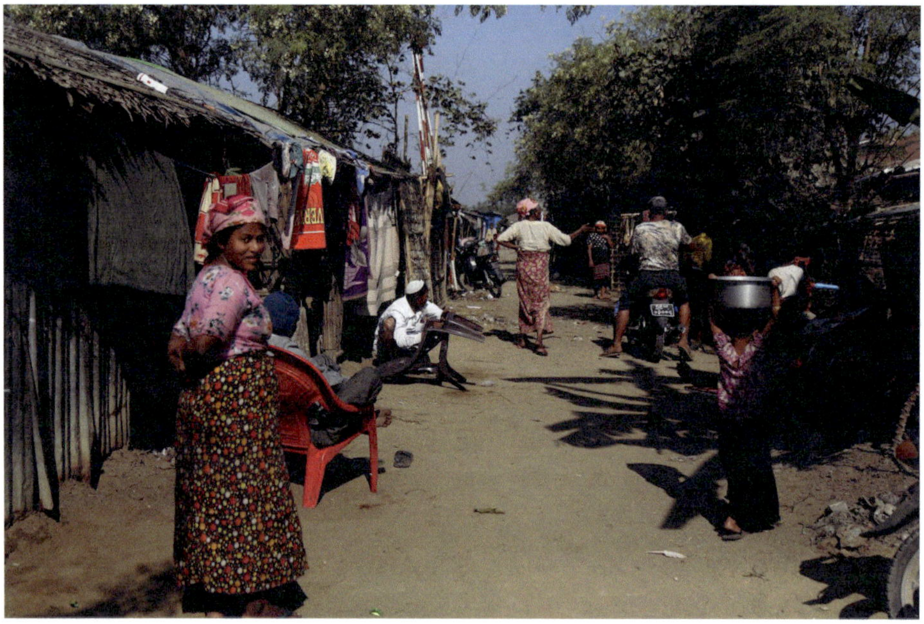

Figure 1.6. Challenges faced by forensic pathologists.

Source: https://minorityrights.org/app/uploads/2023/12/56667438.jpg.

1.1.8. Future Directions in Forensic Pathology

Forensic pathology is using new technology and this is greatly improving its accuracy and efficiency. Artificial intelligence (AI) sits right at the center of this shift—not merely a flashy upgrade, but a tool that's reshaping many aspects in forensic medicine, from spotting key identifiers to pinning down post-mortem timeframes. Generally speaking, it cuts down on human bias and slashes errors, offering a cost-friendly path to improved decision-making (Piraianu et al., 2023). At the same time, the use of CT and MR scans is making it possible to record crime scenes in greater detail which helps investigators analyze them more easily. And then there's the rise of multi-modal methods that let experts build virtual 3D reconstructions, which in turn help uncover the flow of crime scenes and even lend a fresh spin to courtroom visuals—methods including, for instance, virtual reality (Villa et al., 2023). Taken all together, these tech breakthroughs hint at a future where forensic pathology might very well redefine its methods and results, opening up new avenues for precision and innovation (Figure 1.7).

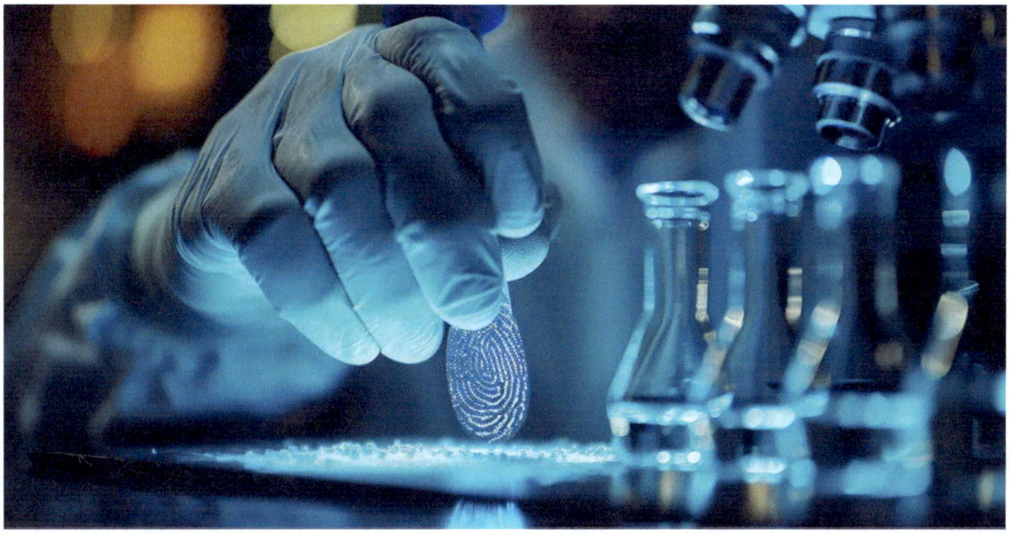

Figure 1.7. Forensic pathology is now weaving in new technologies, and you can see its accuracy and efficiency getting a real boost.

Source: https://www.lablynx.com/wp-content/uploads/2022/07/On-the-Hunt-The-Ideal-LIMS-for-Forensic-Labs-Medical-Examiners.jpg.

Test Your Knowledge

1. Explain the role of forensic pathologists.
2. Write a short note on post-mortem computed tomographic angiography (PMCTA).
3. What is exhumation?

1.2. Forensic Toxicology

Learning Outcome

1. Give the definition and importance of forensic toxicology;
2. Identify types of substances analyzed;
3. Explain methods of toxicological analysis;
4. Learn interpretation of toxicology reports;
5. Know legal implications of toxicology findings;
6. Identify challenges in forensic toxicology;
7. Describe advances in toxicological research.

Toxicology and forensic science join forces to deal with messy criminal cases. They analyze biological samples to see if drugs, alcohol or poisons were involved in the death or impairment of the person. Sometimes, the same tests are used to guide decisions in court and also to safeguard public health. It's many straightforward lab work and unexpected detective tricks.

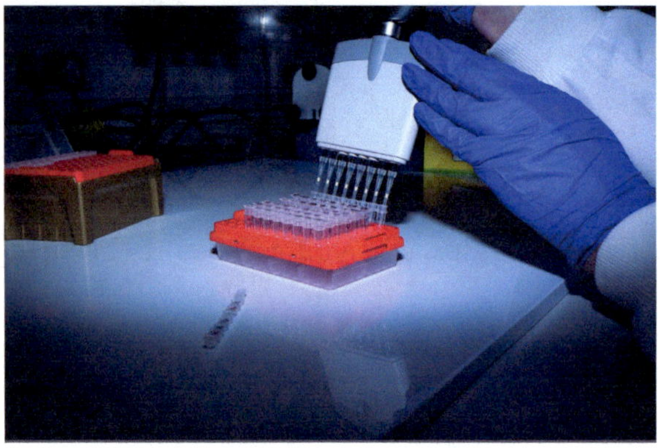

Figure 1.8. Toxicology and forensic science.

Source: https://www.rcpath.org/static/319f42e4-854b-48bd-b195c9dcaf934b9f/1440x960_highestperformance_4a7c7e45a350/Pipetting-image-7-North-West-Cancer-Research-Centre-112019.jpg.

Modern tech has shaken things up. Experts now use advanced tools like mass spectrometry and gas chromatography, which help sharpen their readings from samples (Balhareth et al., 2024). In most cases, adding artificial intelligence into the mix speeds things up further—offering rapid analyses and even predictive models on how toxic substances might behave (Singh et al., 2023). Generally speaking, these shifts not only quicken the pace of investigations but also stress just how critical forensic toxicology is to serving justice and keeping our communities safe (Figure 1.8).

1.2.1. Definition and Importance of Forensic Toxicology

It is often hard to understand how substances affect human health and it is in these situations that the study of drugs or forensic toxicology, becomes very important. In other words, it looks at the movement and effects of drugs in the body when legal matters are involved, to explain causes of death, accidents on the road or poisoning cases.

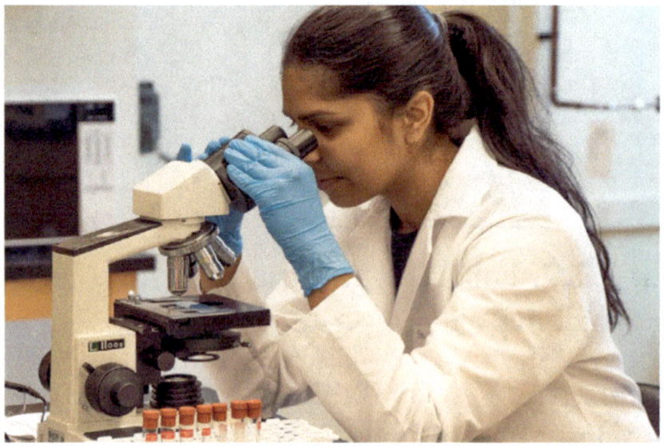

Figure 1.9. Importance of forensic toxicology.

Source: https://cdn.prod.website-files.com/627cdcca8bc0d22df9b2672f/64b51db3d97c954b4aee54f0_Forensic%20Pathologist%20Interview%20Questions.webp.

Novel psychoactive substances are causing new issues which are pushing the field to change and try new ways of dealing with them. Quick access to emergency data is, in most cases, important too; recent studies have even highlighted how these new substances can wreak unexpected havoc on public health (Logan et al., 2017). To summarize, forensic toxicology isn't just about running tests—it's a key element in boosting safety and even guiding legal standards in our society (Zeppenfeld et al., 2022) (Figure 1.9).

1.2.2. Types of Substances Analyzed

Looking at the substances in forensic medicine allows us to understand how poisonings and sudden deaths happen. For example, alcohol keeps appearing in these studies; some researchers say it's responsible for over 60% of fatal poisonings in certain areas which shows how much it affects public health. Beyond that, labs also check for other offenders like carbon monoxide and narcotic drugs, and these too frequently show up in poisoning cases, mirroring broader social and medical challenges (Ebeneezar et al., 2025).

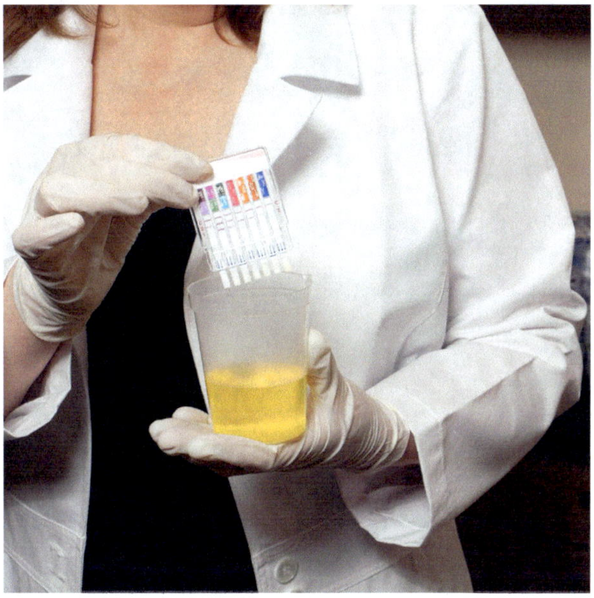

Figure 1.10. Examining the substances tested in forensic medicine turns out to be key—it helps us piece together how poisoning cases and unexpected fatalities actually unfold.

Source: https://knowledge.carolina.com/wp-content/uploads/2022/07/forensic-toxicology-106582985.jpg.

Looking into the numbers, it seems that drug-related poisoning tends to hit males between 25 and 50 years old more often, pointing to a clear need for targeted interventions (Ebeneezar et al., 2025). To summarize, knowing these substances inside and out not only sharpens forensic analysis but also paves the way for developing better prevention and treatment strategies in the field of forensic medicine (Figure 1.10).

1.2.3. Methods of Toxicological Analysis

The process of forensics depends on correctly spotting and measuring toxic substances which can make it possible to solve cases of death or crimes involving substances. Tests for toxicology have existed for a long time, but now there are some surprising new methods used. In most cases, bioanalytical methods have recently gotten a boost, letting laboratories quickly extract and examine substances think atypical antidepressants, which have been misused more and more (Roszkowska et al., 2022). They are applied both in clinical labs and in forensic investigations to make sure the results are accurate. Using modern steps before testing and new detection tools helps make the assessments more accurate. Forensic experts now lean heavily on understanding these hands-on processes, as they've become key in medico-legal autopsies – a point that emphasizes how important it is to keep training and education on point (Kakkeri et al., 2020) (Figure 1.11).

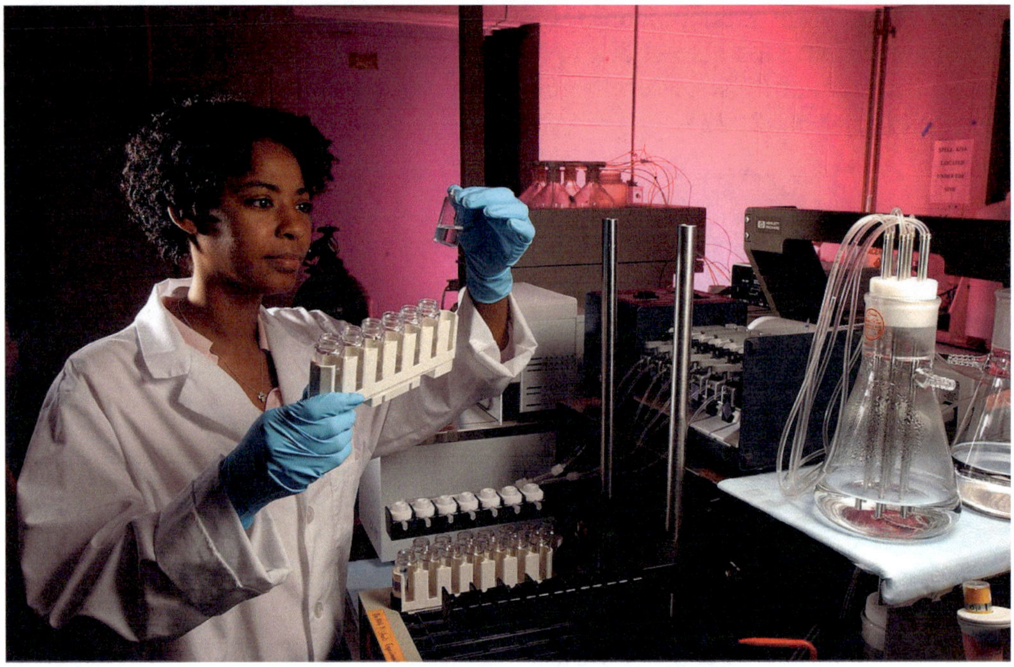

Figure 1.11. Traditional tests have long been around, but there's now a surprisingly inventive side to toxicological analysis.

Source: https://upload.wikimedia.org/wikipedia/commons/thumb/d/d3/USAPHC_TOX_Lab_%286129598147%29.jpg/1200px-USAPHC_TOX_Lab_%286129598147%29.jpg.

1.2.4. Role in Drug-Related Deaths

Investigating drug-related fatalities isn't a neat, one-size-fits-all scenario. Forensic experts usually start by sorting through a mix of clues, running tests for toxins and considering many details that might not be easy to spot. More and more people believe that higher death rates are caused by mixing drugs and the fact that the risks of some drugs are not always easy to notice which makes it harder to investigate. It is sometimes found in labs that when opioids are mixed with benzodiazepines or stimulants, the harmful effects of both drugs increase. And when someone's body gets used to drugs, the usual overdose signs can get fuzzy, making it all the more challenging to nail down the real cause—so in most cases, forensic pros end up doing very thorough, if not slightly uneven, autopsies while keeping an eye on the ever-shifting scene of drug interactions and personal histories (Zeppenfeld et al., 2022; Zhang et al., 2022) (Figure 1.12).

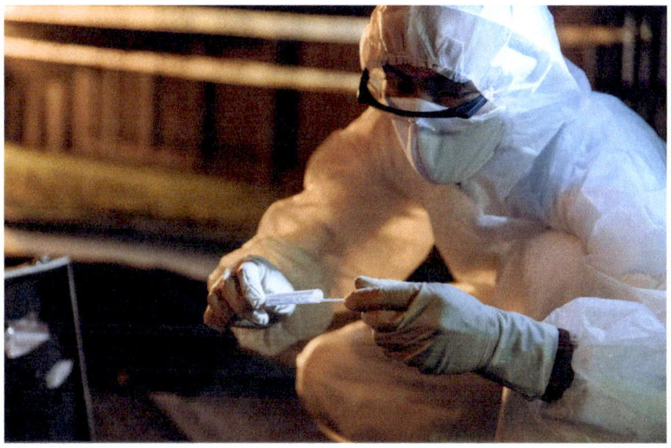

Figure 1.12. Forensic experts often dive straight into a jumble of clues—running toxin tests while also weighing many surrounding details that aren't always obvious.

Source: https://ejournals.eu/uploads/files/6721e685ad7b4_670fd382a45df-pexels-cottonbro-studio-10481324-jpg-6721e685a3ccf.jpg.

1.2.5. Interpretation of Toxicology Reports

Toxicology reports are hard to interpret mainly because forensic cases often include a wide variety of substances. Take synthetic cathinones, for example; chloromethcathinone (CMC) shows why analyses need to be spot on. Research generally points out that its tendency to become unstable in bodily samples muddles up our ability to judge its toxicity, especially in overdose situations that sometimes turn fatal (Romańczuk et al., 2023).

Often, labs end up leaning on biomarkers that hold steady; dihydro-CMC, for instance, sticks around in biological matrices even when its parent compound has already faded away (Romańczuk et al., 2023). More often than not such findings lead us to review our risks carefully, since the results may be hard to predict. To summarize, getting a genuine grip on these toxic interactions is key to piecing together what causes fatalities (Figure 1.13).

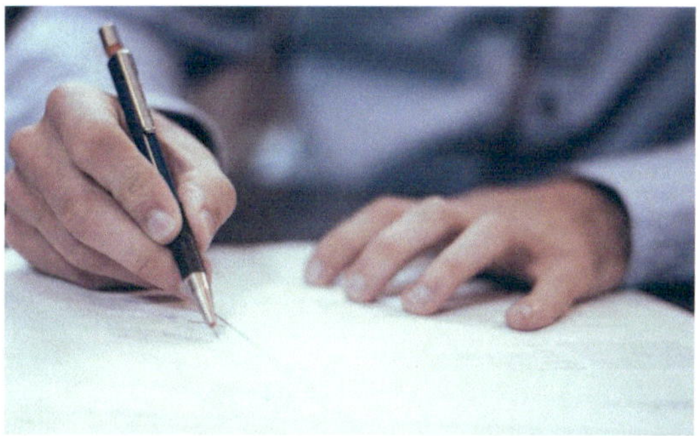

Figure 1.13. Interpreting toxicology reports is a tough nut to crack—primarily because forensic cases involve such a wild mix of substances.

Source: https://www.dnalegal.com/sites/default/files/styles/content_image/public/blog-images/scott-graham-OQMZwNd3ThU-unsplash_0.jpg?itok=CCxTOC0t.

1.2.6. Legal Implications of Toxicology Findings

Solid evidence is often crucial in courtrooms when they decide cases involving dangerous substances. In one murder case in South Korea, the absence of usual nicotine toxic signs made it harder to solve the case. They found that nicotine which is usually predictable, could sometimes lead to death without the typical stomach symptoms which confused the way things were understood.

That twist not only helped nail the case but also underscored how forensic science can untangle perplexing toxic details (Yoo et al., 2024). Old methods rubbing shoulders with modern techniques further deepen our view on the legal side of toxic exposure; sometimes, ancient know-how still speaks volumes in today's labs (Yoo et al., 2024). To summarize, these cases show that even when science is full of unexpected turns, the legal system leans on every scientific crumb to work through the tangled reality of poisoning cases (Figure 1.14).

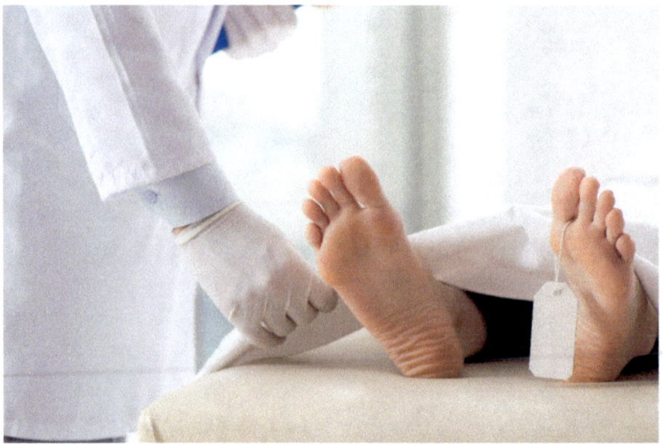

Figure 1.14. Legal implications of toxicology findings.

Source: https://godoymedical.net/wp-content/uploads/2022/08/shutterstock_1054195061-5559x3706.jpg.

1.2.7. Challenges in Forensic Toxicology

Technology and science are constantly blending in forensic toxicology which leads to both great opportunities and serious obstacles now. Many labs trying to improve substance detection and measurement have to deal with the unpredictable nature of biological samples. Because drugs often break down and form different metabolites in the body, this usually makes it harder for researchers, so they must use creative and sometimes easy approaches to distinguish them and learn about their effects.

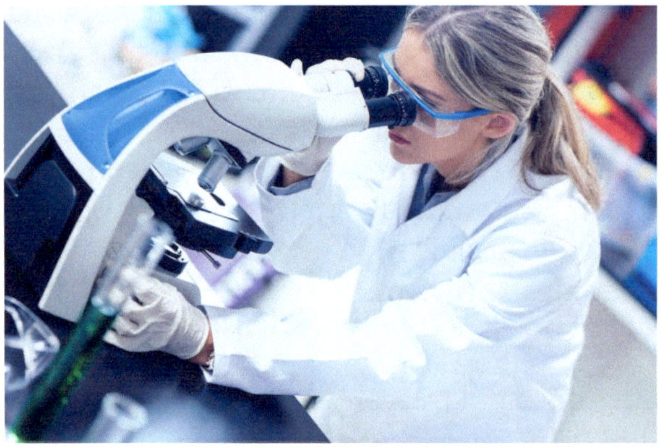

Figure 1.15. Tech and science in forensic toxicology keep intertwining—these days, they bring both exciting possibilities and some pretty tough hurdles.

Source: https://www.atascientific.com.au/wp-content/uploads/2020/01/Forensic-Sciences.jpg.

Take new tech like wearable electrochemical sensors, for example; they're starting to offer a way to get non-invasive, real-time data on everything from therapeutic drugs to substances of abuse (Teymourian et al., 2020). Such progress usually leads to customized medicine and, in a way, could help law enforcement stop drug smuggling. Still, mixing these innovations with traditional forensic methods isn't straightforward; folks often wonder about their overall reliability, the need for standard protocols, and even some legal complications that might pop up during investigations (Zeppenfeld et al., 2022). To summarize, the field finds itself in a balancing act, trying to embrace fresh ideas while keeping tests as accurate and trustworthy as possible (Figure 1.15).

1.2.8. Advances in Toxicological Research

New advances in technology have helped toxicologists find and study dangerous substances in many different places. The use of advanced AI in toxicology has generally made it easier to process and interpret data which helps detect dangerous substances more quickly. Machine learning allows scientists to identify detailed patterns in messy data which can sometimes lead to discoveries about how toxins work and how they might be stopped. Forensic review of toxic evidence in courts is also helped by these innovations, not just the work done in labs. As many would note, a solid collaboration between toxicologists and data scientists is pretty crucial for making the most of these advances, ultimately improving public health outcomes and safety measures (Poalelungi et al., 2023; Zeppenfeld et al., 2022). Overall, these developments illuminating the ever-changing realm of forensic medicine, paving the way for more precise assessments in toxicological cases (Figure 1.16).

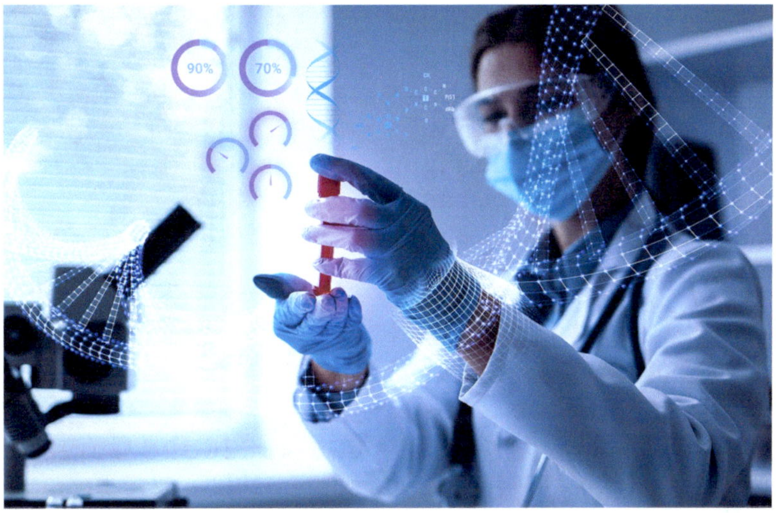

Figure 1.16. Integrating cutting-edge AI tools into toxicology has, in most cases, made data crunching and interpretation much faster, which in turn speeds up the spotting of dangerous compounds.

Source: https://www.freyrsolutions.com/sites/default/files/blog-thumbnails/Pharmacovigilance%20Redefining%20Drug%20Safety%20with%20AI%20and%20Technological%20Innovations.webp.

Test Your Knowledge

1. Name common poisons detected in forensic cases.
2. How can poisons get into the body?

1.3. Forensic Anthropology

Learning Outcome

1. Understand the definition and role of forensic anthropology;
2. Learn techniques for identifying human remains;
3. Discuss estimating age, sex, and ancestry;
4. Describe the analysis of skeletal trauma;
5. Focus on recovery and preservation of remains;
6. Discuss collaboration with law enforcement;
7. Identify ethical issues in forensic anthropology;
8. Know future trends in forensic anthropology.

Forensic anthropology and legal investigations are linked in ways that may not be clear at first and this connection leads to forensic medicine. Forensic anthropologists rely on advanced techniques to determine what remains are which may influence the outcome of a criminal trial. Take skull sex estimation, for example; using wavelet and Fourier transform methods, results have hit roughly 90.9% accuracy for males and about 94.4% for females (Yang et al., 2020)—a notable leap over the old ways. Also, the role in disaster victim identification (DVI) has changed quite a bit by drawing on lessons from recent large-scale tragedies to bring forensic teams closer together (de Boer et al., 2018). In short, this hands-on method makes identifications easier and helps improve the field of forensic medicine, proving the importance of forensic anthropology to justice and public safety.

1.3.1. Definition and Role of Forensic Anthropology

Forensic science is sometimes hard to follow and forensic anthropology is one of the most eye-catching areas. Forensic anthropologists study human bones to figure out who a person was and this area is important in the legal field. Often, you see these experts in action during disaster situations like DVI events, where they're busy piecing together fragmented remains and using imaging tricks that boost identification (de Boer et al., 2018). In most cases, as the challenges in forensic work evolve, it's not just about the latest gadgets; instead, the focus shifts to why we reconstruct scenes, keep track of details, and even ward off crimes (Roux et al., 2021). To summarize, by mixing different approaches, forensic anthropology (yes, sometimes a tiny slip in spelling reminds us of our human side) lends real support to the broader goals of forensic science, leaving its own mark on the world of forensic medicine (Figure 1.17).

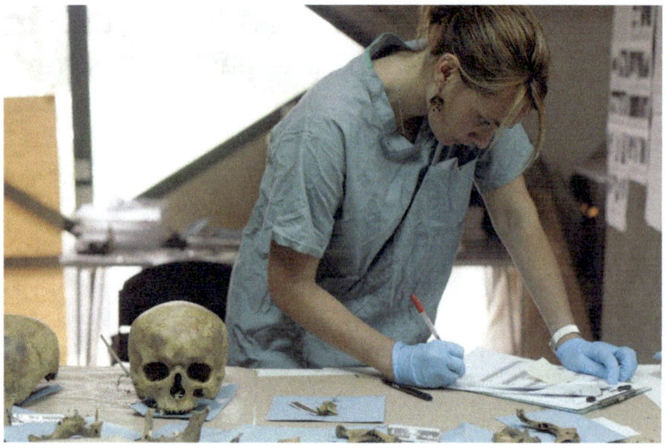

Figure 1.17. Forensic science can be a bit of a maze, and one branch that jumps out is forensic anthropology.

Source: https://cdn.britannica.com/92/91892-050-43C2CBD8/Forensic-anthropologist-human-skull-grave-Bosnia-and-2005.jpg.

1.3.2. Techniques for Identifying Human Remains

There are always new difficulties in working with human remains—every case is different. Many times, the best way is to use different methods instead of just one. In particular, forensic dentistry is now very useful since it uses unique dental details to help discover a person's identity. Besides taking dental impressions, radiographs and cheiloscopy help by giving more information when traditional methods don't work as well, especially in situations where many people are involved. Digital tech, like 3D modeling, also gives these methods a boost by providing swifter, reliable outcomes that become crucial during emergencies (Sanzyapova, 2025). When forensic dentists join forces with the police, the approach is often more complete and ethical, even if the process looks rough sometimes which highlights how important their work is. Overall, this mix of human know-how, cutting-edge techniques, and sometimes unexpectedly casual collaboration confirms that forensic dentistry remains a major pillar in modern forensic medicine (Figure 1.18).

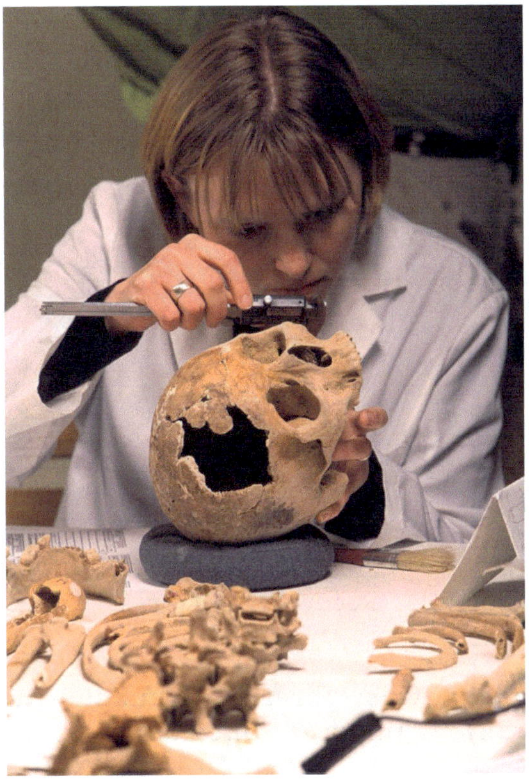

Figure 1.18. Forensic dentistry has stepped up as a particularly useful tool because its focus on unique dental records and features helps pinpoint an individual's identity.

Source: https://wp.stu.ca/forensicscience/wp-content/uploads/sites/22/2015/04/Forensic-Anthropology-forensic-anthropology-6380688-1200-1783-689x1024.jpg.

1.3.3. Estimating Age, Sex, and Ancestry

Correctly identifying someone is very important in forensic medicine because it helps solve cases and maintain justice. The first things looked at are age, gender and ancestry since they quickly help narrow the list of suspects. Generally speaking, looking at cranial suture closure can give you an age estimate with roughly a ±10-year margin, offering useful insight during autopsy investigations (Buzdar et al., 2024). Even tiny variations in body composition related to age, gender or ethnicity affect the accuracy of assessments. Many predictive formulas—built on extensive analyses—often guide experts in estimating traits tied to sex and ancestry from various physical measurements (Campa et al., 2024). To summarize, these methods show that careful forensic analysis is key to piecing together identities and ensuring accountability in legal matters (Figure 1.19).

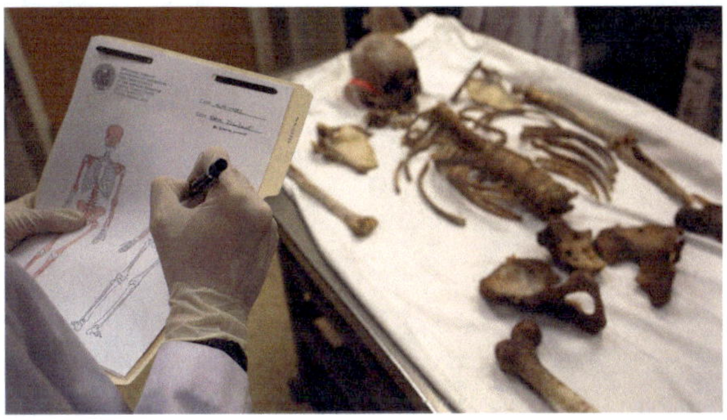

Figure 1.19. Age, gender, and ancestry are usually the first clues checked because they quickly narrow down the possibilities.

Source: https://cropper.watch.aetnd.com/cdn.watch.aetnd.com/sites/4/2021/07/GettyImages-460247660-resize.jpg.

1.3.4. Analysis of Skeletal Trauma

In many forensic investigations, skeletal trauma analysis is central—it helps to explain both violent crimes and sudden accidents. Many cases include injuries like broken bones and joint problems which appear again and again as important clues to the cause of death. Most of the time, forensic anthropologists use their extensive experience to tell apart injuries that happened before death, during it or after it which helps to create a basic timeline and guess at possible motives. Lately, there's been a noticeable twist: modern transport options like electric scooters are adding a new chapter to trauma studies, with recent research generally showing a marked rise in fractures—especially those impacting the legs (Siedin et al., 2024). To summarize, merging these skeletal clues into investigations not only aids in piecing together a sequence of events, but also broadens our overall insight into human behavior and evolving societal trends (Yadav et al., 2023) (Figure 1.20).

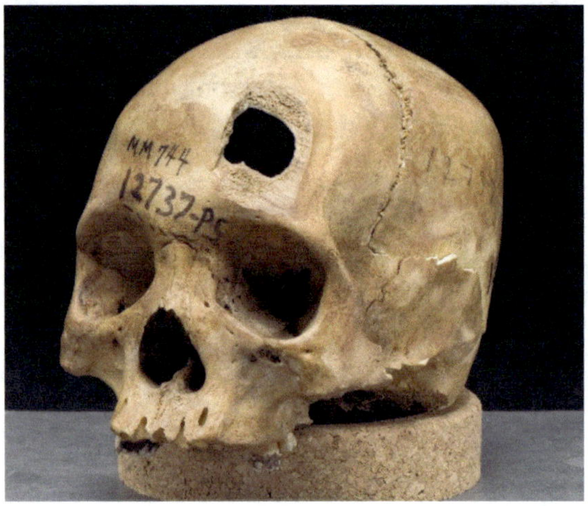

Figure 1.20. Skeletal trauma analysis is a key element when examining both violent acts and unexpected accidents.

Source: https://pressbooks.ccconline.org/ppscant2315introtoforensicanthropology/wp-content/uploads/sites/131/2023/04/image1.jpeg.

1.3.5. Recovery and Preservation of Remains

It is very hard to identify human remains, so forensic experts must be very careful. Since decomposition happens in several steps, it is important to recover and keep the fragments safe, sometimes more than you would think. Some cases, like when loads of lower limbs turned up along North American coasts, highlight just how messy it can be connecting bits to a single individual, especially since little attention has been given to methods for matching feet (Barrett et al., 2014). Some new ways to preserve samples have appeared and these usually help keep them in good condition for analysis; even if the results aren't always major, they make a difference. Most studies agree that how samples are kept can influence microbial analysis which is important for building a biological profile. It appears that narrowing down which storage methods work best is quickly becoming a hot spot for future forensic research (Figure 1.21).

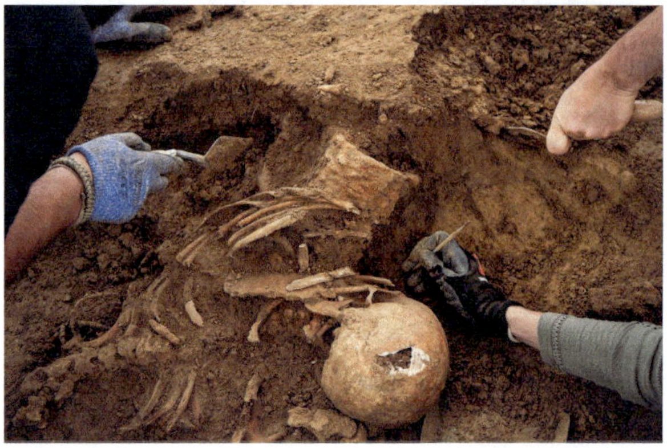

Figure 1.21. Recovery and preservation of remains.

Source: https://breakinggroundheritage.org.uk/____impro/1/onewebmedia/027_EX%20JOAN%20OF%20ARC%202018_DSC_0335_%C2%A9%20HARVEY%20MILLS%202018.jpg?etag=%22348b98-5ceff8f1%22&sourceContentType=image%2Fjpeg&ignoreAspectRatio&resize=2000,1331&quality=85.

1.3.6. Collaboration with Law Enforcement

There is a lot of overlap between forensic medicine and law enforcement which can be confusing. A mix of old and new technology makes the industry full of surprises. Take forensic DNA work—you see many liberal and community-focused thinking, especially in places like Singapore (Toom et al., 2014) where safety often wins over personal rights. Then there are fresh approaches like forensic epigenetics and genetic genealogy that blur the lines between what's strictly medical, commercial, or forensic (Granja et al., 2024); suddenly, everyone has to rethink their role. Having these areas overlap leads to teamwork, but also causes arguments about who is responsible for different tasks. Overall, understanding these ever-changing dynamics is, generally speaking, essential for moving forensic medicine forward and for trying to use new technology ethically in policing contexts (Figure 1.22).

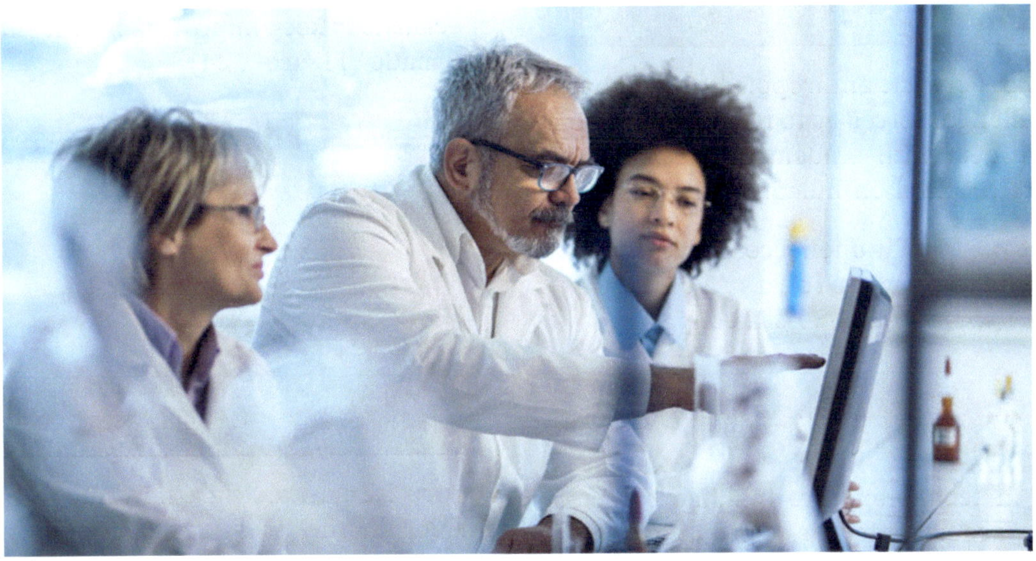

Figure 1.22. Forensic medicine and law enforcement come together in a way that feels pretty muddled.

Source: https://online.campbellsville.edu/wp-content/uploads/2019/04/Modern-Forensic-Technology-header-CU-1024x544.jpg.

1.3.7. Ethical Issues in Forensic Anthropology

Because of the ethical issues involved, forensic anthropology makes us pay closer attention to the way we handle unidentified remains. Every year, many people pass away without ever being identified, usually because economic struggles in low- and middle-income regions leave little room for proper resources; in most cases, this means a lack of attention that not only robs individuals of a dignified burial but also leaves their families battling a deep, unresolved pain (Suwalowska et al., 2023). New tech like 3D printing is showing some promise in reconstructing or visualizing remains, yet it also brings up tricky questions about how these remains should be put on display in court settings (Carew et al., 2020). To summarize, tackling these ethical dilemmas is absolutely crucial if we want to honor the departed while still pushing the boundaries in forensic anthropology (Figure 1.23).

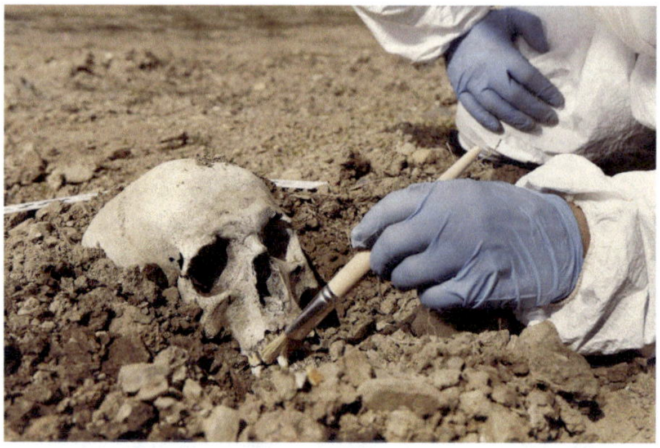

Figure 1.23. Forensic anthropology mixed with ethical challenges forces us to take a closer look at how we deal with unidentified remains as these cases hit hard on human rights issues.

Source: https://www.openaccessgovernment.org/wp-content/uploads/2022/04/dreamstime_xxl_116794080-scaled.jpg.

1.3.8. Future Trends in Forensic Anthropology

Advances in technology are making it easier and more accurate to do work in forensic anthropology. AI tools, for instance, are now nudging decision-making in ways that can change how experts examine bones and piece together crime scenes (Mariani et al., 2021). Machine learning is able to notice small details in bones that might go unnoticed by a doctor. Forensic science is now used more often to identify disaster victims which demonstrates its growing role in areas where many different fields meet. Recent events have also stressed the need for solid techniques in tissue sampling for DNA work—especially in large disaster scenes where remains end up scattered and broken apart (de Boer et al., 2018). In most cases, as these trends catch on, forensic anthropologists will probably have to mix new technologies with good old teamwork among different forensic specialists to keep improving how identifications are made (Figure 1.24).

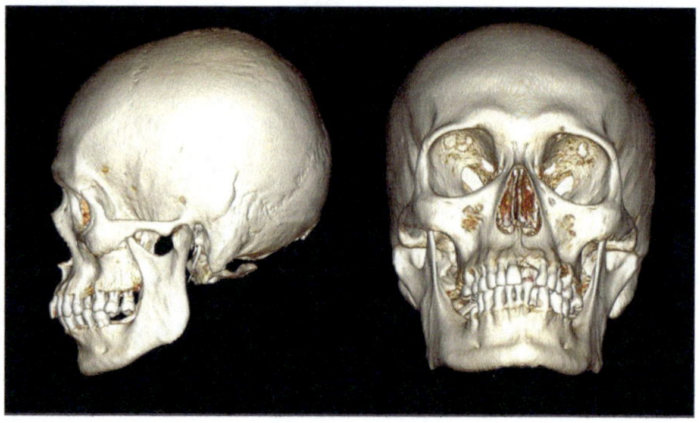

Figure 1.24. AI tools are now nudging decision-making in ways that can change how experts examine bones and piece together crime scenes.

Source: https://www.csiro.au/-/media/News-releases/2025/February/CSIRO-develops-AI-tool-for-rapid-identification-in-forensic-investigations/Volume-rendered-CT-scan-visualised-in-OsiriX.jpg?mw=1200&hash=70932766A2D7B7F47C51F606961AF6CC.

Test Your Knowledge

1. What is using dental examination in forensic anthropology?
2. Name the bones commonly used to determine age.

1.4. Forensic Psychology

Learning Outcome

1. Explain the definition and scope of forensic psychology;
2. Know its role in criminal profiling;
3. Learn assessment of competency to stand trial;
4. Understand criminal behavior;
5. Give expert testimony in court;
6. Discuss psychological evaluations of victims;
7. Identify challenges in forensic psychology;
8. Know future directions in forensic psychology.

When the law meets unusual human behavior, many people become interested in how forensic psychology fits into forensic medicine. This area of study which looks at the mindset of criminals, also helps us decide on the mental fitness and guilt of those facing legal charges. Generally speaking, a broad approach known as Behavior Analysis in Medicine shows that mixing forensic psychology with other areas—like health law and deception detection—can sharpen clinical reviews (Domínguez-Muñoz et al., 2024). It becomes clear that looking at mental health and crime together can reveal that a simple approach in court may result in errors. Usually, forensic psychologists help clear up these difficult relationships which greatly influences how mental health and the justice system work together.

1.4.1. Definition and Scope of Forensic Psychology

Forensic psychology is where mental health and the law meet and it's not limited to only what happens in a clinic. It involves many aspects, for example, looking at whether someone could be violent, testing if people are able to understand what they do and closely examining the effects crimes have on both the offenders and the victims. Generally speaking, it also peeks into cases of missing persons, stressing that mental health angles here still don't get enough attention (Dickens et al., 2019). The field, in many situations, wrestles with those ethical and practical challenges that come up when making clinical calls despite shaky empirical backup (Barlow et al., 2018). By mixing what we know about psychology with legal reviews, forensic psychology helps out in courtrooms while also shaping ways to prevent issues and guide rehab efforts within forensic medicine (Figure 1.25).

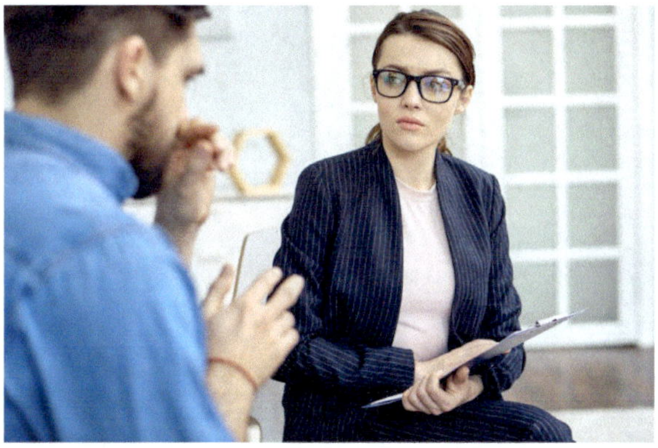

Figure 1.25. Forensic psychology sits squarely at the crossroads of mental health ideas and the legal world—it's not just about what happens in a clinic.

Source: https://online.maryville.edu/wp-content/uploads/sites/97/2023/09/forensic-psychologist.jpg.

1.4.2. Role in Criminal Profiling

It is very important in profiling which is a major part of forensic medicine, to understand the different aspects of criminal behavior. Experts use what they learn from psychology and from hands-on investigations to build profiles of people who repeatedly show certain behaviors and traits. When different fields are put together, police can narrow their list of suspects and also learn more about what motivates someone which can stop future problems. Today, using technology and smart data processing has made profiling much more precise. It is now much easier for researchers to look through a lot of information quickly. By tapping into genomic clues about behavior, they can spot connections that often went unnoticed before, drawing biology and criminal psychology a little closer together (Satam et al., 2023). To summarize, this evolving scene reminds us that keeping different fields in touch—collaborating constantly—is pretty much key to refining profiling methods, which in turn can lead to better legal outcomes (Luíz César Peres, 2017) (Figure 1.26).

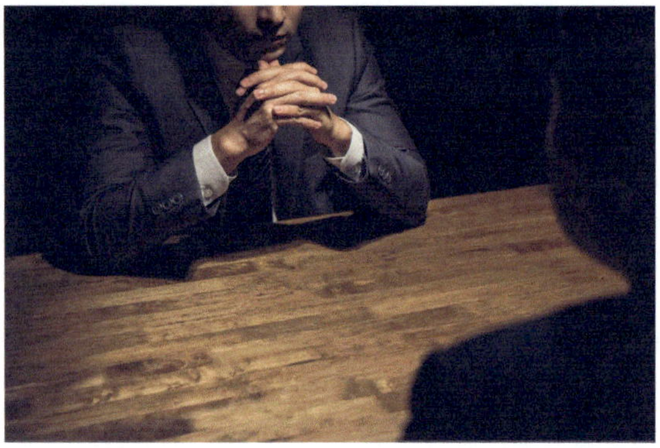

Figure 1.26. Grasping the twists of criminal behavior matters—a lot—in the realm of profiling, which plays a major role in forensic medicine.

Source: https://blog.ipleaders.in/wp-content/uploads/2021/09/Criminal-Psychologist-scaled.jpg.

1.4.3. Assessment of Competency to Stand Trial

Deciding if someone is fit to go to trial depends on legal and psychological evaluations. The main point is that a person can understand the charges and participate in their defense which is very important. In most cases, about 74.2% of forensic assessments lean on specific structured tools to boost the trustworthiness of expert calls (Neal et al., 2014). Still, hidden cognitive shortcuts in forensic mental health often complicate things and may skew these evaluations a bit (Neal et al., 2014). Generally, seeing and addressing these biases is necessary for assessments to be viewed as fair and accurate. A solid, sometimes even no-nonsense approach to testing competency not only keeps the legal process honest but also takes into account the basic rights of everyone caught up in it (Figure 1.27).

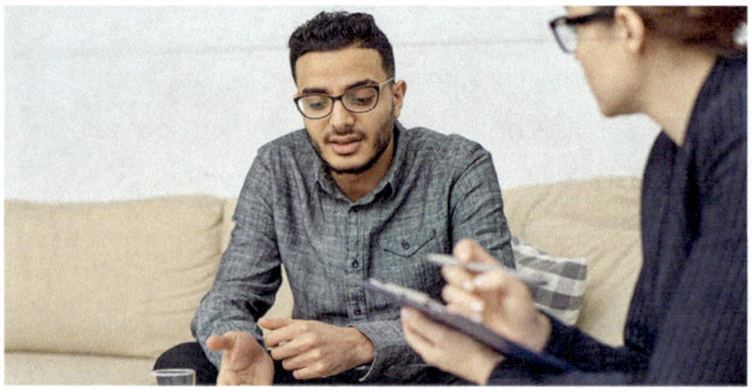

Figure 1.27. Legal and psychological evaluations matter when it comes to figuring out if someone's fit to stand trial.

Source: https://www.apa.org/images/article-psychological-testing-assessment_tcm7-285069.jpg.

1.4.4. Understanding Criminal Behavior

Looking at criminal behavior isn't limited to the crime itself; it makes us explore what is happening in the brain and mind. For example, forensic psychology often notes that mental health problems, for example schizophrenia, can change the way people think and make decisions which can lead to more complex everyday decisions. Recognizing these brain-based influences is key since it helps legal professionals build a more detailed insanity defense that, in most cases, tries to balance upholding justice with understanding mental health concerns (Moriarty et al., 2016). At the same moment, new findings in genetics and the discussions over DNA databases introduce new ideas about inherited tendencies toward certain behaviors. It appears that linking specific genetic markers with criminal actions muddies the waters between nature and nurture, and, generally speaking, calls for sticking to rigorous ethical standards in forensic studies (Kaye et al., 2006). To summarize, taking a varied, multifaceted approach is essential if we want to untangle the many layers that make up criminal behavior (Figure 1.28).

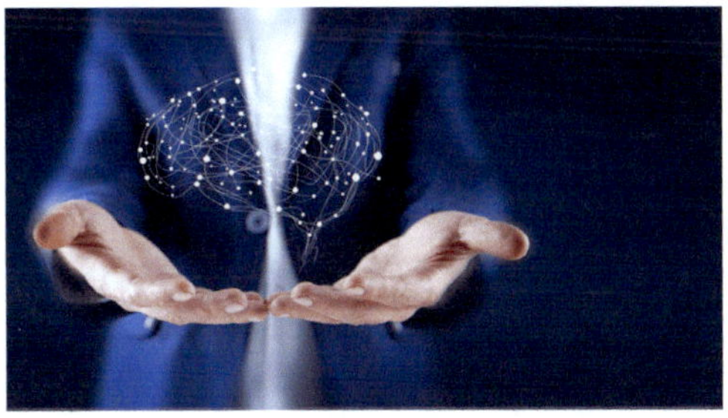

Figure 1.28. Criminal behavior isn't just about the act itself—it invites us to dig into what's happening in the brain and the mind.

Source: https://www.easyprey.com/wp-content/uploads/2023/06/PNG-image-2.png.

1.4.5. Expert Testimony in Court

Forensic medicine relies heavily on expert testimony which should never be ignored. Forensic physicians and pathologists are responsible for giving unbiased and independent results to the courts which usually ensures justice is given in most cases. They often work closely with law enforcement and stick to accepted forensic standards, a practice that naturally boosts trust in the evidence (Cusack, 2025). In many situations, the way courts take in this testimony depends on a set of specific criteria intended to keep these expert opinions reliable—this is especially important since many judges might not have a deep background in forensic science (Smith et al., 2025). Because legal systems can be complicated, taking time for thorough checks and questioning adds fairness and reliability. Ultimately, expert testimony ties together the world of science and the realm of law, playing a key role in shaping major judicial decisions (Figure 1.29).

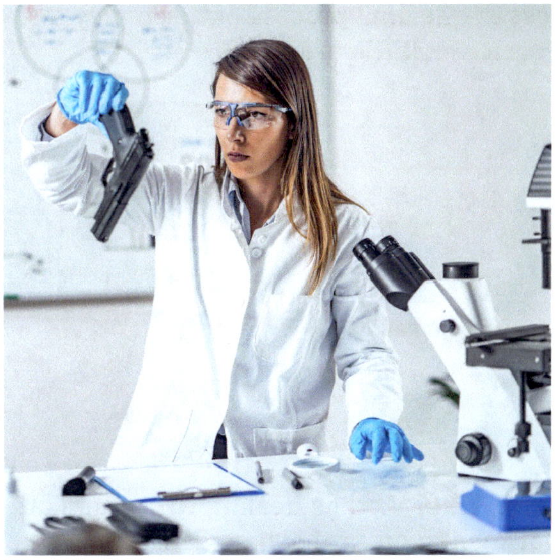

Figure 1.29. Expert testimony is a big deal in forensic medicine.

Source: https://thefernandezfirm.com/wp-content/uploads/2023/09/forensic-science-expert-examining-gun-collected-at-2021-08-26-16-53-21-utc.jpg.

1.4.6. Psychological Evaluations of Victims

Forensic medicine now sees that psychological evaluations and the aftermath of trauma are more closely related than was believed before. People who go through traumatic events usually feel many different emotions and knowing what they are thinking is important for both the legal process and personal care. Sometimes, experts who examine these psychological effects notice small changes in behavior and perception that people might not notice. In cases like cyberbullying, for example, forensic psychology teams up with law enforcement to figure out just how much emotional strain is being put on victims, which can help steer the right kind of intervention (Kian et al., 2025). Sometimes, even examining injuries—say, to the mouth or teeth—can reveal patterns that guide medical treatment and shape legal records (Saker et al., 2025). To summarize, these evaluations not only boost the healing process but also play a significant role in piecing together the bigger picture in forensic work (Figure 1.30).

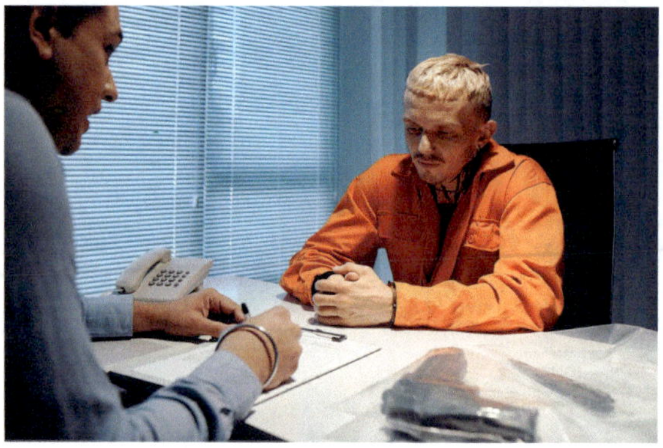

Figure 1.30. Victims dealing with traumatic events often face a storm of emotions, and knowing what's going on in their minds is key for both legal steps and personal support.

Source: https://thefernandezfirm.com/wp-content/uploads/2023/08/penitent-criminal-testifying-as-witness-2023-08-15-22-04-31-utc.jpg.

1.4.7. Challenges in Forensic Psychology

Forensic psychology involves both the law and mental health which leads to many challenges that should be addressed quickly. A major concern is the weak educational setup for newcomers—though forensic medicine now shows up in many medical programs, fresh grads still often stumble when it comes to crafting solid medico-legal reports (Atreya et al., 2025). Since there is no standard way to train, the issue is made worse by inconsistencies in the practice that may affect the reliability of legal evaluations.

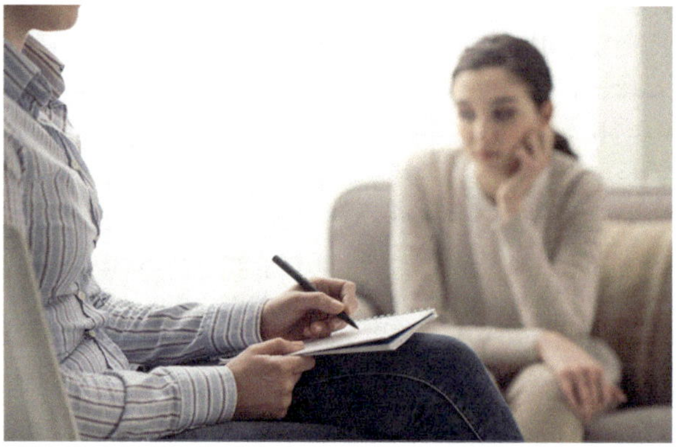

Figure 1.31. Legal systems and mental health mix in forensic psychology.

Source: https://www.medpsych.net/wp-content/uploads/2021/01/forensic-psychology.jpg.

In response, inventive approaches like the System for Analysis of Validity in Evaluation (SAVE) (Domínguez-Muñoz et al., 2024) have cropped up, aiming to refine assessment accuracy and encourage a looser, cross-disciplinary teamwork. To summarize, ramping up curricula and mixing in advanced methods appear, in most cases, absolutely essential for forensic psychology to navigate its layered and complex challenges (Figure 1.31).

1.4.8. Future Directions in Forensic Psychology

Forensic psychology is being altered by the use of new technology. Instead of staying rigid, the field now sees tools like Explainable AI (XAI)—a concept meant to show how AI reaches its decisions—in a light that's refreshingly open and, generally speaking, more trustworthy. This is very important when real situations such as justice and legal responsibilities, are involved; the stress is high. In many cases, using XAI lets experts dig into messy data from psychological tests and criminal records, often coming up with recommendations that hold up better in court (Longo et al., 2024). Some believe these new methods might even iron out old problems—like giving explanations that fit different audiences—which, in turn, ups the value of forensic insights in various legal setups (Ali et al., 2023). In short, using modern technology with traditional skills appears to be pushing forensic psychology toward a time when people's insights and new methods work hand in hand.

Test Your Knowledge

1. What is criminal profiling?
2. What is an expert witness in forensic psychology?

Summary

Looking into forensic medicine can reveal ideas that go further than a simple medical review—usually it proves that we should follow the same methods and ethical rules always. Look at Bulgaria's use of the Abbreviated Injury Scale (AIS); this example kind of demonstrates how one framework might merge different practices and even make trauma checks feel more balanced (Dokov et al., 2014). Sometimes, confirmation bias stubbornly reappears, hinting at deeper issues that, generally speaking, jeopardize the trust we place in forensic science; in most cases, this calls for a little extra effort to raise awareness and adopt better habits to fight against these recurring problems (McGowan et al., 2017). All in all, using standardized tools to fight biases improves the forensic process and makes our justice system more reliable, keeping forensic medicine true to its main promises of truth and fairness.

Since forensic medicine involves medical work and legal issues, specialists must be familiar with both areas. Digital tech, now stepping into telemedicine, has stirred up many fresh regulatory challenges – which clearly shows that our legal rules ought to catch up (Jordi, 2024). Groups like the Carers Forum remind us that pooling different expert views is pretty important; after all, many insights proves key when helping those with forensic backgrounds, and it boosts the whole care setup (Hickman et al., 2025). Most of the time, these bits show us how forensic medicine keeps changing, relying on teamwork and new ideas to solve modern legal and ethical issues. Being able to use both medical and legal knowledge makes forensic practitioners more successful in our ever-changing medical world.

KEY TERMS FROM THIS CHAPTER

- Accidents
- Autopsy
- Cause of Death
- Civil litigation
- Entomology
- Exhumation
- Forensic anthropologists
- Forensic odontologists
- Manner of Death
- Pathology
- Poisonings
- Precision
- Samples
- Toxicology

Short Answer Questions

1. How does forensic toxicology help in criminal investigations?
2. How do toxicological reports affect legal cases in court?
3. Outline how chain of custody matters in the management of toxicology samples.
4. Explain the difference between homicidal, suicidal, and accidental poisoning.
5. In what ways does a toxicology report affect insurance and civil litigation cases?
6. Describe the methods used to estimate age from bones.
7. Outline the way forensic psychologists handle interviews with witnesses and victims.

Critical Thinking Questions

1. **Forensic pathology primarily deals with:**
   a. Treating living patients
   b. Analyzing tissue cultures
   c. Investigating causes of death
   d. Psychological profiling
2. **The main tool of a forensic pathologist is the:**
   a. Autopsy
   b. Polygraph
   c. Microscope
   d. DNA sequencer
3. **Which of these is not one of the tasks that a forensic pathologist does?**
   a. Performing postmortem examinations
   b. Testifying in court as an expert witness
   c. Conducting psychological therapy for victims
   d. Determining time and cause of death
4. **In medico-legal autopsies, the minimum requirement is to examine:**
   a. Only the chest cavity
   b. Only the suspected area
   c. The entire body (head to toe)
   d. Only external injuries
5. **Who should record the injuries and how they relate to the main cause of death?**
   a. Forensic psychologist
   b. Forensic pathologist
   c. Crime scene investigator
   d. Radiologist

Answers to Critical Thinking Questions

1. (c); 2. (a); 3. (c); 4. (c); 5. (b)

References

1. Adel, A. (2023). Unlocking the future: Fostering human–machine collaboration and driving intelligent automation through Industry 5.0 in smart cities. *Smart Cities, 6*, 2742–2782. https://doi.org/10.3390/smartcities6050124.
2. Aggarwal, A., Mittal, M., & Battineni, G. (2021). Generative adversarial network: An overview of theory and applications. *International Journal of Information Management Data Insights, 1*, 100004. https://doi.org/10.1016/j.jjimei.2020.100004.
3. Aimar, A., Palermo, A., & Innocenti, B. (2019). The role of 3D printing in medical applications: A state of the art. *Journal of Healthcare Engineering, 2019*, 5340616. https://doi.org/10.1155/2019/5340616.
4. Ali, S., Abuhmed, T., El-Sappagh, S., Muhammad, K., Alonso, J. M., Confalonieri, R., Guidotti, R., et al. (2023). Explainable artificial intelligence (XAI): What we know and what is left to attain trustworthy artificial intelligence. *Information Fusion, 99*, 101805. https://doi.org/10.1016/j.inffus.2023.101805.
5. Atreya, A., Rajbanshi, R., Menezes, R. G., et al. (2025). Evaluation of undergraduate forensic medicine education in Nepal: A critical analysis using Schwab's five commonplaces and Schubert's curriculum images. *BMC Medical Education, 25*, 147. https://doi.org/10.1186/s12909-025-06741-7.
6. Awan, E. A., Afzal, H., Yousfani, G. M., Imran, S., Memon, A. A., & Pehlwani, H. A. (2023). Retrospective analysis of 258 consecutive forensic exhumations with emphasis on causative agents/cause of death. *Deleted Journal, 13*(1), 9–12. https://doi.org/10.62118/jmmc.v13i1.254.
7. Bairoch, A. (2018). The Cellosaurus, a cell-line knowledge resource. *Journal of Biomolecular Techniques, 29*, 25–38. https://doi.org/10.7171/jbt.18-2902-002.
8. Balhareth, A. A. S., Jamesh, M., Zabarah, G. A., Almotlaq, M. M., Alabaaltahin, M. A. M., Al Jaarah, A. H. A., Aldawsari, A. G. A., et al. (2024). The role of forensic medicine in modern criminal justice: A review of current practices and innovations. *Journal of Eco Humanism, 3*(7). https://doi.org/10.62754/joe.v3i7.4669
9. Barlow, E. M., & Dickens, G. L. (2018). Systematic review of therapeutic leave in inpatient mental health services. https://core.ac.uk/download/228178293.pdf (accessed on 29 May 2025).
10. Barrett, J., Bidmos, G., Bilge, Y., et al. (2014). The foot in forensic human identification–A review. https://core.ac.uk/download/30660095.pdf (accessed on 29 May 2025).
11. Bartoshyk, N. (2024). Analysis of the number of deaths due to poisoning by the most common poisonous substances in the LVIV region in 2018–2023. *Forensic-Medical Examination*. https://www.semanticscholar.org/paper/11ab7886efe10b9fb28d671682ea7cd842c27417 (accessed on 29 May 2025).
12. Brassett, C., Cosker, T., Davies, D. C., Dockery, P., Gillingwater, T. H., Lee, T. C., Milz, S., et al. (2020). COVID-19 and anatomy: Stimulus and initial response. *Journal of Anatomy, 237*(3), 393–403. https://doi.org/10.1111/joa.13274.

13. Buzdar, Z. A., Murad, T., Shabbir, S., Ahmed, A., Soomro, T. A., & Masood, R. (2024). Estimating age on the autopsy table: A postmortem study of forensic investigations. *JSMC, 14*(4), 353–358. https://jsmc.pk/index.php/jsmc/article/view/995 (accessed on 29 May 2025).

14. Campa, F., Coratella, G., Cerullo, G., Noriega, Z., Francisco, R., Charrier, D., Irurtia, A., et al. (2024). High-standard predictive equations for estimating body composition using bioelectrical impedance analysis: A systematic review. *Journal of Translational Medicine, 22*. https://www.semanticscholar.org/paper/f744b316b1eed48b81522277b42cdaef522c1094 (accessed on 29 May 2025).

15. Carew, R. M., & Errickson, D. (2020). An overview of 3D printing in forensic science: The tangible third-dimension. *Journal of Forensic Sciences, 65*, 1752–1760. https://doi.org/10.1111/1556-4029.14442.

16. Cusack, D. A. (2025). The European Council of Legal and Forensic Medicine: Its role and work in progressing harmonized standards and recommendations in forensic and legal medicine investigation procedures, training and teaching through pursuit of internationally agreed and peer-reviewed published guidelines. *International Journal of Legal Medicine*. https://www.semanticscholar.org/paper/719183438f940c331c215a64484cbb4530b3379e (accessed on 29 May 2025).

17. de Boer, H. H., Blau, S., Delabarde, T., & Hackman, L. (2018). The role of forensic anthropology in disaster victim identification (DVI): Recent developments and future prospects. *Forensic Sciences Research, 4*(4), 303–315. https://doi.org/10.1080/20961790.2018.1480460.

18. Di Candia, D., Giordano, G., Boracchi, M., & Zoja, R. (2022). Postmortem forensic toxicology cases: A retrospective review from Milan, Italy. *Journal of Forensic Sciences, 67*(5), 1640–1650. https://doi.org/10.1111/1556-4029.15050.

19. Dickens, G. L., Taylor, C., & Woolnough, P. (2019). Adult missing persons: A concept analysis. https://core.ac.uk/download/237029619.pdf (accessed on 29 May 2025).

20. Dixit, P., Sinha, U. S., Kumar, R., Kumari, M., Chawla, H., Chandra, V., & Anand, A. (2024). Digital detectives: Exploring the integration of artificial intelligence in Indian forensic medicine. *IP International Journal of Forensic Medicine and Toxicological Sciences*. https://www.semanticscholar.org/paper/aa0c9ba499c77035d31fcfb3728d42a3d691e981 (accessed on 29 May 2025).

21. Dokov, W., & Radoinova, D. (2014). Applicability of the abbreviated injury scale in forensic medical practice in Bulgaria. https://core.ac.uk/download/389003102.pdf (accessed on 29 May 2025).

22. Domínguez-Muñoz, A., de la Fuente Madero, J. L., Burgos Moreno, J. M., Sotoca Plaza, A., Juárez Bielsa, A., & López Pérez, R. M. (2024). Behavioral analysis in forensic setting with the SAVE method. *South Florida Journal of Health*. https://www.semanticscholar.org/paper/f3ec7fe30fb8ebb2c934cb024e8f9c691b4d856e (accessed on 29 May 2025).

23. Ebeneezar, S., & Vannya, M. S. (2025). Clinical and epidemiological profile of cases of poisoning brought to a tertiary care center located in a rural border district of South Kerala. *Indian Journal of Forensic Medicine & Toxicology*. https://www.semanticscholar.org/paper/9db9721d3a0f2d46ffa9272d9faf9548ff13a294 (accessed on 29 May 2025).

24. Edler, C., Schröder, A. S., Aepfelbacher, M., Fitzek, A., Heinemann, A., Heinrich, F., Klein, A., et al. (2020). Dying with SARS-CoV-2 infection—An autopsy study of the first consecutive

80 cases in Hamburg, Germany. *International Journal of Legal Medicine, 134*(4), 1275–1284. https://doi.org/10.1007/s00414-020-02317-w.

25. Evanjelin, J. P., & Umamaheswari, T. N. (2024). Distinctive anatomical patterns of the mandibular coronoid process, condyle, and sigmoid notch: Cone beam computed tomography (CBCT) imaging for advanced personal identification. *Cureus, 16*(2). https://www.semanticscholar.org/paper/470bc1491881e2b86659935bc4bb4caa6cf2a98a (accessed on 29 May 2025).
26. Ferretti, L., Wymant, C., Kendall, M., Zhao, L., Nurtay, A., Abeler-Dörner, L., Parker, M., et al. (2020). Quantifying SARS-CoV-2 transmission suggests epidemic control with digital contact tracing. *medRxiv*. https://doi.org/10.1101/2020.03.08.20032946.
27. Grabherr, S., Egger, C., Vilarino, R., Campana, L., Jotterand, M., & Dédouit, F. (2017). Modern post-mortem imaging: An update on recent developments. *Forensic Sciences Research, 2*, 52–64. https://doi.org/10.1080/20961790.2017.1330738.
28. Grabherr, S., Heinemann, A., Vogel, H., Rutty, G. N., Morgan, B., Woźniak, K., Dédouit, F., et al. (2018). Postmortem CT angiography compared with autopsy: A forensic multicenter study. *Radiology, 288*, 270–276. https://doi.org/10.1148/radiol.2018170559.
29. Granja, R., & Wienroth, M. (2024). Dissolving boundaries, fostering dependencies: The new forensic genetics assemblage. https://core.ac.uk/download/619583579.pdf (accessed on 29 May 2025).
30. Hickman, G., Kooner, G., & Redwood, J. (2025). Reflections on introducing a carers' forum in an intellectual disability secure service. *Forensic Update.* https://www.semanticscholar.org/paper/4e6c7849f6bf3b8e92b7417e1337dcdf9dd01c3b (accessed on 29 May 2025).
31. Hubbard, J. A. (2025). Review on toxicology testing in hair. *The Journal of Applied Laboratory Medicine.* Advance online publication. https://doi.org/10.1093/jalm/jfaf026.
32. Joe, H. S., Horne, J., de Wet, G. J., Singh, M., Zeye, M. M., & Simon, K. (2025). Forensic DNA expert evidence in the South African context. *African Journal of Legal Studies*. Brill | Nijhoff. https://www.semanticscholar.org/paper/9fa53c08cf7a461f9e6d8507abbfc1618f0b2da3 (accessed on 29 May 2025).
33. Jones, A. W. (2024). DuBowski's stages of alcohol influence and clinical signs and symptoms of drunkenness in relation to a person's blood-alcohol concentration—Historical background. *Journal of Analytical Toxicology, 48*(3), 131–140. https://doi.org/10.1093/jat/bkae008.
34. Kaczmarska, A., Juda, P., Wójcik, Ł., Kłaptocz, P., Łukoś-Karcz, K., Pajor, D., Nowak, M., et al. (2024). A study of gunshot wounds associated with communist executions of the Cursed Soldiers: A medical and historical analysis of materials from the Department of Forensic Medicine in Kraków. *Problems of Forensic Sciences.* https://www.semanticscholar.org/paper/c228e958d3919feb5787be02a1ec9932e49ad507 (accessed on 29 May 2025).
35. Kakkeri, S. R., Ahmed, K. M., Ahmad, S. R., & Khan, R. (2020). Knowledge and attitude of medical students toward medico-legal autopsy. *IP International Journal of Forensic Medicine and Toxicological Sciences, 3*, 8–11. https://doi.org/10.18231/2456-9615.2018.0002.
36. Kandeel, F., & Azab, R. (2024). Evaluation of permanent infirmities cases examined at forensic medicine and clinical toxicology department, Faculty of Medicine, Menoufia University. *The Egyptian Journal of Forensic Sciences and Applied Toxicology.* https://www.semanticscholar.org/paper/7e58862ab69c1d140935045c5e3d7f38da8086aa (accessed on 29 May 2025).

37. Kaye, D. H. (2006). Behavioral genetics research and criminal DNA databases. https://core.ac.uk/download/62553467.pdf (accessed on 29 May 2025).

38. Khalil, R., Mansour, A., Fadda, W. A., Almisnid, K., Aldamegh, M. S., Al-Nafeesah, A., Alkhalifah, A., et al. (2020). The sudden transition to synchronized online learning during the COVID-19 pandemic in Saudi Arabia: A qualitative study exploring medical students' perspectives. *BMC Medical Education, 20*. https://doi.org/10.1186/s12909-020-02208-z.

39. Klinkner, M. (2009). Forensic science expertise for international criminal proceedings: An old problem, a new context and a pragmatic resolution. *The International Journal of Evidence & Proof, 13*(2), 102–129. https://doi.org/10.1350/ijep.2008.12.1.284.

40. Laot Kian, A. M., Karauwan, D., Hartini, S. I., & Herniati, H. (2025). Forensic psychological analysis of criminal offenses cyberbullying in Indonesia (Case study of the cyberbullying phenomenon among public figures). *Formosa Journal of Multidisciplinary Research*. https://www.semanticscholar.org/paper/2a47d42516d65a42401ae286f00859b19e8c9442 (accessed on 29 May 2025).

41. Lechien, J. R., Chiesa-Estomba, C. M., Hans, S., Barillari, M. R., Jouffe, L., & Saussez, S. (2020). Loss of smell and taste in 2013 European patients with mild to moderate COVID-19. *Annals of Internal Medicine, 173*(8), 672–675. https://doi.org/10.7326/M20-2428.

42. Logan, B. K., Mohr, A. L. A., Friscia, M., Krotulski, A. J., Papsun, D. M., Kacinko, S. L., Ropero-Miller, J. D., et al. (2017). Reports of adverse events associated with use of novel psychoactive substances, 2013–2016: A review. *Journal of Analytical Toxicology, 41*, 573–610. https://doi.org/10.1093/jat/bkx031.

43. Longo, L., Brčić, M., Cabitza, F., Choi, J., Confalonieri, R., Del Ser, J., Guidotti, R., et al. (2024). Explainable artificial intelligence (XAI) 2.0: A manifesto of open challenges and interdisciplinary research directions. *Information Fusion, 106*, 102301. https://doi.org/10.1016/j.inffus.2024.102301.

44. Lutz, L., Zehner, R., Verhoff, M. A., Bratzke, H., & Amendt, J. (2021). It is all about the insects: A retrospective on 20 years of forensic entomology highlights the importance of insects in legal investigations. *International Journal of Legal Medicine, 135*, 2637–2651. https://doi.org/10.1007/s00414-021-02628-6.

45. Mariani, M. M., Perez-Vega, R., & Wirtz, J. (2021). AI in marketing, consumer research and psychology: A systematic literature review and research agenda. *Psychology and Marketing, 39*, 755–776. https://doi.org/10.1002/mar.21619.

46. McGowan, M. (2017). Forensics' fight: A need for aggressive strategies against confirmation bias. *Themis: Research Journal of Justice Studies and Forensic Science, 5*(1), Article 11. https://doi.org/10.31979/THEMIS.2017.0511.

47. Moriarty, J. C. (2016). Seeing voices: Potential neuroscience contributions to a reconstruction of legal insanity. *Fordham Law Review, 85*(2), 599–642. https://ir.lawnet.fordham.edu/flr/vol85/iss2/10 (accessed on 29 May 2025).

48. Neal, T. M. S., & Grisso, T. (2014). Assessment practices and expert judgment methods in forensic psychology and psychiatry. *Criminal Justice and Behavior, 41*, 1406–1421. https://doi.org/10.1177/0093854814548449.

49. Neal, T. M. S., & Grisso, T. (2014). The cognitive underpinnings of bias in forensic mental health evaluations. *Psychology, Public Policy, and Law, 20*, 200–211. https://doi.org/10.1037/a0035824.

50. Peres, L. C. (2017). Post-mortem examination in the United Kingdom: Present and future. *Autopsy and Case Reports, 7*, 1–3. https://doi.org/10.4322/acr.2017.017.

51. Piraianu, A. I., Fulga, A., Mușat, C. L., Ciobotaru, O. R., Poalelungi, D. G., Stamate, E., Ciobotaru, O. C., et al. (2023). Enhancing the evidence with algorithms: How artificial intelligence is transforming forensic medicine. *Diagnostics, 13*, 2992. https://doi.org/10.3390/diagnostics13182992.

52. Poalelungi, D. G., Mușat, C. L., Fulga, A., Neagu, M., Neagu, A. I., Piraianu, A. I., & Fulga, I. (2023). Advancing patient care: How artificial intelligence is transforming healthcare. *Journal of Personalized Medicine, 13*(8), 1214. https://doi.org/10.3390/jpm13081214.

53. Prahladh, S., & Van Wyk, J. (2020). Protocol for a scoping review of the current data practices in forensic medicine. *Systematic Reviews, 9*. https://doi.org/10.1186/s13643-020-01308-7.

54. Prajapati, G., Sarode, S. C., Sarode, G. S., Shelke, P., Awan, K. H., & Patil, S. (2018). Role of forensic odontology in the identification of victims of major mass disasters across the world: A systematic review. *PLoS ONE, 13*(6), e0199791. https://doi.org/10.1371/journal.pone.0199791.

55. Qayyum, A., Qadir, J., Bilal, M., & Al-Fuqaha, A. (2020). Secure and robust machine learning for healthcare: A survey. *IEEE Reviews in Biomedical Engineering, 14*, 156–180. https://doi.org/10.1109/rbme.2020.3013489.

56. Ranjan, A., Kumar, P., & Verma, A. (2024). An analysis of medicolegal autopsies conducted at Patna Medical College, Patna (Bihar)—A mortuary-based study. *Global Journal for Research Analysis*. https://www.semanticscholar.org/paper/a60a0794b0cbd51c85a0134391381bd0ed94cd6f (accessed on 29 May 2025).

57. Rodda, L. N., Candela, K. E., Hart, A. P., Moffatt, E. G., Pearring, S., & Scott, K. S. (2025). Bladder wash as an alternative postmortem toxicology specimen: Forensic pathologists' perspectives. *The American Journal of Forensic Medicine and Pathology*. https://www.semanticscholar.org/paper/249a8a04b2c49d319667dbb39c4c79f2ec06668e (accessed on 29 May 2025).

58. Romańczuk, A., Rojek, S., Synowiec, K., Maciów-Głąb, M., & Kula, K. (2023). Interpretative problems due to the presence of chloromethcathinone isomers in the biological material from postmortem cases. *Journal of Analytical Toxicology, 47*, 797–806. https://doi.org/10.1093/jat/bkad070.

59. Roszkowska, A., Plenis, A., Kowalski, P., Bączek, T., & Olędzka, I. (2022). Recent advancements in techniques for analyzing modern, atypical antidepressants in complex biological matrices and their application in biomedical studies. *TrAC Trends in Analytical Chemistry, 152*, 116609. https://doi.org/10.1016/j.trac.2022.116609.

60. Roux, C., Willis, S., & Weyermann, C. (2021). Shifting forensic science focus from means to purpose: A path forward for the discipline? *Science & Justice, 61*(6), 678–686. https://doi.org/10.1016/j.scijus.2021.08.005.

61. Saker, L., Gharbi, M., Mellouki, Y., Sellami, L., & Zerairia, Y. (2025). Oral and dental trauma in forensic medicine. *Batna Journal of Medical Sciences*. https://www.semanticscholar.org/paper/fc308514f604049133dfd17543e3bea9261c0a92 (accessed on 29 May 2025).

62. Sallam, M. (2023). ChatGPT utility in healthcare education, research, and practice: Systematic review on the promising perspectives and valid concerns. *Healthcare, 11*, 887. https://doi.org/10.3390/healthcare11060887.

63. Samir, A., Ashour, F. H., Abdel Hakim, A. A., & Bassyouni, M. (2022). Recent advances in biodegradable polymers for sustainable applications. *npj Materials Degradation, 6*. https://doi.org/10.1038/s41529-022-00277-7.

64. Sane, M. R., Kapoor, N., & Badiye, A. (2023). Introduction to forensic medicine and pathology. https://doi.org/10.1007/978-981-99-1377-0_20.

65. Sanz-García, A., Gesteira, C., Sanz, J., & García-Vera, M. P. (2021). Prevalence of psychopathy in the general adult population: A systematic review and meta-analysis. *Frontiers in Psychology, 12*. https://doi.org/10.3389/fpsyg.2021.661044.

66. Sanzyapova, R. R. (2025). The role of dentistry in forensic medicine: Identification of human remains. *Patient-Oriented Medicine and Pharmacy*. https://www.semanticscholar.org/paper/d8db5ae62d74c13d619c3b0324e081b54abd3399 (accessed on 29 May 2025).

67. Satam, H., Joshi, K., Mangrolia, U., Waghoo, S., Zaidi, G., Rawool, S., Thakare, R. P., et al. (2023). Next-generation sequencing technology: Current trends and advancements. *Biology, 12*(7), 997. https://doi.org/10.3390/biology12070997.

68. Shivakumar, D. K. (2024). Forensic medicine and toxicology: A fusion of science and mythology in Indian context. *Annals of Advanced Biomedical Sciences*. https://www.semanticscholar.org/paper/92925aaad86e2fa6d424e6a65031fc667c0d8b1b (accessed on 29 May 2025).

69. Siedin, M. S., Plis, S. S., Klevno, V. A., Maksimov, A. V., & Plashchinskiy, A. A. (2024). Retrospective analysis of nonfatal skeletal injuries sustained in road incidents involving electric scooters. *Russian Journal of Forensic Medicine, 10*(2), 160–170. https://doi.org/10.17816/fm15597.

70. Singh, W. U., & Singh, K. P. (2023). The transformative role of artificial intelligence in forensic medicine and toxicology. *Journal of Medical Society, 37*, 101–102. https://doi.org/10.4103/jms.jms_54_24.

71. Suwalowska, H., Ali, J., de Almeida, J. R., Fonseca, S. A., Heathfield, L. J., Keyes, C. A., Lukande, R., et al. (2023). "The nobodies": Unidentified dead bodies—A global health crisis requiring urgent attention. *The Lancet Global Health, 11*(12), e1691–e1693. https://doi.org/10.1016/S2214-109X(23)00420-5.

72. Teymourian, H., Parrilla, M., Sempionatto, J. R., Montiel, N. F., Barfidokht, A., Van Echelpoel, R., De Wael, K., et al. (2020). Wearable electrochemical sensors for the monitoring and screening of drugs. *ACS Sensors, 5*(9), 2679–2700. https://doi.org/10.1021/acssensors.0c01318.

73. Toom, V. (2014). Trumping communitarianism: Crime control and forensic DNA typing and databasing in Singapore. *East Asian Science, Technology and Society: An International Journal, 8*(3), 273–296. https://doi.org/10.1215/18752160-2416805.

74. Villa, C., Lynnerup, N., & Jacobsen, C. (2023). A virtual, 3D multimodal approach to victim and crime scene reconstruction. *Diagnostics, 13*(17), 2764. https://doi.org/10.3390/diagnostics13172764.

75. Volobuyeva, O. (2024). About the determinants of sexual crimes and their consideration in criminal proceedings. *Uzhhorod National University Herald. Series: Law*. https://www.semanticscholar.org/paper/8998e06fbbd289853ef61f9b5eff22fc4dec8574 (accessed on 29 May 2025).

76. Yadav, S., Kulshreshtha, N., Sharma, S., & Joshi, T. (2023). Victim identification through skeletal remains: A review. *IP International Journal of Forensic Medicine and Toxicological Sciences*. https://www.semanticscholar.org/paper/8d6b18b90c46e911e5d6a1a412908a00865d5a3c (accessed on 29 May 2025).

77. Yang, W., Zhou, M., Zhang, P., Geng, G., Xiaoning, L., & Zhang, H. (2020). Skull sex estimation based on wavelet transform and Fourier transform. *BioMed Research International, 2020*, Article 8608209. https://doi.org/10.1155/2020/8608209.

78. Yoo, S. H., Lee, W. T., & Lee, J. (2024). Evaluating the forensic inferences of oral nicotine ingestion: Autopsy case review, animal experimentation, and legal implications. *Korean Journal of Legal Medicine*. https://www.semanticscholar.org/paper/bef3c6d5f655f507e7ff17ce67f0bbea83c64386 (accessed on 29 May 2025).

79. Zeppenfeld, K., Tfelt-Hansen, J., Riva, M., Winkel, B. G., Behr, E. R., Blom, N. A., Charron, P., et al. (2022). 2022 ESC guidelines for the management of patients with ventricular arrhythmias and the prevention of sudden cardiac death. *European Heart Journal, 43*, 3997–4126. https://doi.org/10.1093/eurheartj/ehac262.

80. Zhang, Z., Qin, S., Chen, Y., Zhou, L., Yang, M., Tang, Y., Zuo, J., et al. (2022). Inhibition of NPC1L1 disrupts adaptive responses of drug-tolerant persister cells to chemotherapy. *EMBO Molecular Medicine, 14*, e14903. https://doi.org/10.15252/emmm.202114903.

LEGAL PROCEDURES IN FORENSIC MEDICINE

2

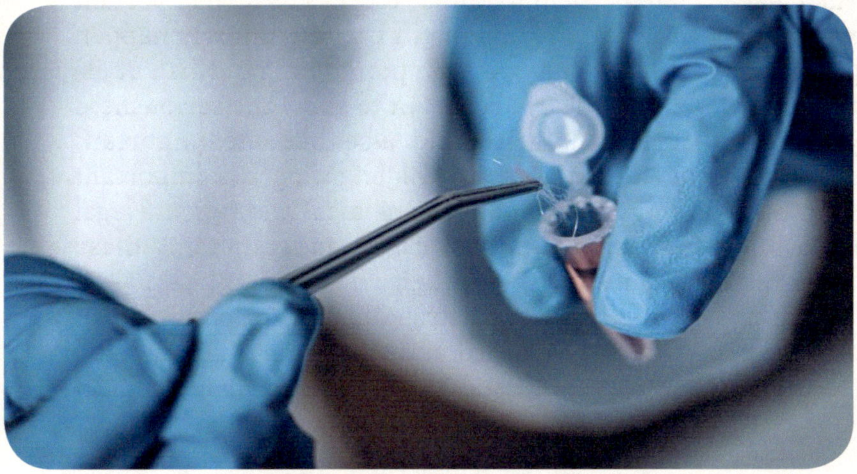

LEARNING OBJECTIVES

After studying this chapter, you will be able to:

1. Describe the part forensic medicine plays in legal cases;
2. Understand the legal framework governing forensic medicine;
3. Learn procedures for evidence collection and analysis;
4. Know ethical and professional considerations in forensic medicine.

Introduction

Forensic medicine is now experiencing changes because of the merging of technology and law and the outcomes are not the same as before. Because of AI and new imaging techniques, legal processes now have to keep up with the rapid changes happening around us. AI-driven autopsy methods, for instance, are stepping into the spotlight: they can boost both how effective and fair forensic analysis feels, yet they also spark fresh debates over ethics and legal responsibility (Kumar et al., 2024). Most of the time, the law is carefully working to blend new technologies into old ways of doing things which can be difficult but is necessary. In general, using both innovation and careful supervision is necessary to maintain the reliability of forensic work and the justice system. As forensic medicine wrestles with these evolving challenges, a careful, and sometimes uneven, look at legal routines becomes even more crucial (Pereira et al., 2024).

Importance of Legal Procedures in Forensic Medicine

Investigations rely on the combination of legal rules and forensic medicine to be solid. If medical-legal decisions depend on clear science, it is necessary to follow set guidelines. Experts in biomechanics—take Dr. Eng. Marco Bernardini, for instance—have shown that sharing rigorous research with lawmakers highlights why we need to keep to these standards in medicolegal situations (Bernardini, 2024). This is clear when examining detailed dental trauma cases; it shows that using a step-by-step approach is important in forensics. Forensic odontologists, for example, have to run both steady clinical checks and thorough radiographic assessments so their results come off as both spot-on and defensible in court (Khan et al., 2024). Most of the time, these legal actions help maintain the quality of evidence and also increase public trust in our justice system, even if things get complicated—since every case must meet strict legal requirements.

Overview of the Relationship between Law and Medicine

There are many ways law and medicine are connected and this is especially true in forensic science, where a doctor's knowledge is often central to solving legal cases. You can see this in international criminal cases, where every bit of forensic evidence, like that from exhumations done through forensic archaeology, gets disturbed under intense scrutiny to prove its worth (Klinkner et al., 2009). DNA used in disaster victim identifications isn't just about pinpointing who's who; it also stumbles into murky territory about family ties and ethical dilemmas (Haimes et al., 2014). Most of the time, this mix of law and medicine demonstrates that both fields must cooperate to achieve justice which can be a bit messy but very interesting.

Scope of Legal Procedures in Forensic Medicine

Forensic medicine procedures in law are not simple because they require a detailed analysis of different injuries and their legal meaning. For example, traumatic nerve damage gets a lot of scrutiny since it needs detailed record-keeping to back legal claims, especially in risky jobs like security; after all, one study examined over 393 cases (Emre Gürkan Bulutluöz et al., 2025). Dental trauma, too, has its own important role by shedding light on how injuries happen and even helping pinpoint victims (Khan et al., 2024). They are meant to show the seriousness of the injuries and also become important evidence in court, highlighting the important relationship between medical findings and legal decisions. In most cases, understanding these connections—though a bit complicated—is generally seen as strengthening the credibility of forensic evidence, and that, in turn, helps fortify the overall legal framework used in medical investigations (Figure 2.1).

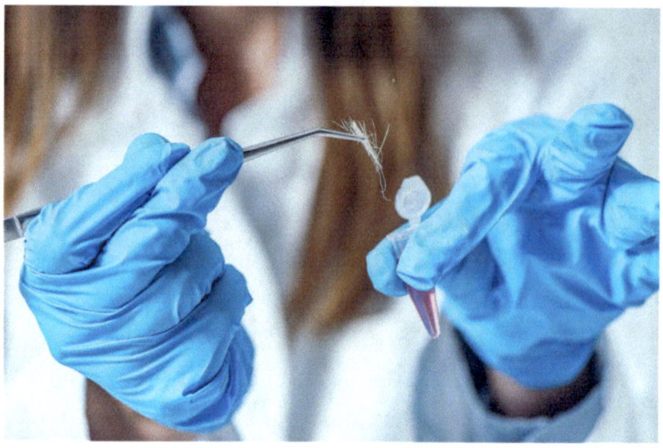

Figure 2.1. Legal procedures in forensic medicine.

Source: https://www.dawelllifescience.com/wp-content/uploads/2024/08/13.jpg.

Relevance to Current Legal and Medical Practices

The fast progress of technology is linking medicine and law in surprising ways, mainly in forensic investigations. Both areas now rely on artificial intelligence which improves results and saves time. Still, many AI systems work like black boxes, leaving us uncertain about just how clear or reliable their decisions are; this naturally drives a push for eXplainable AI (XAI) that fits legal standards and ensures proper accountability and understanding in court (Ali et al., 2023). Meanwhile, therapeutic drug monitoring is reshaping drug treatments in forensic psychiatry by offering more tailored approaches for individuals with unique needs (Hiemke et al., 2017). In short, these steps underline that a strong, almost married cooperation between fresh laws and medical progress is necessary to maintain the strength, trustworthiness and effectiveness of forensic science.

2.1. The Role of Forensic Medicine in Legal Proceedings

Learning Outcome

1. Know the types of cases involving forensic medicine;
2. Explain the role of forensic experts in court;
3. Discuss the importance of evidence collection;
4. Know the chain of custody in forensic evidence;
5. Explain how the results of forensic investigations affect legal decisions;
6. Focus on ethical considerations in forensic medicine;
7. Find out what problems forensic experts encounter when working in legal cases.

Forensic medicine connects science and the law and greatly affects legal outcomes. While a case is being investigated, experts slowly put together a story from the scientific clues, much like putting together a puzzle. As an example, international criminal tribunals use the process of digging up mass graves to uncover facts and find important details about the victims which support the claims of war crimes. Usually, this results in what people call a "forensic truth," which is then put to the test in court and can receive uneven and tough review. In most cases, it is during expert testimony in court that the connection between law and science is most obvious and tough questioning and opposing opinions are often needed to check the expert's credibility and relevance. To summarize, this messy interaction underlines the need for a solid, adaptable framework to direct the role of forensic scientists in legal proceedings (Klinkner et al., 2009).

Forensic medicine is very important in solving legal problems at the intersection of health and law. It uses medical knowledge to help settle legal issues, whether in criminal or civil cases and makes sense of confusing evidence. People working in this field review medical signs, try to find out the cause of death or the severity of injuries and most of the time, their findings influence the court's decisions. At times, going through physical evidence helps them find clear facts that support the case in court. Because of advancements in technology, especially artificial intelligence, forensic medicine is not staying the same. The new rules, like the AI Act (Veale et al., 2021; (Ali et al., 2023), hint at fresh legal responsibilities tied to these innovations, showing just how much the field is evolving. In short, being aware of what forensic medicine involves is very important for understanding its role in legal cases.

2.1.1. Types of Cases Involving Forensic Medicine

When science and law meet in a legal case, forensic medicine becomes very important. In homicide investigations, forensic pathologists are used to find out the cause of death and also to detect any signs that the death was not natural. Think about the exhumations tied to the Srebrenica events; that evidence played a major role in the Krstic trial and showed just how messy the mix of forensic know-how and international law can be (Klinkner et al., 2009). Moving on to another subject, child abuse cases with shaken baby syndrome claims can be very surprising. Often, pediatricians and experts in forensic medicine examine the same evidence such as subdural bleeding or damaged retinal vessels. Basically, these issues make it clear that forensic medicine involves both finding hidden facts and ensuring fairness in the law. Sometimes the process feels a tad uneven, but in most cases, that very unpredictability is what makes it so crucial to our legal system (Duncea et al., 2017) (Figure 2.2).

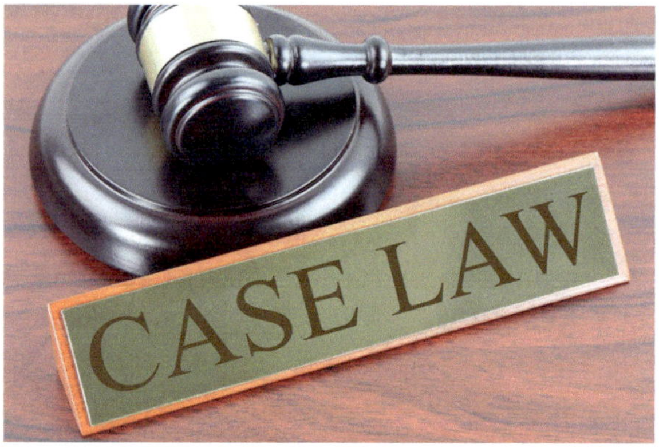

Figure 2.2. Legal cases can get tricky when science and law overlap.

Source: https://blog.ipleaders.in/wp-content/uploads/2021/07/case-law-2.jpg.

2.1.2. The Role of Forensic Experts in Court

Since legal cases can be very confusing, experts are brought in to explain the details. Their judgments help make the facts clear and they can also have a strong impact on the results. Take juvenile cases, for instance: psychologists are often called on to explain behaviors sometimes tagged as demoralization or delinquency, all while sticking to the strict methods set by legal authorities (Rode et al., 2023). Then there are administrative matters where forensic specialists toss in crucial evidence that backs up the claims from all sides, further deepening how decisions get made (Lunina et al., 2023). To summarize, mixing in these expert insights usually means the process is better informed, which is pretty essential for serving justice—despite the occasional minor inconsistency in style (Figure 2.3).

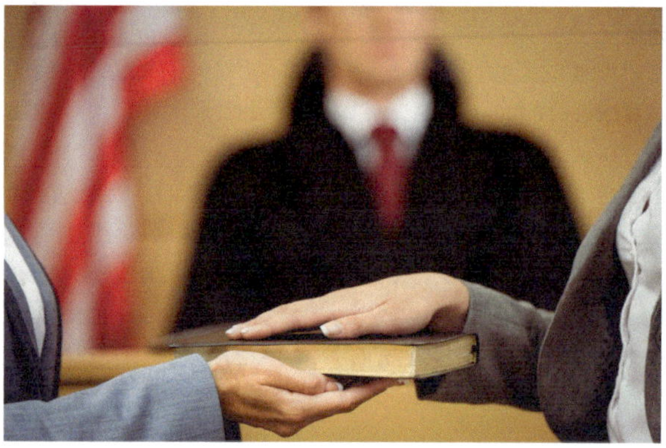

Figure 2.3. The role of forensic experts in court.

Source: https://www.mdd.com/wp-content/uploads/2012/02/iStock-537972247.jpg.

2.1.3. Importance of Evidence Collection

The success of a forensic case depends on careful evidence collection which affects how the case is handled legally. When investigations move forward, the way facts are organized does not only record events; it also builds a narrative that links science with legal rules and may present important details in a different way. Take, for example, what happened at the International Criminal Tribunal for the former Yugoslavia, where digging up and analyzing mass graves shows, in most cases, how forensic techniques meet judicial demands (Klinkner et al., 2009). Such careful work, with its mix of precise detail and natural human error, means expert testimony often stands up under close trial scrutiny—think about how forensic archaeology gets called upon for those particularly knotty legal questions (Klinkner et al., 2009). To summarize, the fairness of legal processes pretty much relies on thorough evidence collection; it not only helps uncover the truth but also upholds justice, especially in the nuanced world of forensic medicine (Figure 2.4).

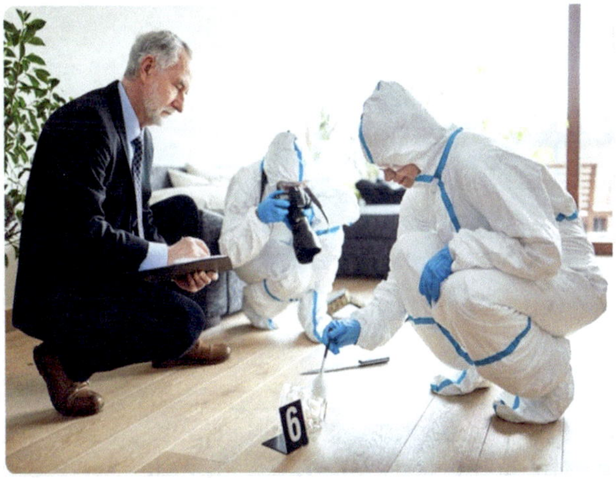

Figure 2.4. Evidence collection.

Source: https://d1g9yur4m4naub.cloudfront.net/image-handler/picture/2021/8/shutterstock_1400087216.jpg.

2.1.4. Chain of Custody in Forensic Evidence

Forensic work starts with treating evidence with extreme care. All samples, no matter if they are physical, chemical or microbiological, are kept clean and tracked from the beginning until they are used in court. Actually, studies show that even a small lapse in this process can mean evidence gets thrown out, which, in most cases, jeopardizes the whole legal case (Appuhamy, 2022). It's important to follow biosecurity rules as well as record every time the sample is passed to someone else. When you combine good record-keeping with safety measures, the outcomes are usually dependable and maintain the public's trust in our courts. To summarize, treating evidence with such attention not only supports dependable forensic outcomes but also reminds us of its crucial role in both civil and criminal investigations (Figure 2.5).

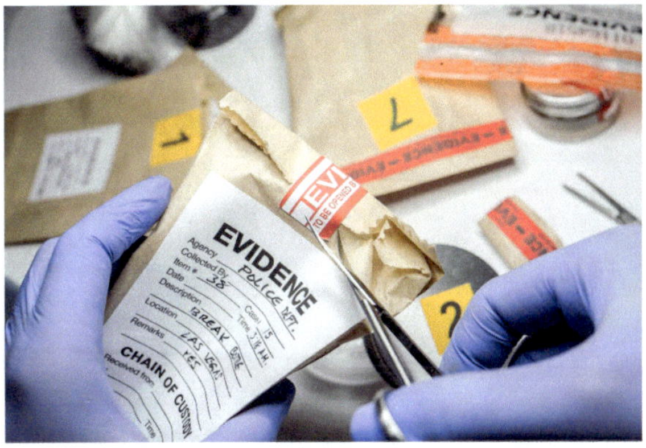

Figure 2.5. Every bit collected—whether it's something physical, a chemical sample, or even a microbiological specimen—is kept pure and tracked from the get-go until it appears in court.

Source: https://i0.wp.com/issglobal.co.uk/wp-content/uploads/2019/11/AdobeStock_268497800.jpeg?fit=5184%2C3535&ssl=1.

2.1.5. The Impact of Forensic Findings on Legal Outcomes

Legal outcomes often hinge on forensic findings. In several criminal cases such details can help one side win by supporting their arguments. If usual types of evidence are not enough, these clues can help confirm the facts, even if they are not direct. Even so, depending so much on forensic science leads to many ethical and procedural concerns, mainly about the way evidence is interpreted and presented in court. Various guidelines, like those proposed for therapeutic drug monitoring in certain groups, generally speak to a need for consistent standardization (so that findings remain both accurate and understandable to juries) (Hiemke et al., 2017). Plus, the emerging trend of shared decision-making in legal settings suggests that, in most cases, there's growing awareness of the messy complexity forensic evidence introduces—and its big impact on justice (Slade, 2017) (Figure 2.6).

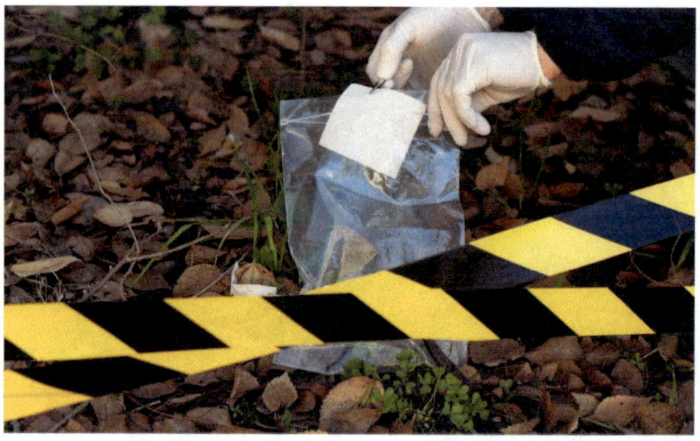

Figure 2.6. The impact of forensic findings on legal outcomes.

Source: https://img.starleaf.com/6rvqnc.jpg.

2.1.6. Ethical Considerations in Forensic Medicine

There are times when medicine and law meet which can raise some tough ethical questions. Experts in forensic psychology such as psychiatrists in legal settings, must handle two very different jobs. They need to examine a case in an unbiased way for the law, but also take care of the people they assess. It is not easy for them to do what's best for the patient and also give a fair evaluation that can be used in court. A good example is the debate on the insanity defense which highlights the conflict between caring for the accused and giving justice. There's also the mess of not having enough reliable data on professional liability claims, which only muddies the ethical waters further (Asokan, 2014). All in all, being aware of these ethical issues is very important for people in forensic medicine.

2.1.7. Challenges Faced by Forensic Experts in Legal Settings

Legal cases can be very complicated and forensic experts often run into many difficulties that affect the outcome. A main problem is making complex scientific findings understandable for judges and jurors who are not experts in technology. The legal process can make it harder when the system's competitive nature can change or misunderstand the evidence. On top of that, new tools like hyperspectral imaging have opened fresh avenues in forensic analysis, yet in most cases, leaning on these methods demands strict checking and standardization to keep things credible in court (Khan et al., 2018). There's also the ethical side: ensuring informed consent while juggling individual rights against public safety – a challenge that, generally speaking, echoes the shared decision-making seen in healthcare (Slade, 2017). In short, forensic experts have to deal with these unexpected situations to make sure their work stays strong in a system that is not simple.

Test Your Knowledge

1. How does forensic medicine assist in criminal investigations?
2. What is a medical expert witness?

2.2. Legal Framework Governing Forensic Medicine

Learning Outcome

1. Understand an overview of relevant laws and regulations;
2. Describe the duties of the judiciary in forensic medicine;
3. Learn standards for forensic evidence admissibility;
4. Be aware of how important court rulings have shaped forensic work;
5. Describe international laws affecting forensic medicine;
6. Discuss the role of professional organizations and guidelines;
7. Identify the legal responsibilities of forensic practitioners;
8. Examine the outcomes of breaking the law in forensic medicine;
9. Learn future trends in legal frameworks.

The rules of law and forensic medicine do not always stay the same, since politics can shift the situation. In many authoritarian places—Singapore, for example—DNA tests and other forensic methods end up being used more for crime control and public safety rather than for guarding individual rights; as a result, privacy and the presumption of innocence can sometimes take a back seat (Toom et al., 2014). On the other hand, arrangements like the Prüm Treaty generally show the European Union leaning toward collective oversight, where member states are expected to share forensic data in a sort of coordinated response to cross-border crime (Prainsack et al., 2012). It influences the way evidence is gathered and applied and it also quietly reflects the main political ideas behind the systems. Forensic medicine relies heavily on legal procedures which help determine justice and affect how society treats individual rights.

2.2.1. Overview of Relevant Laws and Regulations

Forensic medicine law combines scientific accuracy with ethical consideration. The Prüm Treaty is a good example – it makes it necessary for EU countries to exchange important forensic information such as DNA and fingerprints which usually helps them work together against international crime and terrorism. This kind of collaborative legal setup shows, generally speaking, that forensic rules are always evolving to meet new tech challenges and social shifts (Prainsack et al., 2012). In Ukraine, the story changes slightly since reforms are aimed at getting rid of old Soviet-era practices in forensic psychiatry for administrative offenses, yet a few legal gaps still appear. Even with these changes on the horizon, it turns out there's still a need for more reforms to make sure personal rights are fully protected (Butenko et al., 2023). To summarize, these examples remind us that sound laws aren't just about keeping the system in check; they're also key to defending human rights in forensic settings (Figure 2.7).

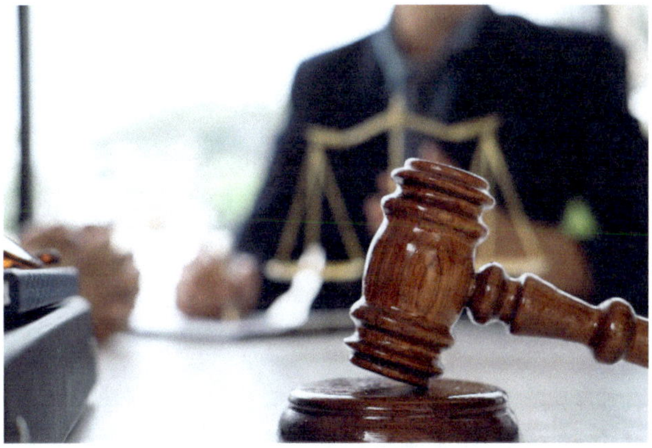

Figure 2.7. Forensic medicine law weaves together a patchwork of rules that mix scientific exactness with ethical care.

Source: https://lighthc.london/wp-content/uploads/2024/10/court-1.png.

2.2.2. The Role of the Judiciary in Forensic Medicine

It often seems that law and science get tangled together in an interesting and sometimes confusing way in forensic medicine. Courts make sure that the evidence from forensics is managed correctly under the law which usually helps maintain a fair process. In many instances, when a sudden cardiac death happens, postmortem genetic tests pop up to reveal hidden causes; such cases stir up ethical and legal dilemmas that the courts have to untangle carefully (Fellmann et al., 2019).

Also, handling cases with mentally disordered offenders calls for a pretty in-depth grasp of forensic psychiatry, balancing public safety with personal rights (Birgit Völlm et al., 2018). To summarize, the legal system isn't only busy interpreting rules—it ends up shaping how forensic methods are practiced, a role that sits at the heart of our whole legal system (Figure 2.8).

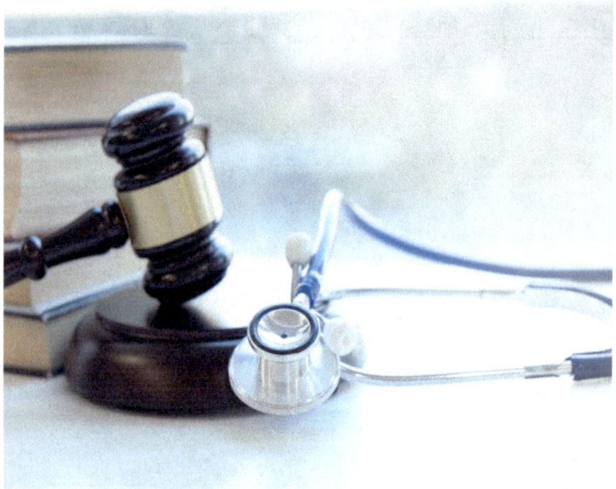

Figure 2.8. The role of the judiciary in forensic medicine.

Source: https://legaldesire.com/wp-content/uploads/2020/06/AdobeStock_182248615-scaled-1.jpeg.

2.2.3. Standards for Forensic Evidence Admissibility

Because of new technology, you need to be familiar with the rules for what the law considers acceptable evidence. Keeping every record exactly as the law requires is crucial – take, for example, South Africa's Electronic Communications and Transactions Act along with the Criminal Procedure Act; they clearly set out what counts as proper electronic evidence in court (Prahladhet al., 2022). These rules are important for trustworthy data, not only for following the law and sometimes they can feel repetitive. Biomarkers – such as the ones checking for alcohol intake – now push forensic methods beyond strictly criminal cases, finding their way into clinical settings to confirm abstinence or even check for misuse (Streichert et al., 2018). All in all, these developments highlight the importance of stronger rules for handling and keeping evidence, so it is legally sound and supports the whole field of forensics.

2.2.4. The Impact of Landmark Cases on Forensic Practices

Landmark legal cases have changed forensic work over time. Because of these high-profile cases, it became obvious that the usual ways of handling things and keeping things private were not enough. Most of the time, people began to rely on data rather than intuition which helped move forensic science toward methods based on real evidence. Many are now talking about the importance of reducing bias, mainly when it comes to serious cases like child abuse, because a single expert's opinion can heavily influence a jury's decision. Experts now frequently find themselves having to juggle uncertainty and keep things objective, even while questions arise over whether their views might be colored by biases or outside pressures (Skellern et al., 2015). Ultimately, those landmark cases have played a big role as change-makers, prompting calls for greater accountability and opening doors for setting stricter, more reliable standards in forensic practices (Garrett et al., 2018) (Figure 2.9).

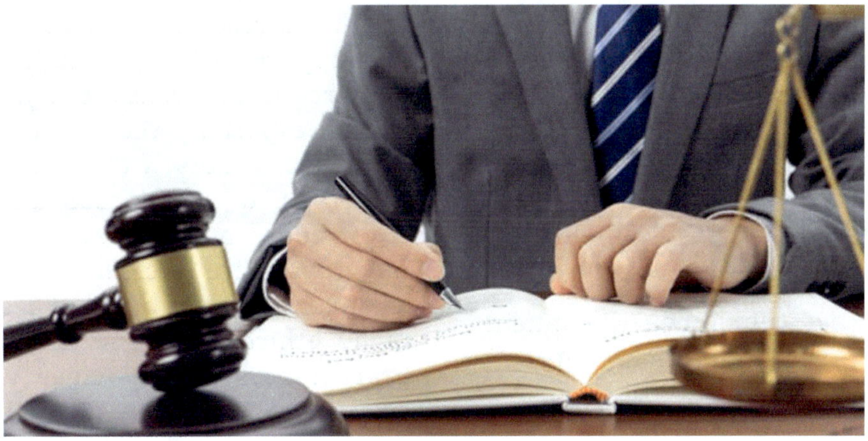

Figure 2.9. Landmark legal cases have changed forensic work over time.

Source: https://cache.careers360.mobi/media/article_images/2023/4/10/landmark-judgments-india.png.

2.2.5. International Laws Affecting Forensic Medicine

International law and forensic medicine can be connected which can affect how legal actions happen in different countries. An example is using genomic data in criminal investigations—Ukraine's Law On State Registration of Human Genomic Information demonstrates how they want to include both local and global guidelines. It tries to ensure that DNA is used ethically, that the law is clear and that personal rights are protected. Over in Switzerland, the rules for checking if a person's eyesight is good enough for driving point to an idea that every driver should get equal treatment; they're pushing for more standardized medical tests (Blaser et al., 2025). All in all such collaborations are important because they ensure that daily practices are just and ethical which makes the evidence used in court cases more reliable.

2.2.6. The Role of Professional Organizations and Guidelines

Professional organizations play a huge role in forensic medicine. They establish rules and also support practitioners in dealing with difficult legal matters—usually, they are more than just people who make laws. Many times, these groups influence daily activities and give assistance when dealing with legal matters becomes complicated. Take psychological evaluations, for example. Guidelines provided by bodies such as the Committee on Professional Practice and Standards (COPPS) often serve as a kind of playbook for carrying out careful, ethical assessments in work environments (American Psychological Association et al., 2018). At the same time, when forensic medicine bumps up against broad societal challenges—say, issues like gender-based violence (GBV)—the same protocols step in to guide efforts across areas like justice and health (Morrison et al., 2004). It's generally true that these organizations don't simply regulate; they also nurture smarter, well-informed practices that, in most cases, mix legal and ethical standards into every decision (Figure 2.10).

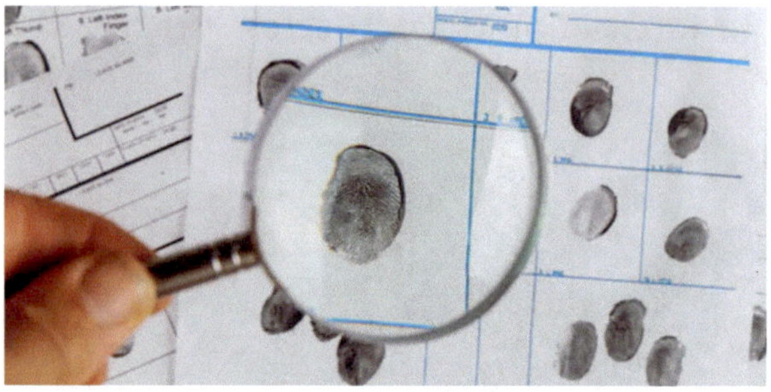

Figure 2.10. Professional organizations play a huge role in forensic medicine.

Source: https://www.ncuindia.edu/wp-content/uploads/2024/06/Legal-Education.webp.

2.2.7. Legal Responsibilities of Forensic Practitioners

Forensic practitioners have to handle many legal duties in addition to the work they do in the lab. In the justice system, these experts are not only scientists but also important people who ensure their findings are correct and follow the rules for evidence and testimony. This duty gets even more crucial in tough cases like abusive head trauma (AHT), where even a tiny misstep in expert testimony (Lucas et al., 2017) can tip the scales. Lately, there's been a clear trend towards relying on structured assessment tools; this shift shows just how much-standardized methods play a role in forensic evaluations (Neal et al., 2014).

They strengthen the outcomes of investigations and also hold practitioners responsible, so that everyone's rights are respected in court. In short, combining forensic skills with following the law helps shape the justice system, often proving how important these professionals are for maintaining proper standards.

2.2.8. Consequences of Legal Violations in Forensic Medicine

Mistakes in the law and in forensic work can cause unexpected problems in our courts and daily routines. If legal rules are ignored, the way evidence is dealt with is usually disorganized which can result in both wrongful convictions and opportunities for justice being missed. Research from forensic examiners shows that biases, especially those stacking up against victims, can mess with both how evidence is gathered and how it's read, ultimately twisting courtroom outcomes and keeping systemic unfairness alive (McMillan et al., 2015). When legal rules are not closely observed, there are many ethical problems that arise, pushing practitioners to pay close attention. With the world in a bit of turmoil – think rising geopolitical tensions and ever-changing public health issues – it seems clear that forensic practices might need a fresh, more culturally tuned-up approach to ensure fairness (Smith et al., 2024). All in all, understanding these mixed-up outcomes is important for trusting forensics and for smooth legal operations.

2.2.9. Future Trends in Legal Frameworks

The legal part of forensic medicine is going through major changes in response to new social issues. Because of rising political and environmental problems, laws in forensic work need to be adaptable and aware of cultural differences to meet new ethical demands. Generally speaking, the bond between forensic psychiatry and our courts calls for guidelines that not only mirror today's ideas about social justice but also encourage more cross-disciplinary teamwork (Smith et al., 2024). Also, emerging quality management models—which stress clear reporting and accountability—mean that agencies will, in many cases, face fresh compliance hurdles under new international mandates, a factor that underlines why sticking to uniform practices in forensic science is so crucial (Heavey et al., 2023). To summarize, this legal shift aims to promote fair outcomes by ensuring that every nuanced part of forensic medicine helps shape a legal process that can keep up with our rapidly changing global landscape (Figure 2.11).

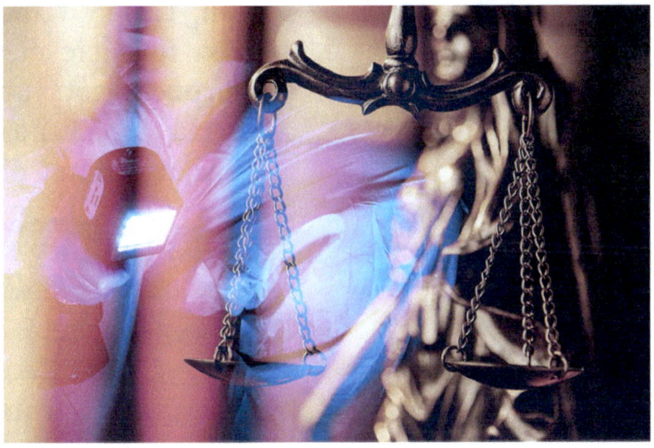

Figure 2.11. Forensic medicine's legal side is on the verge of big changes as it grapples with modern societal challenges.

Source: https://fosterfreeman.com/wp-content/uploads/2024/02/scales-of-justice-comp.jpg.

Test Your Knowledge

1. What is the legal framework in forensic medicine?
2. What is the significance of consent in medico-legal examinations?

2.3. Procedures for Evidence Collection and Analysis

Learning Outcome

1. Perform initial assessment and scene investigation;
2. Explain types of forensic evidence (biological, chemical, etc.);
3. Know techniques for evidence collection;
4. Learn documentation and reporting procedures;
5. Describe laboratory analysis methods;
6. Discuss quality control in forensic analysis;
7. Focus on interpretation of forensic results;
8. Give presentation of evidence in court;
9. Know the limitations and challenges in evidence analysis.

Forensic science and law are closely connected which means investigators must use both planned and unplanned methods to examine and test evidence. Gathering evidence in a loud crime scene or a silent mass grave is very important for forming the "forensic truth" that will be used in court. Take the exhumations following the Srebrenica events of July 1995; generally speaking, expert testimonies paired with hands-on scientific work proved to be quite pivotal in cases such as the Krstic trial (Klinkner et al., 2009). It's worth noting that the strength of evidence often leans on relentless cross-examinations and the occasional presentation of counter-expertise inside trial rooms—especially when there isn't much in the way of clear rules regarding admissibility (Klinkner et al., 2009).

In short, this process which requires careful documentation many times, proves the importance of having written rules to maintain the quality of evidence and increase trust in forensic medicine in legal settings.

2.3.1. Initial Assessment and Scene Investigation

Looking closely at the scene is the first important step in forensic medicine. The initial part of the process sets up the rest and those first steps may affect the analysis and conclusions in ways that are not obvious. From the start, the team works to keep the area safe so nothing is damaged and they take photos, make sketches and jot down a few notes as they go. Cutting-edge approaches, like investigative genetic genealogy, have turned things on their head; by linking clues from distant familial ties based on genetic markers (Kling et al., 2021), experts can now narrow down potential suspects more effectively. It's also important to keep in mind the legal side of things, since how evidence is collected might sway its acceptability in court (Veale et al., 2021). To summarize, a careful yet flexible kick-off not only safeguards the investigation's integrity but also helps sustain the bigger picture of justice within our legal system (Figure 2.12).

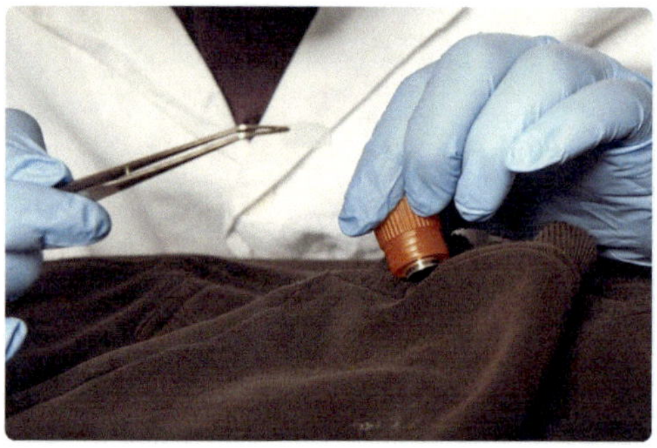

Figure 2.12. Taking a detailed look at the scene is a key starting point in forensic medicine.

Source: https://d1g9yur4m4naub.cloudfront.net/image-handler/picture/2020/2/shutterstock_1275729166.jpg.

2.3.2. Types of Forensic Evidence (Biological, Chemical, etc.)

Organizing evidence is very important in forensic medicine and it plays a major role in legal cases.

There's many clues here, like biological stuff (think DNA, blood, hair) alongside chemical tests that help put together what happened. In many situations, those biological bits help identify someone and also link them to the crime scene; this is what is most important in most cases. People often mention that with DNA, careful sample collection is absolutely key – if the samples degrade, you lose a lot of what makes them useful (Kozma et al., 2018). Chemical tests which detect drugs or toxins, can be used to reconstruct the scene, but sometimes their results are hard to interpret. Still, this kind of evidence comes with its own challenges, and it reminds us that every single step in forensic work needs a lot of scrupulous care (Cole et al., 2020) (Figure 2.13).

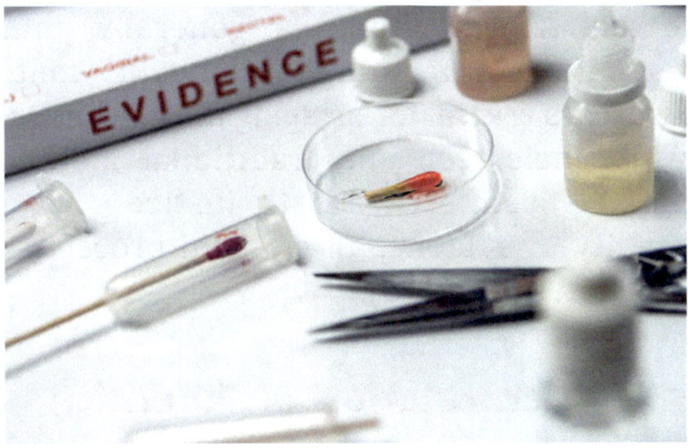

Figure 2.13. Sorting evidence matters a lot in forensic medicine.

Source: https://p39ablog.com/wp-content/uploads/2023/12/Foundational-Validity-in-Forensic-Evidence-India-2-1024x659.png.

2.3.3. Techniques for Evidence Collection

The collection of evidence in forensic medicine matters a lot—it may affect the outcome of a trial. Many different ways are used, sometimes in ways you might not expect, to secure biological, physical and digital evidence; usually, this means sticking to standard protocols to keep samples like DNA uncontaminated. For example, forensic anthropology uses close study of bones to sometimes discover important facts about the person's death. To summarize, these approaches not only bolster investigations but also fortify the legal process by making sure that what's gathered in the field holds up in court, ultimately playing a key role in the quest for justice (Figure 2.14).

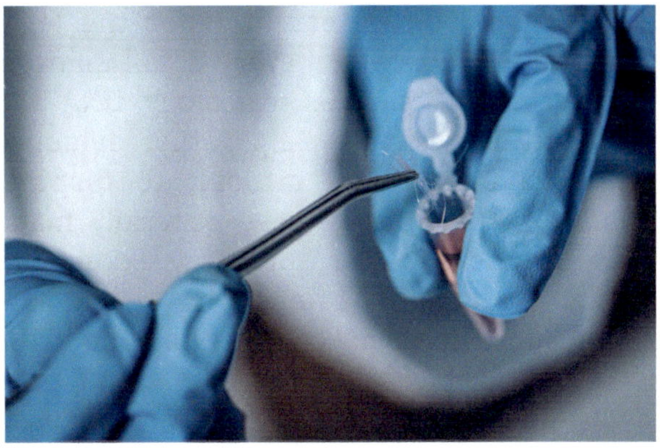

Figure 2.14. Collecting evidence in forensic medicine is absolutely vital.

Source: https://images.ctfassets.net/cnu0m8re1exe/3AqxojG0drM8MqNT5evtvv/680e56943aae20a9dcd983358afd896a/DNA-Forensic-Science-Hair-Sample-Tweezers-Blue-Gloves.jpg.

2.3.4. Documentation and Reporting Procedures

In forensic medicine, detailed record-keeping is important because it can change legal decisions and influence medical studies. Making sure all observations are carefully documented meets the law and also helps investigations use better data. Take national registries, for example; the Swedish Cause of Death Register (Brooke et al., 2017) shows how maintaining careful details offers rich, comprehensive insights into mortality trends and health issues in different communities. Doctors' efforts in spotting and reporting signs of child abuse play a huge role as well—these reports can protect our most vulnerable and help steer legal actions (Christian, 2015). In short, using these procedures ensures the evidence is not altered and supports the whole legal process. In general, keeping records properly is not only about paperwork; it is essential for good clinical work and fair justice in forensic fields.

2.3.5. Laboratory Analysis Methods

Forensic lab work is essential for the legal system to function well – every detail matters. Many techniques such as toxicology, DNA and blood spatter analysis, help gather evidence that most courts find difficult to dispute. Advances in technology have generally made these practices better, allowing experts to examine crime scene samples in great detail. Adding ideas from psychology and medicine also brings in the human side of what happens during difficult investigations. For instance, noticing the unique situations faced by victims has spurred recommendations for clearer steps when figuring out who qualifies as a victim, which, in turn, is pretty important for applying forensic results accurately (Zamani, 2025).

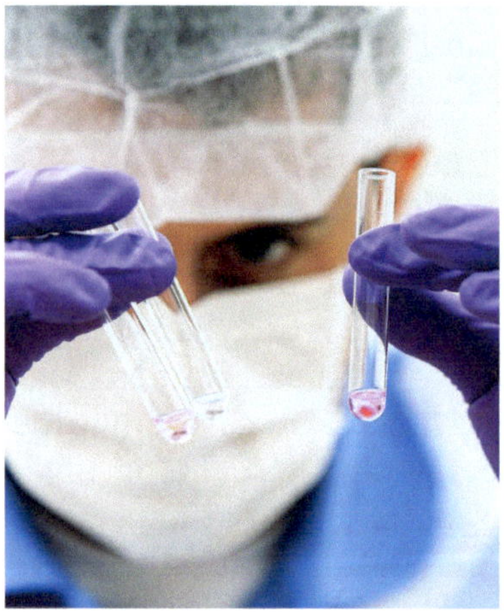

Figure 2.15. Forensic lab work is key to keeping our legal system on track.

Source: https://static01.nyt.com/images/2017/09/06/nyregion/06DNA1/29DNA1-articleLarge.jpg?quality=75&auto=webp&disable=upscale.

Finally, a steady rethinking and tweaking of lab procedures remains essential for keeping these methods both reliable and effective in our justice system (Figure 2.15).

2.3.6. Quality Control in Forensic Analysis

It is important that forensic analysis is solid when the law and order are involved in forensic medicine. Ensuring strict quality checks helps the results be accurate and also makes the evidence more believable in court. Labs check their procedures, use standard methods and train staff well which helps reduce errors and doubts. Regular audits, especially in high-stakes cases like DNA work (where even a tiny misstep can lead to big legal headaches), play a key role too. As the literature generally points out, continually updating these quality control measures is critical for bridging the gap between new forensic tech and traditional methods, ultimately reinforcing both justice and the reliability of evidence in criminal proceedings (Osborne et al., 2018).

2.3.7. Interpretation of Forensic Results

Forensic evidence is interpreted in many ways, not just by analyzing data in a laboratory and it plays a key role in legal cases. Scientific information is turned into clear and personal accounts by experts, so that judges, jurors and others can understand it. It requires you to look closely at every piece of evidence which needs you to understand the science and be able to explain it in a way everyone can understand. In many cases, recent studies have shown that finding SARS-CoV-2 in the central nervous system might lead to pretty complicated neurological issues—a reminder that forensic specialists need to pick up on subtle links between cause and effect (Meinhardt et al., 2020). Similarly, keeping an eye on drug levels in forensic psychiatry makes it clear that accurate measurement is essential when determining things like intent or impairment in a legal setting (Hiemke et al., 2017). Generally speaking, mixing in-depth scientific work with plainspoken explanations is what connects the dots between hard evidence and a case's legal story (Figure 2.16).

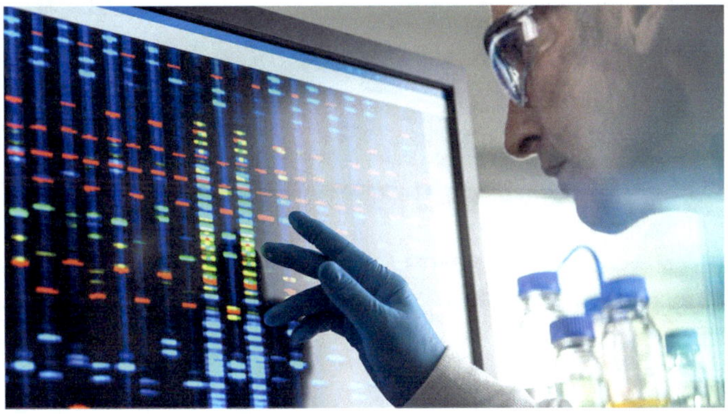

Figure 2.16. Interpreting forensic evidence isn't just about crunching numbers in a lab.

Source: https://media.hswstatic.com/eyJidWNrZXQiOiJjb250ZW50Lmhzd3N0YXRpYy5jb20iLCJrZXkiOiJnaWZcL2dldHR5aW1hZ2VzLTE0Mjg2MTUxMjEuanBnIiwiZWRpdHMiOnsicmVzaXplIjp7IndpZHRoIjoiMTIwMCJ9fX0=.

2.3.8. Presentation of Evidence in Court

How well evidence is presented matters a lot for judicial fairness, as it helps establish who is responsible and the reason for the accident. Forensic medicine understands this well, since it often uses science that must be described in a way everyone can understand to judges and jurors who may not be experts. Take the INFERENCE method, for example; it measures the chances of one event causing another and shows how detailed forensic work can turn complicated medical facts into ideas that make sense in a courtroom context (Meilia et al., 2021). Past cases generally reveal that understanding scientific evidence isn't always straightforward; societal views and courtroom biases sometimes seep in, leaving a lingering tug-of-war between science and law (Diamond et al., 2018). In short, ensuring that forensic evidence is easy to understand and reliable is still essential for fairness in the law.

2.3.9. Limitations and Challenges in Evidence Analysis

Forensic science and the law do not always work together easily. Often, the very methods that claim to reveal "forensic truth" end up showing gaps when they hit a courtroom, where how evidence is seen can shift unexpectedly (Klinkner et al., 2009). It's not easy, —you start to doubt if these techniques really work as well as they claim. Also, the introduction of artificial intelligence in forensic psychiatry introduces its own challenges. A.I. neuroprediction, for instance, can sometimes sharpen risk assessments and tweak intervention plans, but it also stokes deep ethical debates and raises questions over whether courts should trust its results (Tortora et al., 2020). Most of the time, our current practices fall short and new technology keeps advancing, so we have to keep finding new ways to do things. In this tangled mix, pulling together ideas from a range of fields isn't just useful—it's pretty much essential for making sure that our analysis of evidence stays both scientifically solid and legally fair (Figure 2.17).

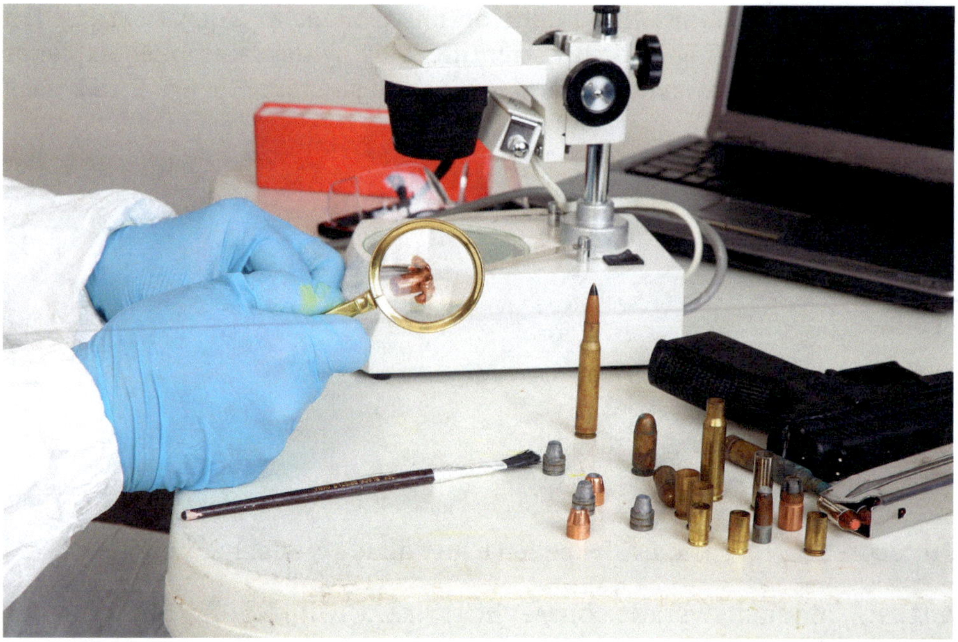

Figure 2.17. Mixing forensic science with the legal world isn't exactly straightforward.

Source: https://www.washingtonpost.com/wp-apps/imrs.php?src=http://www.washingtonpost.com/news/the-watch/wp-content/uploads/sites/22/2015/04/bigstock-forensic-analysis-a-forensic-82606832.jpg&w=1440.

Test Your Knowledge

1. What is the chain of custody in evidence collection?
2. What is contamination in evidence handling?
3. How does the collection of blood happen at the scene of a crime for forensic purposes?

2.4. Ethical and Professional Considerations in Forensic Medicine

Learning Outcome

1. Understand ethical dilemmas faced by forensic practitioners;
2. Focus on informed consent in forensic examinations;
3. Know confidentiality and privacy issues;
4. Explain the role of bias in forensic analysis;
5. Focus on professional conduct and accountability;
6. Discuss continuing education and training requirements;
7. Describe how public opinion affects the way forensic work is done;
8. Describe collaboration between legal and medical professionals;
9. Identify future ethical challenges in forensic medicine.

Forensic medicine is in a position where ethics and the law come into conflict. For example, clinicians should evaluate people without bias and still respect their basic dignity and rights. Patient wellbeing, which traditional medical ethics champions, sometimes gets tangled up with the need for detached, fact based testimony in court; generally speaking, this clash can lead to situations where the drive for justice ends up overshadowing an individual's own needs, as many real-world dilemmas in the field illustrate (Asokan, 2014). There is not enough data on professional liability which makes it hard to design policies that cover everyone. It is clear why it is still very important to learn about the legal results of forensic investigations.

2.4.1. Ethical Dilemmas faced by Forensic Practitioners

People working in forensic medicine regularly face moral dilemmas that challenge their responsibility and personal values. Because of the combination of medical knowledge and strict laws, examiners regularly find themselves managing patient care and following legal rules. As an example, when dealing with late pregnancy terminations, clinicians may experience conflicting emotions: the families are very emotional, but the law may require them to perform feticide after 22 weeks which many find disturbing. Likewise, forensic psychiatrists end up serving as a kind of bridge between medicine and law; they are compelled to maintain impartiality while knowing that their assessments might ripple out to affect lives within the criminal justice system (Bailey, 2011). To summarize, these tangled dilemmas generally highlight the importance of having clear ethical guidelines and ongoing training—as the ever-shifting landscape of forensic practice demands nothing less (Figure 2.18).

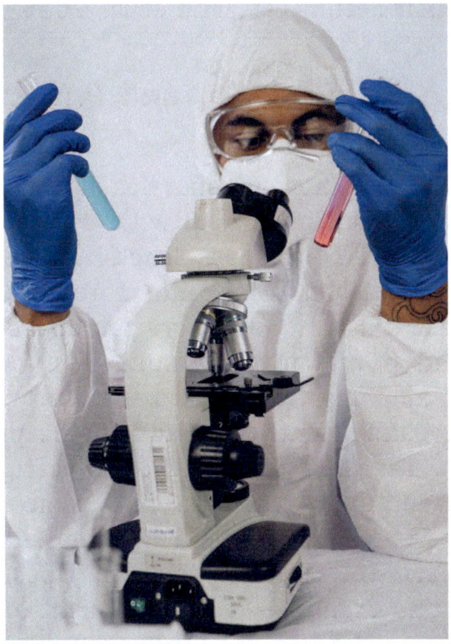

Figure 2.18. Professionals in forensic medicine often confront ethical challenges that test both their sense of duty and personal integrity.

Source: https://wires.onlinelibrary.wiley.com/cms/asset/481846fa-e0f4-464a-aa3e-4c1930d96ad6/wfs21502-toc-0001-m.jpg.

2.4.2. Informed Consent in Forensic Examinations

Forensic exams are not easy which is why a solid consent framework is necessary for all legal actions in forensic medicine. Proper consent protects people's rights and also helps everyone know what they are agreeing to. Take, for instance, cases where alcohol is involved: when biomarker tests get used for legal records—be it in a child custody dispute or checking abstinence after a driver's license suspension (Streichert et al., 2018)—nailing down consent correctly becomes extra important. At the same time, as these methods keep changing, many neuropsychologists believe that strong testing should be used in evaluations, even if the details are sometimes complicated. All of this points to a broader view of consent ethics and highlights the need for clear, honest communication to help avoid any mix-ups or misinterpretations in forensic settings (Martin et al., 2015).

2.4.3. Confidentiality and Privacy Issues

Forensic medicine now relies heavily on genetic profiling which must deal with both shifting laws and privacy issues. Genetic information which scientists now look into more frequently, can make it hard to tell where personal secrets end and public investigations begin; these details, showing what makes a person unique and revealing family ties, add to the privacy debate. In most cases, when investigators handle and study this data, they come across ethical issues that should be handled with care. Take the ALRC Report 96 (Opeskin et al.) as one example—it shines a light on how widespread the impact of these genetic details can be and points out that, in most cases, a tougher, more thoughtful legal setup is needed. Because genome sequencing is now so common, it's almost as easy as checking emails which means the chance of someone getting into the data without permission has gone up. This isn't just about spotting a disease risk or a unusual trait; it's about seeing whole family stories laid out where they might complicate a case (Ayday et al., 2015). To summarize, it seems clear that clear, well-considered policies must be put into place—ones that protect individual privacy while still letting forensic evidence play its crucial role in the legal process (Figure 2.19).

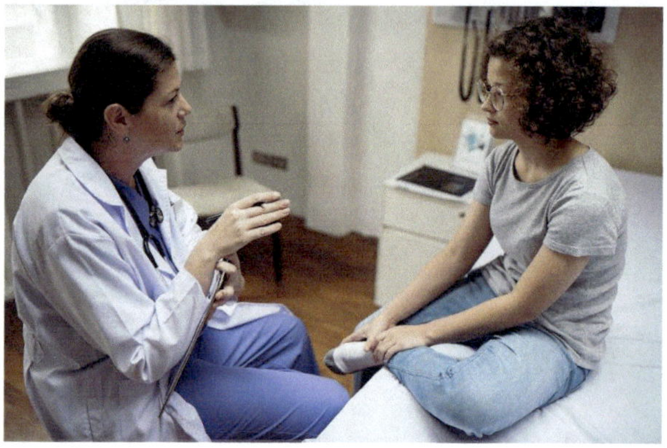

Figure 2.19. Confidentiality and privacy issues.

Source: https://s3.amazonaws.com/utep-uploads/wp-content/uploads/DUQ-MIG/2019/09/13094445/SANE-sitting-with-patient.jpg.

2.4.4. The Role of Bias in Forensic Analysis

Forensic medicine can become complicated when mental factors are not easy to spot. Sometimes, forensic pathologists let their own thoughts or past experiences about how a death happened affect their findings. Ironically, the very decision-making frameworks designed to keep these biases in check can, in many cases, end up intensifying the issue (Al-Saif, 2024). With the changes happening, artificial intelligence is now being seen as a promising solution. AI-powered autopsies and advanced imaging tools—take VIRTOPSY, for instance—bring in dependable data that, generally speaking, works to dilute these subjective influences and pave the way for sharper, more efficient investigations (Kumar et al., 2024). Addressing bias directly is necessary to maintain the honesty of legal processes and to make sure justice is given equally.

2.4.5. Professional Conduct and Accountability

Today, forensic medicine requires people to be truly ethical and responsible—it should not be treated lightly. It is common for professionals to face a mix of legal rules and community standards; being honest, even when it is challenging, is very important. Forensic work now includes technology and AI which usually make things more efficient but can also introduce risks such as bias or misuse. Take the proposed AI Act (Veale et al., 2021) for example; it lays out different rules for various risk levels, subtly pointing to the ethical quagmires that can arise when modern tools are used. Stakeholders, eager to build public trust, are increasingly aware that even unintentional slip-ups can have serious fallout (Schwartz et al., 2022). At the end of the day, sticking to long-standing ethical standards is key—it keeps forensic practices both legally solid and truly accountable (Figure 2.20).

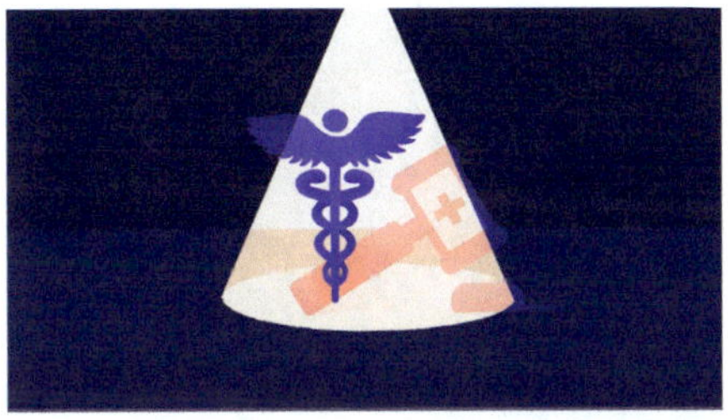

Figure 2.20. Forensic medicine today demands a real commitment to ethics and accountability.

Source: https://www.sermo.com/wp-content/uploads/2022/03/resource-ethical-issues-in-healthcare.jpg.

2.4.6. Continuing Education and Training Requirements

Because forensic medicine is changing rapidly, experts have to keep learning new things to meet both legal and ethical standards. Learning all the time is important, not just a saying, since it involves handling new challenges such as advanced DNA analysis and the effects of genetics on court cases. Often, these training efforts lean on an unexpected mix of teamwork; several associations, for example, host workshops that tweak and refine guidelines, stressing the power of shared knowledge in boosting forensic methods (Wilks et al., 2016). In addition, detailed reviews—such as those carried out by the ALRC—generally point out the pressing need for ethical training about genetic information, reinforcing that forensic practitioners must keep learning to navigate these multifaceted challenges effectively (Opeskin et al., 2025).

2.4.7. The Impact of Public Perception on Forensic Practices

Conversations in daily life can affect the way forensic medicine professionals do their jobs. People in the media, law and other interested groups are always paying attention and their interest can lead to changes in the usual ways of doing things. Increased attention even tends to make practitioners more alert to their own mental shortcuts—some studies have shown that analysts, fixated on case details, sometimes end up chasing confirmation bias (Cooper et al., 2019). When community voices get woven into decision-making, it adds an extra ethical twist that many see as boosting genuine credibility (Slade, 2017). Having public input increases trust and can lead to changes in how the method is used to fit what society wants. It is generally very important to pay attention to what the public thinks, since this helps keep forensics and the law fair and effective.

2.4.8. Collaboration Between Legal and Medical Professionals

It is important to handle oral and dental injuries fast which requires close cooperation between healthcare experts and lawyers. Plenty of evidence shows that many of these cases stem from deliberate actions, which means keeping detailed records and some legal backup is often necessary to support a victim's claim (Saker et al., 2025). Although it may seem unusual for forensic doctors and dentists to work together, their teamwork helps patients and meets all the legal requirements. It is obvious from the reports that combining medical and legal knowledge helps identify who is responsible, mainly when there are signs of malpractice. Working together in this way helps ensure accurate facts and also builds trust in our legal system and helps protect the public. In short, combining law and medicine in forensic medicine improves both areas and makes it more effective.

2.4.9. Future Ethical Challenges in Forensic Medicine

Forensic medicine is expanding rapidly, but it also brings some difficult ethical issues. AI and data analysis are now part of the process which makes some people doubt if the evidence is still reliable. Many people also find themselves involved in consent debates, mainly when dealing with biological samples, because genetic data is used more frequently in investigations. Sometimes the data is not handled correctly which can lead to new concerns about privacy and discrimination. Since a little mistake could shake people's trust in the system, it is important to keep things clear and open. In many cases, sorting out these issues isn't just about modernizing forensic techniques; it's a key step toward protecting justice and keeping legal proceedings on the straight and narrow, as seen in recent talks on ethical responsibilities in scientific research and analysis (Adeniyi et al., 2024; Bulska, 2024) (Figure 2.21).

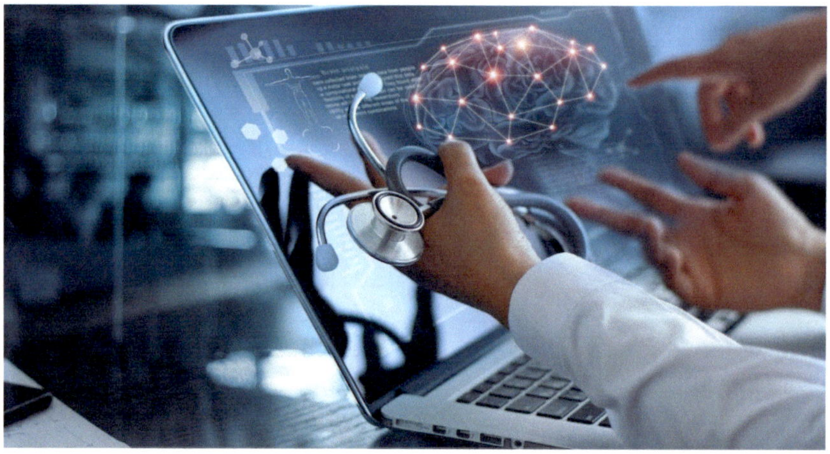

Figure 2.21. Advanced tools like AI and data crunching mix into the work, sparking doubts about whether the evidence stays rock-solid.

Source: https://aranca.com/assets/uploads/blogs/virtual_blog_healthcare.jpg.

Test Your Knowledge

1. Define informed consent. Why is it important in medico-legal examinations?
2. What is confidentiality and how are confidentiality rules followed in forensic cases?

Summary

Legal systems play a big role, as clearly shown by the constant changes in forensic medicine. Even though routine evaluations were disrupted by COVID-19, this proved that unexpected events can disrupt established processes. One study Soni et al. (2024) revealed that during the lockdown autopsy numbers took a sharp dive at first, then slowly bounced back as restrictions eased; a pattern both surprising and telling. The messy details in cases of people dying from guns suggest that our laws about gun ownership and mental health could be reviewed. Most of the time, these insights encourage us to understand that legal procedures should adapt as times and problems change. In the end, understanding these changes well helps forensic medicine play a stronger role in ensuring justice in our legal system.

At the meeting point of law and science, people are now discussing the role of forensic medicine in legal cases. International criminal tribunals rely on expert testimony which is very complex and requires strict rules when examining forensic evidence. Sometimes, evidence from mass grave digs has been important in trials because it proves that experts need solid methods to support their opinions. In several international cases, both the big ideas and the everyday challenges of forensic science were looked into, which, in most cases, revealed issues when it came to admitting and interpreting evidence (Klinkner et al., 2009). Also, piecing together what's often called "forensic truth" becomes a key task as this evidence winds its way through the legal maze, facing intense cross-examination and scrutiny (Klinkner et al., 2008). All in all, these mixed views help explain the delicate and sometimes confusing link between forensic science and the law in seeking justice.

KEY TERMS FROM THIS CHAPTER

- AI-driven autopsy
- Clinical checks
- Dental trauma
- Ethics
- Imaging
- Innovation
- Investigations
- Justice system
- Lawmakers
- Legal accountability
- Legal responsibility
- Radiographic assessments
- Security

Short Answer Questions

1. What is the role of autopsy in medico-legal cases?
2. How is injury documentation useful in court?
3. What does "chain of custody" mean in forensic evidence?
4. Differentiate between *cause of death* and *manner of death*.
5. What is the legal significance of a toxicology report?
6. How can forensic medicine help establish identity?

Critical Thinking Questions

1. **Which document is needed to give permission for an autopsy when someone dies in an unusual way?**
   a. Informed consent from the family
   b. Court order
   c. Police request or Magistrate's order
   d. Written permission from the deceased's employer
2. **Which of these is not included in the usual way evidence is collected in forensic medicine?**
   a. Sealing evidence in tamper-proof packaging
   b. Maintaining the chain of custody
   c. Discussing the findings with the defense lawyer
   d. Documenting all evidence with proper labeling and signatures
3. **When someone is suspected of sexual assault, medical examination is mainly done to:**
   a. Determine the identity of the assailant
   b. Treat the victim's injuries
   c. Collect evidence for the court
   d. Provide psychological counseling
4. **What are the legal rules for a forensic pathologist to give testimony in court?**
   a. They must have a medical degree
   b. They must have specific forensic pathology training and experience
   c. They need to have a license to practice in the place where the case is taking place.
   d. They must be referred by the defense lawyer
5. **Which of these is the top legal concern for a forensic medical practitioner working with a victim's body?**
   a. Ensuring the victim's family is present
   b. Seeking permission from the nearest police station
   c. Making sure evidence is properly stored and handled to keep it unchanged
   d. Publicly announcing the findings to the press

Answers to Critical Thinking Questions

1. (c); 2. (c); 3. (c); 4. (b); 5. (c)

References

1. Adel, A. (2023). Unlocking the future: Fostering human–machine collaboration and driving intelligent automation through Industry 5.0 in smart cities. *Smart Cities, 6*, 2742–2782. https://doi.org/10.3390/smartcities6050124.
2. Aggarwal, A., Mittal, M., & Battineni, G. (2021). Generative adversarial network: An overview of theory and applications. *International Journal of Information Management Data Insights, 1*, 100004. https://doi.org/10.1016/j.jjimei.2020.100004.
3. Aimar, A., Palermo, A., & Innocenti, B. (2019). The role of 3D printing in medical applications: A state of the art. *Journal of Healthcare Engineering, 2019*, 5340616. https://doi.org/10.1155/2019/5340616.
4. Ali, S., Abuhmed, T., El-Sappagh, S., Muhammad, K., Alonso, J. M., Confalonieri, R., Guidotti, R., et al. (2023). Explainable artificial intelligence (XAI): What we know and what is left to attain trustworthy artificial intelligence. *Information Fusion, 99*, 101805. https://doi.org/10.1016/j.inffus.2023.101805.
5. Atreya, A., Rajbanshi, R., Menezes, R. G., et al. (2025). Evaluation of undergraduate forensic medicine education in Nepal: A critical analysis using Schwab's five commonplaces and Schubert's curriculum images. *BMC Medical Education, 25*, 147. https://doi.org/10.1186/s12909-025-06741-7.
6. Awan, E. A., Afzal, H., Yousfani, G. M., Imran, S., Memon, A. A., & Pehlwani, H. A. (2023). Retrospective analysis of 258 consecutive forensic exhumations with emphasis on causative agents/cause of death. *Deleted Journal, 13*(1), 9–12. https://doi.org/10.62118/jmmc.v13i1.254.
7. Bairoch, A. (2018). The Cellosaurus, a cell-line knowledge resource. *Journal of Biomolecular Techniques, 29*, 25–38. https://doi.org/10.7171/jbt.18-2902-002.
8. Balhareth, A. A. S., Jamesh, M., Zabarah, G. A., Almotlaq, M. M., Alabaaltahin, M. A. M., Al Jaarah, A. H. A., Aldawsari, A. G. A., et al. (2024). The role of forensic medicine in modern criminal justice: A review of current practices and innovations. *Journal of Eco Humanism, 3*(7). https://doi.org/10.62754/joe.v3i7.4669
9. Barlow, E. M., & Dickens, G. L. (2018). Systematic review of therapeutic leave in inpatient mental health services. https://core.ac.uk/download/228178293.pdf (accessed on 29 May 2025).
10. Barrett, J., Bidmos, G., Bilge, Y., et al. (2014). The foot in forensic human identification–A review. https://core.ac.uk/download/30660095.pdf (accessed on 29 May 2025).
11. Bartoshyk, N. (2024). Analysis of the number of deaths due to poisoning by the most common poisonous substances in the LVIV region in 2018–2023. *Forensic-Medical Examination*. https://www.semanticscholar.org/paper/11ab7886efe10b9fb28d671682ea7cd842c27417 (accessed on 29 May 2025).
12. Brassett, C., Cosker, T., Davies, D. C., Dockery, P., Gillingwater, T. H., Lee, T. C., Milz, S., et al. (2020). COVID-19 and anatomy: Stimulus and initial response. *Journal of Anatomy, 237*(3),

393–403. https://doi.org/10.1111/joa.13274.

13. Buzdar, Z. A., Murad, T., Shabbir, S., Ahmed, A., Soomro, T. A., & Masood, R. (2024). Estimating age on the autopsy table: A postmortem study of forensic investigations. *JSMC, 14*(4), 353–358. https://jsmc.pk/index.php/jsmc/article/view/995 (accessed on 29 May 2025).

14. Campa, F., Coratella, G., Cerullo, G., Noriega, Z., Francisco, R., Charrier, D., Irurtia, A., et al. (2024). High-standard predictive equations for estimating body composition using bioelectrical impedance analysis: A systematic review. *Journal of Translational Medicine, 22*. https://www.semanticscholar.org/paper/f744b316b1eed48b81522277b42cdaef522c1094 (accessed on 29 May 2025).

15. Carew, R. M., & Errickson, D. (2020). An overview of 3D printing in forensic science: The tangible third-dimension. *Journal of Forensic Sciences, 65*, 1752–1760. https://doi.org/10.1111/1556-4029.14442.

16. Cusack, D. A. (2025). The European Council of Legal and Forensic Medicine: Its role and work in progressing harmonized standards and recommendations in forensic and legal medicine investigation procedures, training and teaching through pursuit of internationally agreed and peer-reviewed published guidelines. *International Journal of Legal Medicine*. https://www.semanticscholar.org/paper/719183438f940c331c215a64484cbb4530b3379e (accessed on 29 May 2025).

17. de Boer, H. H., Blau, S., Delabarde, T., & Hackman, L. (2018). The role of forensic anthropology in disaster victim identification (DVI): Recent developments and future prospects. *Forensic Sciences Research, 4*(4), 303–315. https://doi.org/10.1080/20961790.2018.1480460.

18. Di Candia, D., Giordano, G., Boracchi, M., & Zoja, R. (2022). Postmortem forensic toxicology cases: A retrospective review from Milan, Italy. *Journal of Forensic Sciences, 67*(5), 1640–1650. https://doi.org/10.1111/1556-4029.15050.

19. Dickens, G. L., Taylor, C., & Woolnough, P. (2019). Adult missing persons: A concept analysis. https://core.ac.uk/download/237029619.pdf (accessed on 29 May 2025).

20. Dixit, P., Sinha, U. S., Kumar, R., Kumari, M., Chawla, H., Chandra, V., & Anand, A. (2024). Digital detectives: Exploring the integration of artificial intelligence in Indian forensic medicine. *IP International Journal of Forensic Medicine and Toxicological Sciences*. https://www.semanticscholar.org/paper/aa0c9ba499c77035d31fcfb3728d42a3d691e981 (accessed on 29 May 2025).

21. Dokov, W., & Radoinova, D. (2014). Applicability of the abbreviated injury scale in forensic medical practice in Bulgaria. https://core.ac.uk/download/389003102.pdf (accessed on 29 May 2025).

22. Domínguez-Muñoz, A., de la Fuente Madero, J. L., Burgos Moreno, J. M., Sotoca Plaza, A., Juárez Bielsa, A., & López Pérez, R. M. (2024). Behavioral analysis in forensic setting with the SAVE method. *South Florida Journal of Health*. https://www.semanticscholar.org/paper/f3ec7fe30fb8ebb2c934cb024e8f9c691b4d856e (accessed on 29 May 2025).

23. Ebeneezar, S., & Vannya, M. S. (2025). Clinical and epidemiological profile of cases of poisoning brought to a tertiary care center located in a rural border district of South Kerala. *Indian Journal of Forensic Medicine & Toxicology*. https://www.semanticscholar.org/paper/9db9721d3a0f2d46ffa9272d9faf9548ff13a294 (accessed on 29 May 2025).

24. Edler, C., Schröder, A. S., Aepfelbacher, M., Fitzek, A., Heinemann, A., Heinrich, F., Klein, A., et al. (2020). Dying with SARS-CoV-2 infection—An autopsy study of the first consecutive 80 cases in Hamburg, Germany. *International Journal of Legal Medicine, 134*(4), 1275–1284. https://doi.org/10.1007/s00414-020-02317-w.

25. Evanjelin, J. P., & Umamaheswari, T. N. (2024). Distinctive anatomical patterns of the mandibular coronoid process, condyle, and sigmoid notch: Cone beam computed tomography (CBCT) imaging for advanced personal identification. *Cureus, 16*(2). https://www.semanticscholar.org/paper/470bc1491881e2b86659935bc4bb4caa6cf2a98a (accessed on 29 May 2025).

26. Ferretti, L., Wymant, C., Kendall, M., Zhao, L., Nurtay, A., Abeler-Dörner, L., Parker, M., et al. (2020). Quantifying SARS-CoV-2 transmission suggests epidemic control with digital contact tracing. *medRxiv*. https://doi.org/10.1101/2020.03.08.20032946.

27. Grabherr, S., Egger, C., Vilarino, R., Campana, L., Jotterand, M., & Dédouit, F. (2017). Modern post-mortem imaging: An update on recent developments. *Forensic Sciences Research, 2*, 52–64. https://doi.org/10.1080/20961790.2017.1330738.

28. Grabherr, S., Heinemann, A., Vogel, H., Rutty, G. N., Morgan, B., Woźniak, K., Dédouit, F., et al. (2018). Postmortem CT angiography compared with autopsy: A forensic multicenter study. *Radiology, 288*, 270–276. https://doi.org/10.1148/radiol.2018170559.

29. Granja, R., & Wienroth, M. (2024). Dissolving boundaries, fostering dependencies: The new forensic genetics assemblage. https://core.ac.uk/download/619583579.pdf (accessed on 29 May 2025).

30. Hickman, G., Kooner, G., & Redwood, J. (2025). Reflections on introducing a carers' forum in an intellectual disability secure service. *Forensic Update.* https://www.semanticscholar.org/paper/4e6c7849f6bf3b8e92b7417e1337dcdf9dd01c3b (accessed on 29 May 2025).

31. Hubbard, J. A. (2025). Review on toxicology testing in hair. *The Journal of Applied Laboratory Medicine.* Advance online publication. https://doi.org/10.1093/jalm/jfaf026.

32. Joe, H. S., Horne, J., de Wet, G. J., Singh, M., Zeye, M. M., & Simon, K. (2025). Forensic DNA expert evidence in the South African context. *African Journal of Legal Studies*. Brill | Nijhoff. https://www.semanticscholar.org/paper/9fa53c08cf7a461f9e6d8507abbfc1618f0b2da3 (accessed on 29 May 2025).

33. Jones, A. W. (2024). DuBowski's stages of alcohol influence and clinical signs and symptoms of drunkenness in relation to a person's blood-alcohol concentration—Historical background. *Journal of Analytical Toxicology, 48*(3), 131–140. https://doi.org/10.1093/jat/bkae008.

34. Kaczmarska, A., Juda, P., Wójcik, Ł., Kłaptocz, P., Łukoś-Karcz, K., Pajor, D., Nowak, M., et al. (2024). A study of gunshot wounds associated with communist executions of the Cursed Soldiers: A medical and historical analysis of materials from the Department of Forensic Medicine in Kraków. *Problems of Forensic Sciences*. https://www.semanticscholar.org/paper/c228e958d3919feb5787be02a1ec9932e49ad507 (accessed on 29 May 2025).

35. Kakkeri, S. R., Ahmed, K. M., Ahmad, S. R., & Khan, R. (2020). Knowledge and attitude of medical students toward medico-legal autopsy. *IP International Journal of Forensic Medicine and Toxicological Sciences, 3*, 8–11. https://doi.org/10.18231/2456-9615.2018.0002.

36. Kandeel, F., & Azab, R. (2024). Evaluation of permanent infirmities cases examined at forensic medicine and clinical toxicology department, Faculty of Medicine, Menoufia University. *The*

Egyptian Journal of Forensic Sciences and Applied Toxicology. https://www.semanticscholar.org/paper/7e58862ab69c1d140935045c5e3d7f38da8086aa (accessed on 29 May 2025).

37. Kaye, D. H. (2006). Behavioral genetics research and criminal DNA databases. https://core.ac.uk/download/62553467.pdf (accessed on 29 May 2025).

38. Khalil, R., Mansour, A., Fadda, W. A., Almisnid, K., Aldamegh, M. S., Al-Nafeesah, A., Alkhalifah, A., et al. (2020). The sudden transition to synchronized online learning during the COVID-19 pandemic in Saudi Arabia: A qualitative study exploring medical students' perspectives. *BMC Medical Education, 20.* https://doi.org/10.1186/s12909-020-02208-z.

39. Klinkner, M. (2009). Forensic science expertise for international criminal proceedings: An old problem, a new context and a pragmatic resolution. *The International Journal of Evidence & Proof, 13*(2), 102–129. https://doi.org/10.1350/ijep.2008.12.1.284.

40. Laot Kian, A. M., Karauwan, D., Hartini, S. I., & Herniati, H. (2025). Forensic psychological analysis of criminal offenses cyberbullying in Indonesia (Case study of the cyberbullying phenomenon among public figures). *Formosa Journal of Multidisciplinary Research.* https://www.semanticscholar.org/paper/2a47d42516d65a42401ae286f00859b19e8c9442 (accessed on 29 May 2025).

41. Lechien, J. R., Chiesa-Estomba, C. M., Hans, S., Barillari, M. R., Jouffe, L., & Saussez, S. (2020). Loss of smell and taste in 2013 European patients with mild to moderate COVID-19. *Annals of Internal Medicine, 173*(8), 672–675. https://doi.org/10.7326/M20-2428.

42. Logan, B. K., Mohr, A. L. A., Friscia, M., Krotulski, A. J., Papsun, D. M., Kacinko, S. L., Ropero-Miller, J. D., et al. (2017). Reports of adverse events associated with use of novel psychoactive substances, 2013–2016: A review. *Journal of Analytical Toxicology, 41*, 573–610. https://doi.org/10.1093/jat/bkx031.

43. Longo, L., Brčić, M., Cabitza, F., Choi, J., Confalonieri, R., Del Ser, J., Guidotti, R., et al. (2024). Explainable artificial intelligence (XAI) 2.0: A manifesto of open challenges and interdisciplinary research directions. *Information Fusion, 106*, 102301. https://doi.org/10.1016/j.inffus.2024.102301.

44. Lutz, L., Zehner, R., Verhoff, M. A., Bratzke, H., & Amendt, J. (2021). It is all about the insects: A retrospective on 20 years of forensic entomology highlights the importance of insects in legal investigations. *International Journal of Legal Medicine, 135*, 2637–2651. https://doi.org/10.1007/s00414-021-02628-6.

45. Mariani, M. M., Perez-Vega, R., & Wirtz, J. (2021). AI in marketing, consumer research and psychology: A systematic literature review and research agenda. *Psychology and Marketing, 39*, 755–776. https://doi.org/10.1002/mar.21619.

46. McGowan, M. (2017). Forensics' fight: A need for aggressive strategies against confirmation bias. *Themis: Research Journal of Justice Studies and Forensic Science, 5*(1), Article 11. https://doi.org/10.31979/THEMIS.2017.0511.

47. Moriarty, J. C. (2016). Seeing voices: Potential neuroscience contributions to a reconstruction of legal insanity. *Fordham Law Review, 85*(2), 599–642. https://ir.lawnet.fordham.edu/flr/vol85/iss2/10 (accessed on 29 May 2025).

48. Neal, T. M. S., & Grisso, T. (2014). Assessment practices and expert judgment methods in forensic psychology and psychiatry. *Criminal Justice and Behavior, 41*, 1406–1421. https://doi.org/10.1177/0093854814548449.

49. Neal, T. M. S., & Grisso, T. (2014). The cognitive underpinnings of bias in forensic mental health evaluations. *Psychology, Public Policy, and Law, 20*, 200–211. https://doi.org/10.1037/a0035824.

50. Peres, L. C. (2017). Post-mortem examination in the United Kingdom: Present and future. *Autopsy and Case Reports, 7*, 1–3. https://doi.org/10.4322/acr.2017.017.

51. Piraianu, A. I., Fulga, A., Mușat, C. L., Ciobotaru, O. R., Poalelungi, D. G., Stamate, E., Ciobotaru, O. C., et al. (2023). Enhancing the evidence with algorithms: How artificial intelligence is transforming forensic medicine. *Diagnostics, 13*, 2992. https://doi.org/10.3390/diagnostics13182992.

52. Poalelungi, D. G., Mușat, C. L., Fulga, A., Neagu, M., Neagu, A. I., Piraianu, A. I., & Fulga, I. (2023). Advancing patient care: How artificial intelligence is transforming healthcare. *Journal of Personalized Medicine, 13*(8), 1214. https://doi.org/10.3390/jpm13081214.

53. Prahladh, S., & Van Wyk, J. (2020). Protocol for a scoping review of the current data practices in forensic medicine. *Systematic Reviews, 9*. https://doi.org/10.1186/s13643-020-01308-7.

54. Prajapati, G., Sarode, S. C., Sarode, G. S., Shelke, P., Awan, K. H., & Patil, S. (2018). Role of forensic odontology in the identification of victims of major mass disasters across the world: A systematic review. *PLoS ONE, 13*(6), e0199791. https://doi.org/10.1371/journal.pone.0199791.

55. Qayyum, A., Qadir, J., Bilal, M., & Al-Fuqaha, A. (2020). Secure and robust machine learning for healthcare: A survey. *IEEE Reviews in Biomedical Engineering, 14*, 156–180. https://doi.org/10.1109/rbme.2020.3013489.

56. Ranjan, A., Kumar, P., & Verma, A. (2024). An analysis of medicolegal autopsies conducted at Patna Medical College, Patna (Bihar)—A mortuary-based study. *Global Journal for Research Analysis*. https://www.semanticscholar.org/paper/a60a0794b0cbd51c85a0134391381bd0ed94cd6f (accessed on 29 May 2025).

57. Rodda, L. N., Candela, K. E., Hart, A. P., Moffatt, E. G., Pearring, S., & Scott, K. S. (2025). Bladder wash as an alternative postmortem toxicology specimen: Forensic pathologists' perspectives. *The American Journal of Forensic Medicine and Pathology*. https://www.semanticscholar.org/paper/249a8a04b2c49d319667dbb39c4c79f2ec06668e (accessed on 29 May 2025).

58. Romańczuk, A., Rojek, S., Synowiec, K., Maciów-Głąb, M., & Kula, K. (2023). Interpretative problems due to the presence of chloromethcathinone isomers in the biological material from postmortem cases. *Journal of Analytical Toxicology, 47*, 797–806. https://doi.org/10.1093/jat/bkad070.

59. Roszkowska, A., Plenis, A., Kowalski, P., Bączek, T., & Olędzka, I. (2022). Recent advancements in techniques for analyzing modern, atypical antidepressants in complex biological matrices and their application in biomedical studies. *TrAC Trends in Analytical Chemistry, 152*, 116609. https://doi.org/10.1016/j.trac.2022.116609.

60. Roux, C., Willis, S., & Weyermann, C. (2021). Shifting forensic science focus from means to purpose: A path forward for the discipline? *Science & Justice, 61*(6), 678–686. https://doi.org/10.1016/j.scijus.2021.08.005.

61. Saker, L., Gharbi, M., Mellouki, Y., Sellami, L., & Zerairia, Y. (2025). Oral and dental trauma in forensic medicine. *Batna Journal of Medical Sciences*. https://www.semanticscholar.org/paper/fc308514f604049133dfd17543e3bea9261c0a92 (accessed on 29 May 2025).

62. Sallam, M. (2023). ChatGPT utility in healthcare education, research, and practice: Systematic review on the promising perspectives and valid concerns. *Healthcare, 11*, 887. https://doi.org/10.3390/healthcare11060887.

63. Samir, A., Ashour, F. H., Abdel Hakim, A. A., & Bassyouni, M. (2022). Recent advances in biodegradable polymers for sustainable applications. *npj Materials Degradation, 6*. https://doi.org/10.1038/s41529-022-00277-7.

64. Sane, M. R., Kapoor, N., & Badiye, A. (2023). Introduction to forensic medicine and pathology. https://doi.org/10.1007/978-981-99-1377-0_20.

65. Sanz-García, A., Gesteira, C., Sanz, J., & García-Vera, M. P. (2021). Prevalence of psychopathy in the general adult population: A systematic review and meta-analysis. *Frontiers in Psychology, 12*. https://doi.org/10.3389/fpsyg.2021.661044.

66. Sanzyapova, R. R. (2025). The role of dentistry in forensic medicine: Identification of human remains. *Patient-Oriented Medicine and Pharmacy*. https://www.semanticscholar.org/paper/d8db5ae62d74c13d619c3b0324e081b54abd3399 (accessed on 29 May 2025).

67. Satam, H., Joshi, K., Mangrolia, U., Waghoo, S., Zaidi, G., Rawool, S., Thakare, R. P., et al. (2023). Next-generation sequencing technology: Current trends and advancements. *Biology, 12*(7), 997. https://doi.org/10.3390/biology12070997.

68. Shivakumar, D. K. (2024). Forensic medicine and toxicology: A fusion of science and mythology in Indian context. *Annals of Advanced Biomedical Sciences*. https://www.semanticscholar.org/paper/92925aaad86e2fa6d424e6a65031fc667c0d8b1b (accessed on 29 May 2025).

69. Siedin, M. S., Plis, S. S., Klevno, V. A., Maksimov, A. V., & Plashchinskiy, A. A. (2024). Retrospective analysis of nonfatal skeletal injuries sustained in road incidents involving electric scooters. *Russian Journal of Forensic Medicine, 10*(2), 160–170. https://doi.org/10.17816/fm15597.

70. Singh, W. U., & Singh, K. P. (2023). The transformative role of artificial intelligence in forensic medicine and toxicology. *Journal of Medical Society, 37*, 101–102. https://doi.org/10.4103/jms.jms_54_24.

71. Suwalowska, H., Ali, J., de Almeida, J. R., Fonseca, S. A., Heathfield, L. J., Keyes, C. A., Lukande, R., et al. (2023). "The nobodies": Unidentified dead bodies—A global health crisis requiring urgent attention. *The Lancet Global Health, 11*(12), e1691–e1693. https://doi.org/10.1016/S2214-109X(23)00420-5.

72. Teymourian, H., Parrilla, M., Sempionatto, J. R., Montiel, N. F., Barfidokht, A., Van Echelpoel, R., De Wael, K., et al. (2020). Wearable electrochemical sensors for the monitoring and screening of drugs. *ACS Sensors, 5*(9), 2679–2700. https://doi.org/10.1021/acssensors.0c01318.

73. Toom, V. (2014). Trumping communitarianism: Crime control and forensic DNA typing and databasing in Singapore. *East Asian Science, Technology and Society: An International Journal, 8*(3), 273–296. https://doi.org/10.1215/18752160-2416805.

74. Villa, C., Lynnerup, N., & Jacobsen, C. (2023). A virtual, 3D multimodal approach to victim and crime scene reconstruction. *Diagnostics, 13*(17), 2764. https://doi.org/10.3390/diagnostics13172764.

75. Volobuyeva, O. (2024). About the determinants of sexual crimes and their consideration in criminal proceedings. *Uzhhorod National University Herald. Series: Law*. https://www.

semanticscholar.org/paper/8998e06fbbd289853ef61f9b5eff22fc4dec8574 (accessed on 29 May 2025).

76. Yadav, S., Kulshreshtha, N., Sharma, S., & Joshi, T. (2023). Victim identification through skeletal remains: A review. *IP International Journal of Forensic Medicine and Toxicological Sciences*. https://www.semanticscholar.org/paper/8d6b18b90c46e911e5d6a1a412908a00865d5a3c (accessed on 29 May 2025).

77. Yang, W., Zhou, M., Zhang, P., Geng, G., Xiaoning, L., & Zhang, H. (2020). Skull sex estimation based on wavelet transform and Fourier transform. *BioMed Research International, 2020*, Article 8608209. https://doi.org/10.1155/2020/8608209.

78. Yoo, S. H., Lee, W. T., & Lee, J. (2024). Evaluating the forensic inferences of oral nicotine ingestion: Autopsy case review, animal experimentation, and legal implications. *Korean Journal of Legal Medicine*. https://www.semanticscholar.org/paper/bef3c6d5f655f507e7ff17ce67f0bbea83c64386 (accessed on 29 May 2025).

79. Zeppenfeld, K., Tfelt-Hansen, J., Riva, M., Winkel, B. G., Behr, E. R., Blom, N. A., Charron, P., et al. (2022). 2022 ESC guidelines for the management of patients with ventricular arrhythmias and the prevention of sudden cardiac death. *European Heart Journal, 43*, 3997–4126. https://doi.org/10.1093/eurheartj/ehac262.

80. Zhang, Z., Qin, S., Chen, Y., Zhou, L., Yang, M., Tang, Y., Zuo, J., et al. (2022). Inhibition of NPC1L1 disrupts adaptive responses of drug-tolerant persister cells to chemotherapy. *EMBO Molecular Medicine, 14*, e14903. https://doi.org/10.15252/emmm.202114903.

IDENTIFICATION IN FORENSIC MEDICINE AND TOXICOLOGY

3

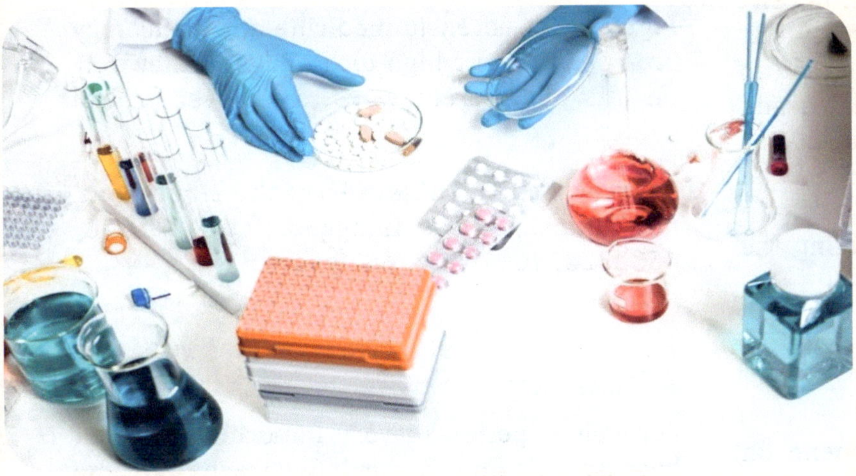

LEARNING OBJECTIVES

After studying this chapter, you will be able to:

1. Identify techniques in forensic identification;
2. Know legal and ethical considerations;
3. Discuss case studies in forensic identification.

Introduction

It is often very hard to identify a person and this is a major problem in forensic medicine and toxicology, especially after huge disasters. When things are messy, knowing a person's height becomes very important for forensic anthropologists as they try to solve the puzzle with the broken parts. Experts typically set up straightforward equations drawn from everyday body measurements—sometimes even using finger lengths as a rough gauge for height—and, generally speaking, the numbers tend to show that male and female figures come out differently (Vadysinghe et al., 2017). In places like Sri Lanka, the push for hands-on training is strong; forensic practitioners are often put through practical tests to see if they can spot subtle postmortem changes and correctly identify skeletal bits (Vadysinghe et al., 2017). All in all, these different methods point out that it is important to use a flexible, layered method when the situation calls for both legal and medical clarity.

Importance of Identification in Forensic Science

Being accurate with the facts helps solve crimes. Forensic science helps experts by using fingerprints, DNA tests and toxicology to determine the substances involved and their effects on the people involved. This careful, sometimes painstaking, process not only clears up why a death occurred but also digs into the odd details behind the incident (Boriwala et al., 2024). Interestingly, forensic work doesn't stop at identifying clues; it also feeds key bits of data into private security measures that, in most cases, help ward off future crimes and keep neighborhoods safer (Saxena et al., 2024). In essence, this approach which is broad and sometimes unpredictable, plays a key role in legal cases and, in general, in protecting the community.

Overview of Methods Used in Identification

Forensic medicine and toxicology depend on many techniques, not only on modern gadgets, to discover important evidence. New tools such as AI, can go through a lot of data to help with diagnoses and post-mortem work, much like having a digital assistant alongside the usual methods. At the same moment, traditional approaches are still very important. Think about toxicology tests that use basic methods to detect dangerous substances. Techniques such as gas chromatography and even spectrophotometry help measure nasty gases like carbon monoxide and hydrogen sulfide in biological samples (Kinoshita et al., 2017). Usually, this combination of new and old techniques shows that a strong forensic setup relies on several different methods. In most cases, mixing these techniques not only sharpens how accurately evidence is identified but also boosts the overall trustworthiness of an investigation (Figure 3.1).

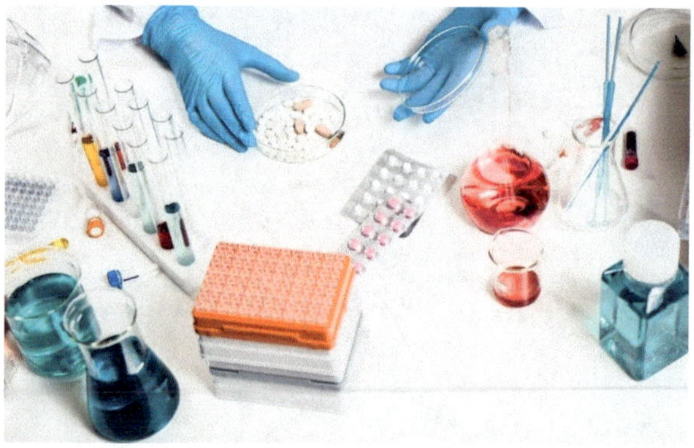

Figure 3.1. Forensic medicine and toxicology aren't just about high-tech gadgets; they rely on lots of different ways to uncover crucial evidence.

Source: https://d2jx2rerrg6sh3.cloudfront.net/images/ news/ImageForNews_671876_4532323740979167782.jpg.

Role of Forensic Experts in Legal Proceedings

Forensic experts are very important in court because their findings can influence the outcome for both juries and judges. It is clear that, over the years, discussions about forensic evidence, especially in cases with arsenic, keep pointing to the importance of solid and skilled work. Long before the Marsh test, many early arsenic detection efforts faced numerous problems which often showed the conflict between new science and old laws.

During many 19thcentury trials, people would argue that some experts were overconfident or unreliable in their work and the tension was clear in those discussions. At the end of the day, forensic experts wrestle not just with the nittygritty of their field but also with farreaching legal consequences, making their work absolutely essential in keeping justice alive and the legal system trustworthy (Caudill et al., 2009).

Ethical Considerations in Forensic Identification

There are many debates about fairness and honesty in our courts because ethics and forensic work often overlap. AI is being used more in traditional forensics and in general, this leads to concerns about privacy, consent and data security. Relying on advanced algorithms might boost efficiency and accuracy—but it can also unintentionally bring in biases or lead to misread details that, To summarize, chip away at what justice is meant to be (Piraianu et al., 2023). At the same moment, using forensic science raises questions about whether those who work with it are always protecting the rights of all individuals, especially those who are more vulnerable. To summarize, balancing the push for scientific progress with our ethical responsibilities remains crucial since forensic identification goes far beyond simple technicalities—it touches on deep-seated human rights and the trustworthiness of our entire legal system (Balhareth et al., 2024).

Challenges Faced in Forensic Identification

Forensic experts regularly deal with problems that can be very difficult and not always easy to solve. In the fast-evolving world of forensic identification, a rising problem is the surge of novel psychoactive substances (NPS), which not only mix up the process of detection but also complicate emergency treatments. For example, one recent study noted that almost half of patients suspected of toxic ingestion ended up testing positive for several substances—a detail that hints, somewhat surprisingly, at how unreliable self-reporting can be (Seyright et al., 2017). Standard ways of screening usually do not keep up with new drugs which makes it harder to spot them accurately. Also, because people react differently to drugs, it becomes even more difficult to plan an effective response. Generally speaking, then, it seems vital to come up with improved ways to track these shifting patterns—ways that support more effective forensic work and ultimately lead to better care for patients in toxic emergencies (Capiau et al., 2016).

3.1. Techniques in Forensic Identification

Learning Outcome

1. Understand DNA profiling and its significance;
2. Explain fingerprinting methods and advancements;
3. Learn ballistics analysis in forensic identification;
4. Discuss toxicological screening methods;
5. Know using digital forensics in identification;
6. Focus on hair and fiber analysis techniques;
7. Discuss the role of autopsy in forensic identification;
8. Describe use of chemical analysis in toxicology;
9. Identify emerging technologies in forensic identification.

Because of the many issues caused by modern drug abuse, advanced forensic methods are very important today. Toxicology tests help in both finding out what is wrong and dealing with legal issues. Generally, forensic toxicology now includes selecting the proper biological samples and checking how the body processes drugs. One striking case involved a 30-year-old man whose death was connected to inhaling psychotropic substances; lab results revealed high fentanyl levels along with small traces of U-47700, a reminder of the risks presented by new, emergent drugs (Coopman et al., 2016). Methods such as gas chromatography-mass spectrometry, with a side of liquid-liquid extraction, have repeatedly proven indispensable in nailing down exactly which substances are present, ultimately supporting the effective management of drug-related forensic cases (Ciobanu et al., 2015).

3.1.1. DNA Profiling and its Significance

Forensic science has developed a lot and DNA profiling, in particular, made it possible to link evidence to suspects in many legal cases. Examiners can sometimes link people to crimes by looking at tiny biological traces found at the scene. In most cases, recent work shows that checking methylation patterns—that is, looking at certain epigenetic markers on DNA—can help distinguish fresh from older semen, which is especially key in sexual assault investigations (Abouelkeir et al., 2022). The field is branching out too; omics technologies are now wedded to forensic methods in a way that usually provides a deeper look into not only what substances are present but also how they interact within different biological settings (Goel et al., 2022). To summarize, DNA profiling not only reinforces the core of forensic work but also opens the door for fresh methods that improve how we interpret evidence, ultimately influencing legal outcomes (Figure 3.2).

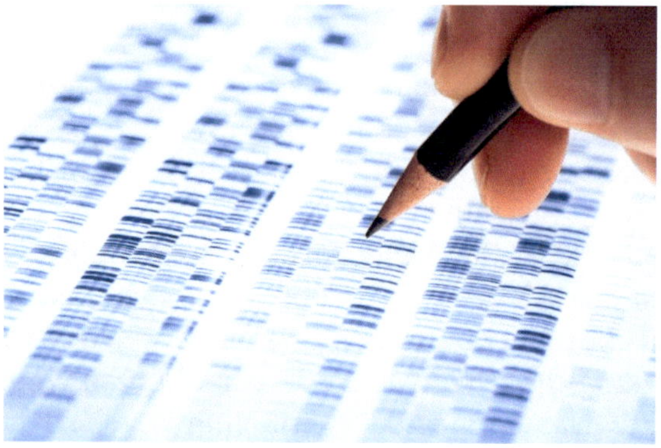

Figure 3.2. DNA profiling.

Source: https://www.yourgenome.org/wp-content/uploads/2024/01/1450-shutterstock_1046584543-1920x1282.jpg.

3.1.2. Fingerprinting Methods and Advancements

Fingerprinting methods have advanced a lot—older approaches are now combined with new technology and affect how we do forensic ID. AI is now being used in labs and this means fingerprint analysis is done more quickly and accurately. These smart algorithms look at every tiny ridge and little bump (yes, the minutiae) to cut down on slip-ups from human reading (Piraianu et al., 2023). Still, it's not all smooth sailing; one study on wrongful convictions shows that a lot of the mix-ups in forensic reports come from fuzzy standards or simple misinterpretations, not from misclassifying the prints (Morgan, 2023). It seems to point out that we should keep working on training, updating technology and making rules clearer. To summarize, mixing these advanced methods into everyday practice not only polishes the identification process but also increases the trust factor of forensic evidence in court (Figure 3.3).

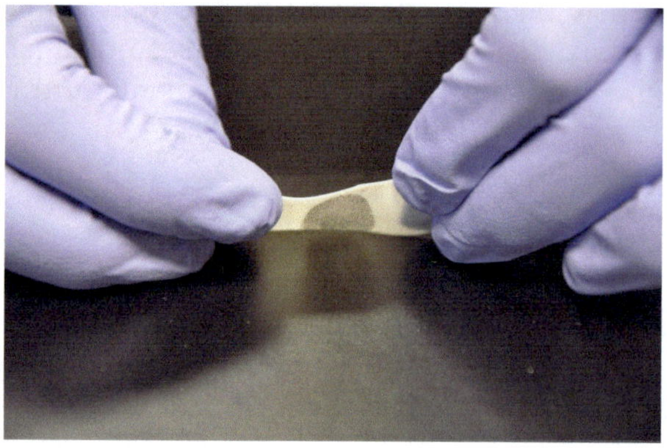

Figure 3.3. Fingerprinting methods.

Source: https://www.nist.gov/sites/default/files/images/2018/03/06/fingerprint_lifting_from_jstaymates.jpg.

3.1.3. Ballistics Analysis in Forensic Identification

Forensics in ballistics relies on evidence integrity, because any small error could result in a wrongful conviction. Ballistics analysis usually looks at small marks on bullets and the unique marks on cartridge cases to link a firearm to a crime scene, but this isn't always easy. Generally, doubts about how reliable such evidence is have grown; critics point out that ever since the Daubert ruling, experts are expected to build their testimony on methods that have proven dependable (Fabricant et al., 2018). Meanwhile, initiatives like Project FORESIGHT are chipping away at lab inefficiencies and bolstering statistical checks, adding extra layers of scrutiny to these techniques (Speaker et al., 2017). To summarize, these efforts not only influence courtroom decisions but also help keep the public's trust in forensic identification intact (Figure 3.4).

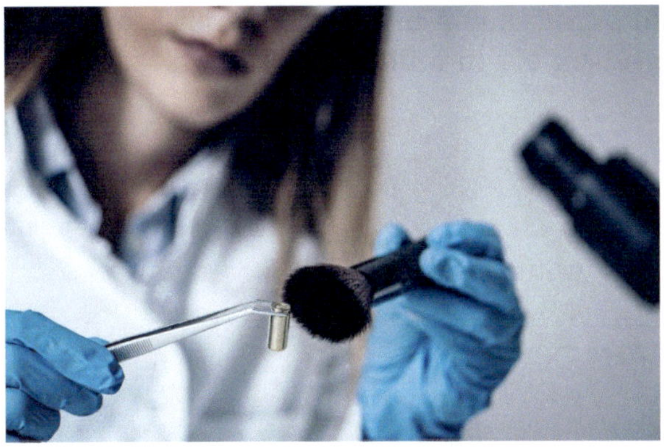

Figure 3.4. Ballistics analysis in forensic science.

Source: https://microscopes.unitronusa.com/wp/wp-content/uploads/2021/08/forensics-feature-image.jpg.

3.1.4. Toxicological Screening Methods

Analytical methods have reshaped toxicology screening in forensic medicine. Take the dilute-and-shoot method paired with liquid chromatography-tandem mass spectrometry (LC–MS-MS)—it's proving to be a solid option for checking out a wide mix of substances in biological samples. In practice, this approach can pick up nearly 95 different illicit drugs and medications in urine; in most cases, that gives us key glimpses into substance use patterns and even backs public health initiatives (dos Santos et al., 2024). One validation study, generally speaking, confirmed the method's reliability by hitting acceptable precision and bias limits, underscoring its fit for both clinical and forensic settings (Zeppenfeld et al., 2022). To summarize, these innovative screening techniques not only sharpen toxicological assessments but also help shape safety policies, making them indispensable tools in the world of forensic toxicology and medicine (Figure 3.5).

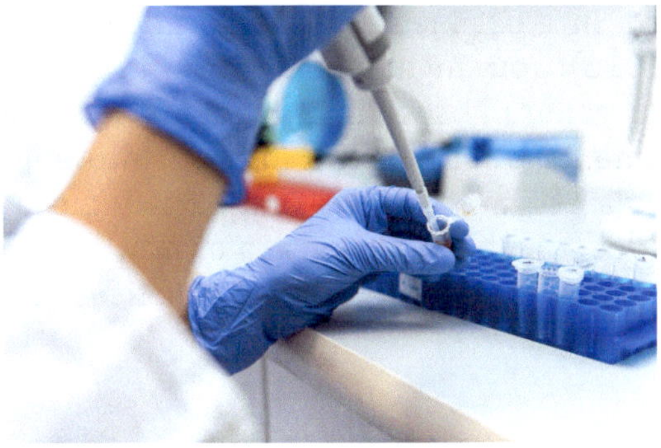

Figure 3.5. Analytical methods have reshaped toxicology screening in forensic medicine.

Source: https://d1g9yur4m4naub.cloudfront.net/images/Article_Images/ImageForArticle_141_17399722768836503.jpg.

3.1.5. Use of Digital Forensics in Identification

Digital forensics has affected the way we identify evidence in forensics. Because of digital traces like emails, social media posts and online transactions, investigators can now understand events much better than they could before. In many situations, this strategy helps solve cases and also helps clear people who were falsely accused. By examining these digital trails, experts can usually construct new timelines and notice details that might have gone unnoticed. Now, AI tools are used in the process which helps sort through a lot of data quickly and with more accuracy, even though the pace can be inconsistent. As our lives get more tangled with digital devices, mixing these fresh techniques with time-honored forensic methods creates a framework that, in most cases, leads to more dependable outcomes in legal contexts (Poalelungi et al., 2023; Zeppenfeld et al., 2022).

3.1.6. Hair and Fiber Analysis Techniques

There have been some interesting interactions between forensic medicine and toxicology lately which have led to new developments in analytical testing, especially in hair and fiber studies. Hair is special in this way; it can be used to monitor drugs and toxins in the body for a long time without being invasive. In many cases, tools such as gas chromatography paired with mass spectrometry (GC-MS/MS) have been fine-tuned to pick up even the tiniest traces of psychoactive substances—which, in most instances, helps uncover drug abuse patterns across different groups (Moreno et al., 2016). You might also notice that the emerging field of hair proteomics is gradually making its mark; generally speaking, it seems set to improve how accurately we diagnose issues and tweak treatments, offering extra insights into both chronic conditions and prolonged substance exposure (Adeola et al., 2018). To summarize, these methods not only play a big role in forensic work but also deepen our overall grasp of how health and diseases unfold in individuals, underscoring their vital place in today's forensic practices (Figure 3.6).

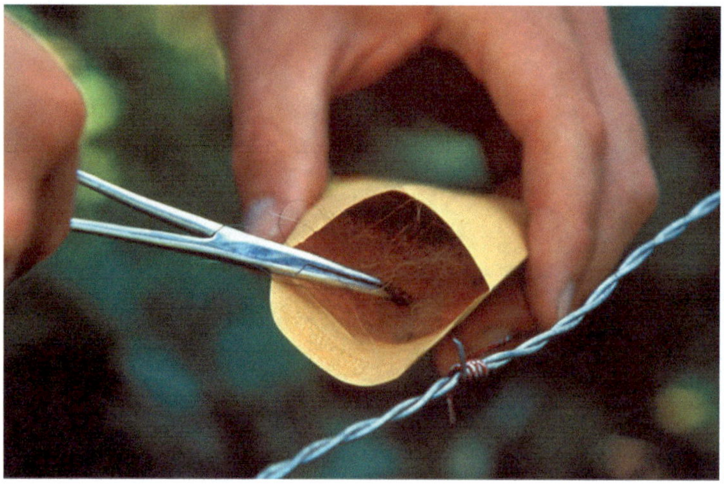

Figure 3.6. Hair and fiber analysis techniques.

Source: https://www.hairphysician.com/wp-content/uploads/sites/77/2018/01/hair-dna-testing-houston-texas.jpg.

3.1.7. The Role of Autopsy in Forensic Identification

Autopsy reports show the cause of death and also help build a clearer picture of what happened around the person's final moments. In a lot of cases, examining the remains allows forensic experts to learn the victim's identity, health and even some details about their interactions with their environment. Consider, for instance, cases marked by repeated offenses, such as those tied to Jeffrey Dahmer; here, an autopsy may spotlight recurring behavioral patterns and even hint at psychological traits (Ho et al., 1994). The diatom test – which looks for tiny algae-like cells – nicely illustrates how a routine procedure can unravel specific scenarios, like confirming drowning when diatoms show up in the victim's organs (Kaushik et al., 2017). To summarize, autopsy work mixes careful scientific analysis with investigative insight, generally speaking, piecing together the intricate narrative behind a tragic event in a manner that's as human as it is methodical (Figure 3.7).

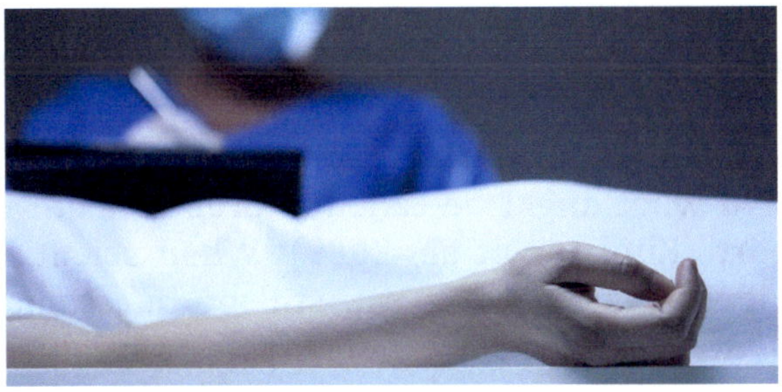

Figure 3.7. The role of autopsy in forensics.

Source: https://images.theconversation.com/files/603657/original/file-20240628-17-p3zsb7.jpg?ixlib=rb-4.1.0&rect=0%2C933%2C5607%2C2799&q=45&auto=format&w=1356&h=668&fit=crop.

3.1.8. Use of Chemical Analysis in Toxicology

It is very important in forensics to accurately identify substances, especially when drugs are involved in misuse or overdose. Testing chemicals in toxicology is not only a standard lab task; it also helps healthcare professionals to find out if someone is addicted and to confirm that the right treatments are being used. Sometimes, by examining biological samples, it is possible to identify which drugs are involved which guides both medical and legal actions. There's one case that stands out: a 30yearold man was found dead after inhaling psychoactive substances, and a thorough lab check revealed not only fentanyl but also traces of U47700, an opioid far stronger than morphine (Coopman et al., 2016). In most cases, these types of evaluations highlight how crucial it is to choose the right sample and the proper analysis method, echoing the core ideas of toxicology (Ciobanu et al., 2015). This way of studying the body helps us understand how drugs move through it which makes it easier to assess drugrelated cases.

3.1.9. Emerging Technologies in Forensic Identification

The use of new technology has changed the ways forensic labs detect different substances. Labs that used to focus on toxicology are now discovering more cases of phenazepam and etizolam which appear to be showing up in the black market regularly. Many studies have found that the Immunalysis® Benzodiazepines ELISA kit detects these new substances in about 79%–107% of cases. Because new psychoactive drugs are always being discovered, it is now necessary to find new ways to screen for them rather than just a helpful option. The Advisory Council on the Misuse of Drugs (ACMD) even stresses that generally speaking, there's a need for government departments to, you know, team up and tackle these complications together (Advisory Council on the Misuse of Drugs, 2011). All in all, using advanced tools together with traditional methods helps solve forensic cases and also improves public health responses to new drug dangers.

Test Your Knowledge

1. What is the role of fingerprint analysis in identification?
2. Define dental identification.
3. What is DNA profiling?

3.2. Legal and Ethical Considerations in Forensic Identification

Learning Outcome

1. Explain the role of forensic evidence in court;
2. Learn standards for admissibility of forensic evidence;
3. Discuss ethical dilemmas in forensic identification;
4. Know the impact of wrongful convictions;
5. Focus on privacy concerns in forensic investigations;
6. Talk about the need to keep a chain of custody in place;
7. Describe the function of expert witnesses in a legal case;
8. Analyse public perception of forensic science;
9. Describe legislative changes affecting forensic practices.

Forensic medicine and toxicology do not have a simple way to identify people; many legal and ethical rules must be followed to ensure dignity and fairness. Respect for someone who has passed is a big deal, especially since their cultural and religious backgrounds often sway how identification goes and, in many cases, affect the justice their next of kin eventually receives (Reid et al., 2025). Fair treatment of those who remain unidentified, regardless of differing economic circumstances, brings to light some pretty glaring gaps in the resources and techniques used during investigations (Balhareth et al., 2024). Another ethical issue arises when a mistake could harm someone's reputation or affect court decisions; this just shows that not causing harm is very important. Since technology is always changing in forensics, we must also update our ethics to cover privacy, consent and proper use of databases so that the law remains fair and respects both science and human rights.

3.2.1. The Role of Forensic Evidence in Court

In legal cases, forensic evidence is very important, proving that careful science is necessary for justice. Those who have witnessed many crimes give expert testimony and forensic science plays a key role in helping shape the events in the courtroom. Take, for instance, those mass grave cases tackled by the International Criminal Tribunal for the former Yugoslavia; here, digging into the past has uncovered key clues that help build what might be called a forensic truth in court (Klinkner et al., 2009). When scientific evidence is strong, it can still be questioned by the court about how reliable it really is. The way law and science mix means there's a lot of probing into methods – through cross-examinations and alternative expert opinions – as seen in many trials (Klinkner et al., 2009). To summarize, presenting and weighing forensic evidence isn't merely a scientific exercise; it stands as a core part of the legal process that can ultimately tip the scales on a verdict (Figure 3.8).

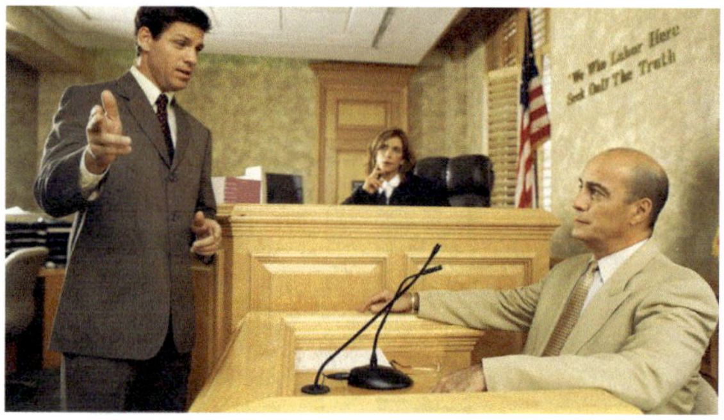

Figure 3.8. Expert testimony.

Source: https://blog.ipleaders.in/wp-content/uploads/2019/09/111-1.jpg.

3.2.2. Standards for Admissibility of Forensic Evidence

Many scholars have studied how courts and forensic evidence interact—major legal rulings have changed the kinds of evidence that courts accept. An important moment was when the U.S. Supreme Court decided Daubert v. Merrell Dow Pharmaceuticals, Inc. which introduced a new standard for judging expert testimony by focusing on its reliability. Even with that change, research generally shows a worrying trend: courts sometimes let in forensic methods that, frankly, don't hold up under close inspection, a misstep that risks convicting innocent folks—DNA exonerations (Fabricant et al., 2018) back this up. Experts, too, are often chosen based merely on their credentials or years on the job; this isn't always a sure sign they truly have the needed skill, bringing their testimonies into question (Garrett et al., 2018). All in all, it is obvious that a clear and orderly review of expert opinions is required for the rules in forensic medicine and toxicology to be just and accurate.

3.2.3. Ethical Dilemmas in Forensic Identification

Forensic technology has advanced a lot, making criminal investigations much different and raising many ethical problems. While AI and biometric ID improve accuracy, they also lead to concerns about privacy, giving consent and possible misuse of data.

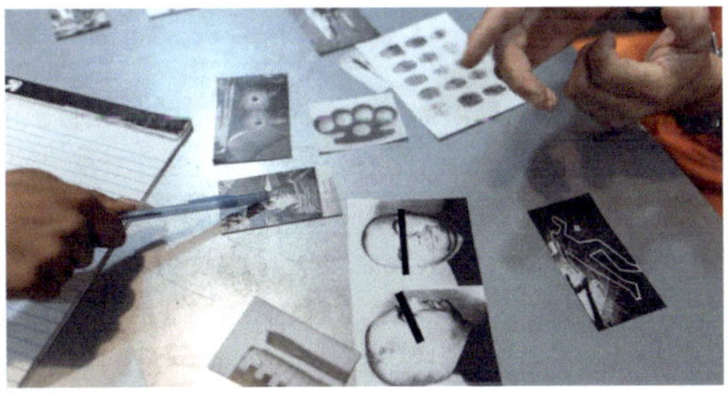

Figure 3.9. Ethical dilemmas in forensic identification.

Source: https://eclipseforensics.com/wp-content/uploads/2024/10/Digital-forensics--720x380.png.

There are times when using these methods too much makes people overconfident, so they overlook the importance of ethical judgment to avoid wrongful convictions or spot misconduct. Recent studies even point out that, in most cases, forensic experts should weave ethical considerations into every step, especially when technical limits or broader system flaws might shake the very core of justice (Ferrara et al., 2018). In short, a deeper grasp of ethical guidelines is key if we want the latest tech advances to back true justice instead of unintentionally undermining it (Llerena et al., 2024) (Figure 3.9).

3.2.4. The Impact of Wrongful Convictions

Wrongful convictions cause trouble for many more people than just the convicted, as they can affect the way forensic science and the law are used. Because forensic medicine is always evolving and AI is now involved in evidence collection, making sure identifications are correct is now very important. However, depending heavily on lab findings can be risky if, for example, toxicology reports are twisted or not well examined. Look at the low conviction numbers in drug-facilitated sexual assault cases; a poor grasp of systematic toxicological reviews not only blocks justice but also fuels more wrongful convictions and chips away at public trust in the courts (Wille et al., 2021). Plus, while using AI in forensic work is meant to boost precision in presenting evidence, it calls for careful checks—because relying on imperfect technology can trigger serious miscarriages of justice (Parmar, 2023). In short, dealing with these issues is necessary for any real progress in legal outcomes.

3.2.5. Privacy Concerns in Forensic Investigations

Forensic investigators have to balance searching for the truth with respecting people's privacy. Many times, AI and digital monitoring are added to the mix and in general, these new technologies make people worry about possible misuse and overstepping. AI, for instance, now plays a big role in sifting through forensic evidence—improving accuracy and speeding up processes—but it also stokes debates over data privacy and, in most cases, the bias that can creep into algorithm-based decisions (Singh et al., 2023). Consider, too, emerging devices such as wearable electrochemical sensors that show promise for personalized medicine and real-time tracking of substance use; they , too, stir up concerns regarding the unauthorized gathering and handling of delicate data (Teymourian et al., 2020). Balancing the power of these forensic methods with the need for solid privacy protections remains, without a doubt, an urgent priority for both practitioners and policymakers alike (Figure 3.10).

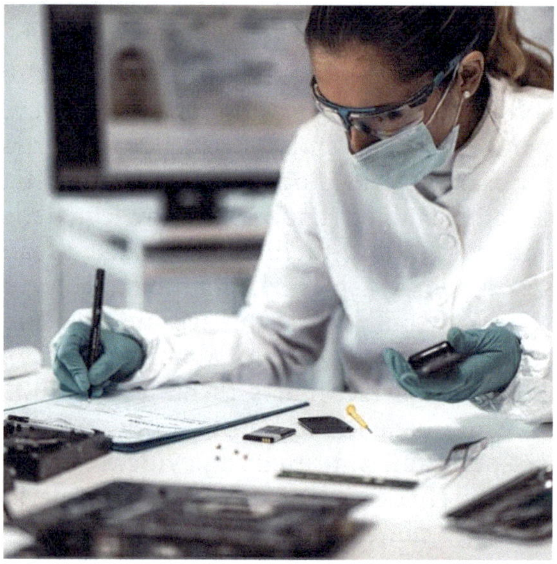

Figure 3.10. Forensic investigations often juggle the demands of finding the truth while keeping personal privacy intact.

Source: https://d3s0v64y40yzea.cloudfront.net/Blogs/Debunking+the+Myths/proaxis+solutions-+Common+Misconceptions+About+Forensic+Science.webp.

3.2.6. The Importance of Maintaining Chain of Custody

The success of every forensic case depends on the evidence which must be handled according to a strict and sometimes odd chain-of-custody process. Whenever evidence is moved or handled, someone carefully records that action; this makes sure the evidence can be trusted in court. A tiny error in the record of a sexual assault case can lead to big changes in the legal process and the help given to the victim. A small mistake or contamination can result in the wrong person being blamed or the actual culprit walking free which explains why proper procedures in forensic medicine and toxicology are so necessary. You often read in the literature that healthcare providers aren't just focused on immediate care; they also get involved in carefully collecting and preserving evidence, making sure the chain of custody remains unbroken throughout the investigative process (Crawford-Jakubiak et al., 2017; Vrees, 2017). In short, a reliable, though sometimes unpredictable, chain of custody supports the trust in forensic evidence and also supports justice and victim protection.

3.2.7. The Role of Expert Witnesses in Legal Proceedings

In some cases, legal disputes change direction and experts in forensic medicine and toxicology become very important. They give explanations that make difficult scientific matters easier for juries to understand and support the evidence in the case. Take DNA experts—they explain how natural decay impacts genetic material; recent work (Bhoyar et al., 2024) even shows that environmental factors play a big part in determining timelines of death and other criminal details. Meanwhile, when forensic pathologists team up with other experts, they cover both the body's inner workings and toxic influences that might have led to someone's passing—even if discussions over autopsies can get a bit messy (Abrol, 2024). Generally speaking, these experts act as a bridge between hard science and courtroom drama, steadily pushing the quest for real justice (Figure 3.11).

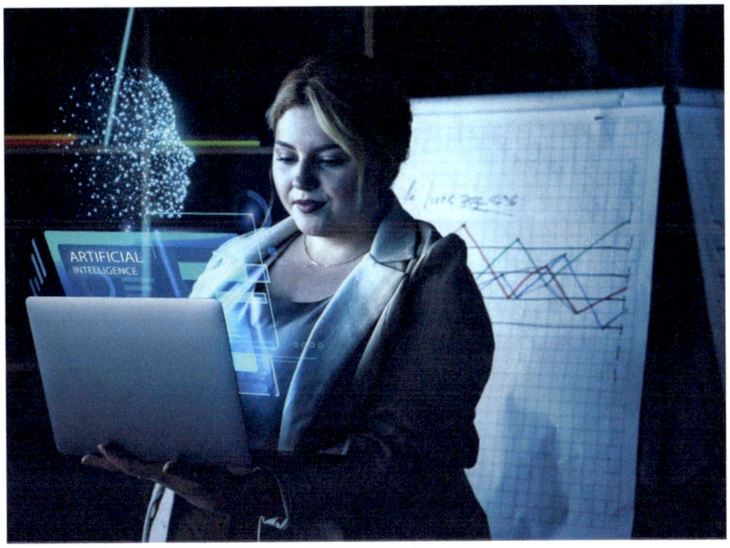

Figure 3.11. The role of expert witnesses in legal proceedings.

Source: https://www.ecsinfotech.com/wp-content/uploads/2024/01/person-using-laptop-using-artificial-intelligence-generate-images-scaled.jpg.

3.2.8. Public Perception of Forensic Science

Forensic science often splits public opinion in odd ways. Because TV shows make forensic tests look flawless, many people think every test is perfect. Even so, the real process behind the scenes is often quite messy. Sometimes, the bright promise of using nanotechnology to boost forensic tests gets drowned out by concerns about worker safety and potential health risks—a point raised in recent studies (Adamec et al., 2019). Further, the rise of new psychoactive substances further complicates matters, challenging how well we understand what forensic science can do (Mannocchi et al., 2015). In general, it appears important to have a more open discussion about how what people expect from forensic medicine and toxicology often differs from the actual realities.

3.2.9. Legislative Changes Affecting Forensic Practices

New laws have been created to deal with the rising number of new psychoactive substances which have affected forensic work. There are so many new drugs showing up that it's hard to keep up and this often leads policymakers to make changes to the laws. A clear sign of this shift is the growing reliance on high-resolution mass spectrometry (HRMS) – a tool now central to spotting these substances quickly and accurately in labs. Recent tweaks in HRMS let experts scoop up tons of data and even look back over past findings, helping police and medical professionals stay a bit ahead of potential dangers (Klingberg et al., 2022). On top of that, the move toward more affordable ambient ionization methods shows an inventive side—it's a clever adaptation under changing legal demands that ultimately boosts how toxicology tests perform in both clinical and forensic settings (Maria del Ena et al., 2021) (Figure 3.12).

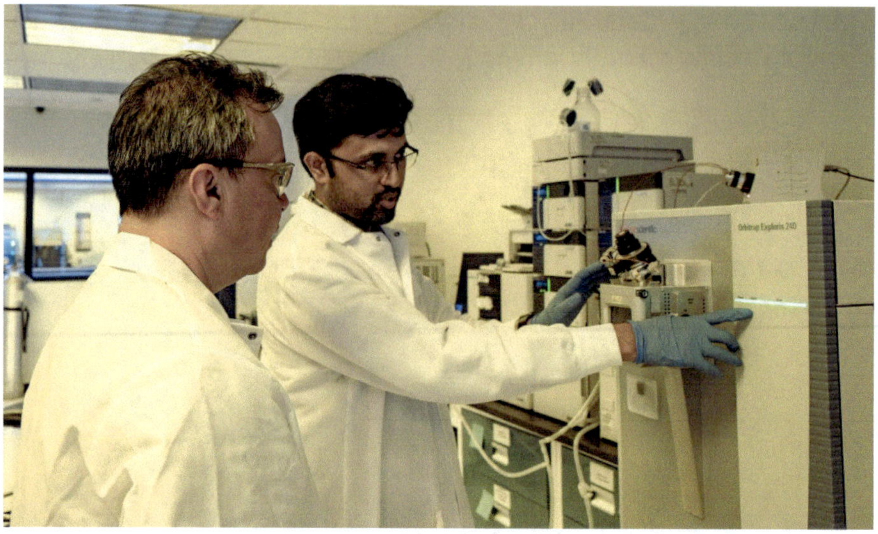

Figure 3.12. A clear sign of this shift is the growing reliance on high-resolution mass spectrometry (HRMS) – a tool now central to spotting these substances quickly and accurately in labs.

Source: https://www.sannova.net/wp-content/uploads/2023/07/Sannova_ImageLibrary-51-scaled-e1690463185164.jpg.

Test Your Knowledge

1. What is the legal importance of forensic identification?
2. Can DNA samples be collected without consent in criminal cases? Justify briefly.
3. What is meant by postmortem privacy?

3.3. Case Studies in Forensic Identification

Learning Outcome

1. Understand notable historical cases and their impact;
2. Know modern cases showcasing forensic advancements;
3. Analysis of high-profile toxicology cases;
4. Discuss lessons learned from forensic failures;
5. Explain the ways forensic identification is used in cold cases;
6. Learn comparative analysis of different forensic techniques;
7. Look at how media coverage affects forensic cases;
8. Describe cross-disciplinary collaboration in forensic investigations;
9. Understand the ways case studies will affect future forensic work.

3.3.1. Notable Historical Cases and Their Impact

Forensic toxicology can be full of surprises. A 30-year-old man died at home after breathing in fumes from a substance burned on aluminum foil which is not a common event. At the scene, examiners collected blood and urine samples (yes, the usual ones) to figure out what had gone wrong. The lab results? Fentanyl was found at 10.9 μg/L which is very high and there were also small amounts of U-47700, a potent opioid analgesic that, in most cases, is stronger than morphine. Even more revealing, he looked up information on new psychotropic drugs which might have been a sign of intentional misuse. Using high-tech methods like gas chromatography and mass spectrometry, investigators confirmed the presence of these substances—making this the first reported fatal intoxication where U-47700 acted as a psychotropic agent—and reminding us just how crucial forensic medicine and toxicology are in unraveling today's drug-related tragedies (Capiau et al., 2016; Coopman et al., 2016).

3.3.2. Modern Cases Showcasing Forensic Advancements

Recently, forensic science has improved a lot—it has made it much easier to find and examine evidence in crimes. In most cases, using advanced DNA profiling and digital investigation has become necessary for solving cases. Take forensic veterinary medicine; this field, drawing on toxicology and genetic analysis know-how, now plays a key role in untangling crimes that involve animal-related clues (Mores et al., 2025). New twists in imaging techniques and AI are further nudging up the accuracy with which we read evidence—a shift that, generally speaking, bears significant weight on justice outcomes (Balhareth et al., 2024). They help both the accuracy of forensic evidence and the way investigations are run, so law enforcement can tackle tough cases more efficiently. As forensic methods keep evolving, their part in upholding justice and supporting legal proceedings is set to become even more crucial in our modern society (Figure 3.13).

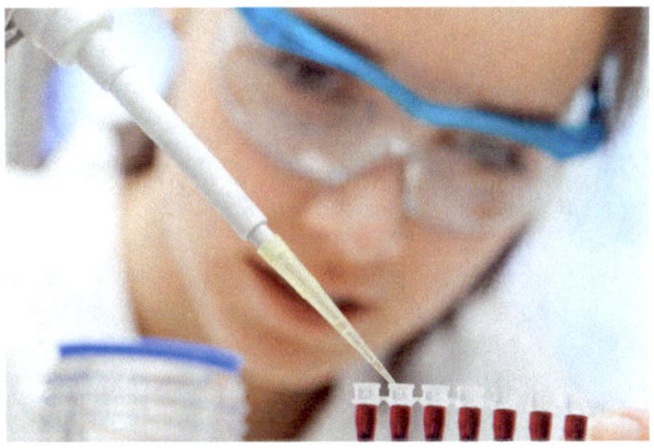

Figure 3.13. Cutting-edge tools like advanced DNA profiling and digital investigation methods have, in most cases, proven indispensable in today's cases.

Source: https://online.maryville.edu/wp-content/uploads/sites/97/2019/12/dna-sampling.jpg?w=750.

3.3.3. Analysis of High-profile Toxicology Cases

In recent years, well-known toxicology cases have led people to talk more about substance abuse and how it should be regulated. It is not uncommon for toxicology testing to be messy and this can happen when new psychoactive substances or legal highs, are present. The ACMD generally notes that these substances tend to appear fast and act unpredictably, giving both users and healthcare providers a whole lot of trouble (Capiau et al., 2016). In many instances, the ACMD even pushes for laws that force vendors to prove their stuff is safe, basically flipping the burden of proof onto them (Advisory Council on the Misuse of Drugs, 2011). Investigating such famous cases gives forensic medicine some useful hints on how to handle new problems in drug culture. To summarize, the mix of toxicology with public health points to the need for a coordinated effort to ease the harms linked to substance use (Figure 3.14).

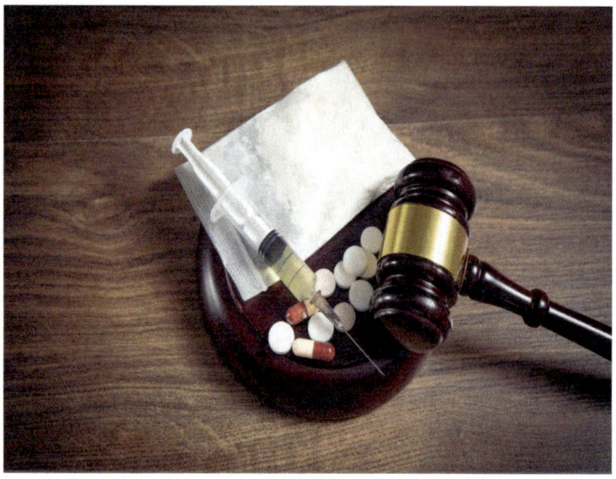

Figure 3.14. The Advisory Council on the Misuse of Drugs (ACMD) generally notes that these substances tend to appear fast and act unpredictably.

Source: https://stepstogether.co.uk/wp-content/uploads/2025/01/shutterstock_2303318971-scaled.jpg.

3.3.4. Lessons Learned from Forensic Failures

There have been many cases where forensic science and the courts clashed and these situations have shown us important lessons from previous errors, especially when people depend too much on anecdotes. There is not always strong scientific support for fingerprint analysis and bitemark comparison which can end up repeating ideas from old and discredited sciences such as phrenology. This kind of reliance, often accepted uncritically by legal practitioners, has in many cases led to some troubling miscarriages of justice (Faigman et al., 2008). Looking at many big errors shows that we need to rethink things, especially in forensic identification and toxicology and move towards practices based on strong evidence. In most cases, by taking a step back and learning from these missteps, future investigations might pick up sharper, more refined methods, similar to how teams tried to comb through the details of the Columbia mishap (Singla et al., 2023). Basically, the forensic field needs to focus on strict scientific rules to regain trust in the legal setting.

3.3.5. The Role of Forensic Identification in Cold Cases

Forensic science has improved a lot recently which is helping solve many cold cases. These methods which use information from molecules and isotopes, can provide key information that changes the outcome of cases that were once considered unsolvable. For example, when experts study synthetic cathinones using chiral analysis, they not only pick out what substances are in play but can also sometimes tie them back to their sources (Morrison et al., 2017). Then there are those creative extraction techniques—like the ones used to pull hazardous substances from old herbarium mount paper—that show, quite clearly, why we need to keep refining our tests to uncover even the tiniest traces of evidence (Chen et al., 2011). In most cases, these approaches work hand in hand to help law enforcement finally bring closure to victims and their families, while also proving that modern forensic methods have come into their own (Figure 3.15).

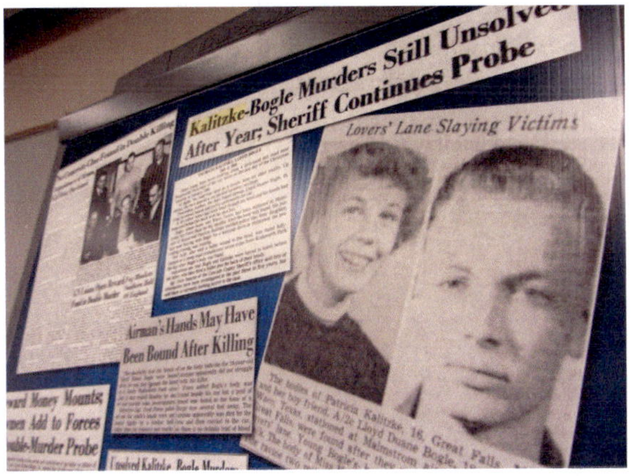

Figure 3.15. The role of forensic identification in cold cases.

Source: https://media.npr.org/assets/img/2021/06/11/2021-06-09t225103z_26680079_mt1usatoday16232141_rtrmadp_3_clippings-from-the-great-falls-tribune-were-part-of-the_custom-d8dfdd909b4dfd0025700ba39bd6f374e9025487.jpg.

3.3.6. Comparative Analysis of Different Forensic Techniques

Forensic approaches have developed a lot, bringing together different ways to help identify people in forensic medicine. For example, forensic dentistry has become very important, especially when large disasters make it hard to use older, traditional approaches. It makes use of dental records which join details about teeth with X-rays, to help professionals identify people even when their bodies are in poor condition. It's clear from examining different techniques that dental exams are rarely done alone; they are often joined by information from molecular genetics and anthropology. And with digital tech advances and AI consistently pushing boundaries—generally speaking, they've given forensic dentistry a serious boost, making it an indispensable part of modern investigations (Sanzyapova, 2025).

3.3.7. The Influence of Media on Forensic Cases

The way media reports on forensic cases has a major impact on the outcomes and this is being noticed more in today's discussions on criminal justice. Sensational news can change how people feel about a case, sometimes affecting how jurors judge which could be unfair. With more new psychoactive substances appearing, the media increases awareness but may also make the details of the cases seem less complicated than they really are. For example, the Advisory Council on the Misuse of Drugs once pointed out that a more unified response is needed to tackle these challenges, hinting that an informed public is key in pushing legislative efforts (Advisory Council on the Misuse of Drugs, 2011). When you check out synthetic cannabinoids like MDMB-CHMICA in a forensic setting, it becomes clear that media stories about drug-related incidents can steer societal reactions and even influence legal outcomes, which underscores why getting the details right is absolutely essential (Seyright et al., 2016) (Figure 3.16).

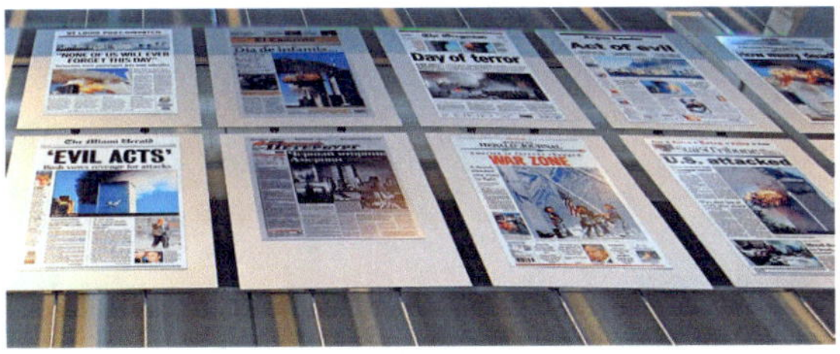

Figure 3.16. Media coverage has become a big player in shaping forensic case outcomes, and it's drawing more attention in today's criminal justice talks.

Source: By Fletcher6 - Own work, CC BY-SA 3.0, https://commons.wikimedia.org/w/index.php?curid=4399457.

3.3.8. Cross-disciplinary Collaboration in Forensic Investigations

Forensic science is most interesting when various kinds of expertise interact in unexpected ways. It is common for toxicologists, doctors and law enforcement experts to be involved in the same case which helps present the evidence in a wider way. Take Canada, for example—there, field professionals and academic folks are increasingly teaming up in a way that, in most cases, kick-starts a lively exchange of ideas essential for pushing forensic methods ahead (Casella et al., 2011). Historical cases—like the John Donald Merrett trial—leave no doubt that when medical insights mix with specialized forensic know-how, our view of evidence gets a serious makeover, with boundaries all but blurred and analysis taking on new layers of depth (Duvall et al., 2016). All in all such teamwork makes forensic investigations more accurate and encourages the development of new solutions for recurring issues.

3.3.9. Future Implications of Case Studies on Forensic Practices

Case studies often share important insights that lead forensic practices to unexpected changes. They not only make us better at forensic science, but they also improve how well we identify cases in forensic medicine and toxicology. As they try out several possibilities, investigators notice similarities and usually come up with new methods that help gather and understand evidence more accurately. Artificial intelligence and other modern tools help make the process more efficient and sometimes they also boost the accuracy of the identifications. As our field shifts to meet fresh challenges, those earlier lessons from past investigations still play a crucial role in helping experts cut down on mistakes and keep the wheels of justice turning in complex legal settings (Lechien et al., 2020; Zeppenfeld et al., 2022).

Test Your Knowledge

1. Why do forensic experts use case studies?
2. Give an example of a situation where forensic odontology was used to find out who a victim was.

Summary

New developments in forensic medicine and toxicology demonstrate, in general, that getting accurate identifications is very important, whether for trials or routine investigations. Take, for instance, the detailed study of animal hair using differential histological methods; local reference databases end up being a real must-have to catch the subtle differences in specimens, ultimately helping with crime scene assessments and suspect recognition (Ahmed et al., 2018). Also, the rising presence of synthetic cathinones pushes us to try out inventive techniques—like chiral and stable isotope analysis—to untangle the messy workings of illicit drug markets and boost overall forensic intelligence (Morrison et al., 2017). All in all, these different ways prove that you have to use both old and new methods together. Overall, as forensic methods improve, they help us rely on evidence more and they are essential in our ongoing pursuit of justice.

Because modern crime is complex, we have to rely on better forensic tools. Forensic identification which uses DNA tests and other methods, can unexpectedly prove that suspects were at the crime scene. At the same time, forensic science isn't limited to matching evidence; it also supports private security agencies which usually helps prevent more crimes. When evidence-based practices are put to work, community safety noticeably improves (Saxena et al., 2024). Such a mix of methods allows for solving cases and helps the public trust security measures more over time. Overall, the partnership between forensic medicine and toxicology clearly shows how key identification techniques are in shaping court outcomes and keeping society secure in an increasingly unpredictable world (Tammi et al., 2021).

KEY TERMS FROM THIS CHAPTER

- Carbon monoxide
- Data security
- Hands-on training
- Investigation
- Spectrophotometry
- Consent
- Fairness
- Honesty
- postmortem changes
- Trustworthiness
- Crimes
- Gas chromatography
- Hydrogen sulfide
- Privacy

Short Answer Questions

1. Explain using fingerprints in forensic identification.
2. Describe the role of dental records in identifying unknown bodies.
3. Write a note on DNA fingerprinting and its importance.
4. Discuss how forensic odontology assists in mass disaster victim identification.
5. Explain the role of radiological methods in forensic identification.

Critical Thinking Questions

1. **The most reliable method of human identification is:**
   a. Fingerprint analysis
   b. Dental records
   c. Facial recognition
   d. DNA profiling
2. **Which of the following techniques is used to compare a skull with a photograph of a person?**
   a. Superimposition
   b. Reconstruction
   c. Radiocarbon dating
   d. Palynology
3. **The uniqueness of fingerprints is due to:**
   a. Age of the individual
   b. DNA structure
   c. Ridge patterns
   d. Blood type
4. **Dental identification is especially useful in cases of:**
   a. Poisoning
   b. Decomposition or burning
   c. Drowning
   d. Suffocation
5. **What is the branch of forensic science that deals with teeth for identification purposes?**
   a. Forensic odontology
   b. Forensic anthropology
   c. Forensic pathology
   d. Forensic entomology

Answers to Critical Thinking Questions

1. (d); 2. (a); 3. (c); 4. (b); 5. (a)

References

1. Abouelkeir, R., Ali, A. A., Abdelsatar, M. F., Rashed, L. A., & Alsaeed, S. A. (2022). Application of the methylated markers (spectrin beta and DEAD-box protein) for definitive differentiation between fresh and aged semen by evaluating their role in identifying semen from mixed body fluids. *International Journal of Medical Toxicology and Forensic Medicine*, *12*(4), 386. https://doi.org/10.32598/ijmtfm.v12i4.38615.
2. Abrol, V. (2024). *Forensic Science: Revealing the Clues*. IntechOpen eBooks. https://doi.org/10.5772/intechopen.1003870.
3. Adamec, V., Köbölová, K., Pavlíková, S., et al. (2019). Current approaches of occupational and safety health management in work environments containing nanoparticles. *Transactions of the VSB–Technical University of Ostrava Safety Engineering Series*, *XIV*(2). https://core.ac.uk/download/287648860.pdf (accessed on 29 May 2025).
4. Adeola, H. A., Van Wyk, J. C., Arowolo, A. T., & Khumalo, N. P. (2018). Human hair as a testing substrate in the era of precision medicine: Potential role of 'omics-based approaches. *IntechOpen*. https://doi.org/10.5772/intechopen.77215.
5. Advisory Council on the Misuse of Drugs. (2011). Consideration of the novel psychoactive substances ('legal highs'). https://core.ac.uk/download/1643031.pdf (accessed on 29 May 2025).
6. Ahmed, Y. A., Ali, S., & Ghallab, A. (2018). Hair histology as a tool for forensic identification of some domestic animal species. *EXCLI Journal*, *17*, 663–670. https://doi.org/10.17179/excli2018-1478.
7. Balhareth, A. A. S., Jamesh, M., Zabarah, G. A., Almotlaq, M. M., Alabaaltahin, M. A. M., Al Jaarah, A. H., Aldawsari, A. G., Almastaneer, K. A. M., Alyami, S. M., & Al Yami, A. S. H. (2024). The role of forensic medicine in modern criminal justice: A review of current practices and innovations. *Journal of Eco Humanism*, *3*(7), 2699–2707. https://doi.org/10.62754/joe.v3i7.4669.
8. Basso, C., Aguilera, B., Banner, J., Cohle, S., d'Amati, G., de Gouveia, R. H., di Gioia, C., Fabre, A., Gallagher, P. J., Leone, O., Lucena, J., Mitrofanova, L., Molina, P., Parsons, S., Rizzo, S., Sheppard, M. N., Mier, M. P. S., Kim Suvarna, S., Thiene, G., van der Wal, A., & Association for European Cardiovascular Pathology. (2017). Guidelines for autopsy investigation of sudden cardiac death: 2017 update from the Association for European Cardiovascular Pathology. *Virchows Archiv*, *471*(6), 691–705. https://doi.org/10.1007/s00428-017-2221-0.
9. Bhoyar, L., Mehar, P., & Chavali, K. (2024). An overview of DNA degradation and its implications in forensic caseworks. *Egyptian Journal of Forensic Sciences, 14*. https://doi.org/10.1186/s41935-024-00389-y.
10. Boriwala, A., & Hankare, M. (2024). Literature review about forensic toxicology and poisoning. *Journal of Ayurveda and Integrated Medical Sciences*, *9*(4), 176–183. https://jaims.in/jaims/article/view/3079 (accessed on 29 May 2025).

11. Boronat Ena, M. del M., Cowan, D., & Abbate, V. (2021). Ambient ionization mass spectrometry applied to new psychoactive substance analysis. *Mass Spectrometry Reviews, 42*, 3–34. https://doi.org/10.1002/mas.21695.

12. Buzdar, Z. A., Murad, T., Shabbir, S., Ahmed, A., Soomro, T. A., & Masood, R. (2024). Estimating age on the autopsy table: A postmortem study of forensic investigations. *Journal of Saidu Medical College, Swat.* https://www.semanticscholar.org/paper/fde681bc296472e9b38d3a4bc9801e2195d2b32b (accessed on 29 May 2025).

13. Capiau, S., Stove, C., & Velghe, S. (2016). Opening the toolbox of alternative sampling strategies in clinical routine: A key role for (LC-)MS/MS. Retrieved from: https://core.ac.uk/download/84043363.pdf (accessed on 29 May 2025).

14. Casparsen, C. (2024). The role of toxicology in forensic investigations. *International Journal of Forensic Medicine*, *6*(1), 31–33.

15. Caudill, D. S. (2009). Arsenic and old chemistry: Images of mad alchemists, experts attacking experts, and the crisis in forensic science. Retrieved from: https://core.ac.uk/download/229258057.pdf (accessed on 29 May 2025).

16. Chango, X., Flor-Unda, O., Gil-Jiménez, P., & Gómez-Moreno, H. (2024). Technology in forensic sciences: Innovation and precision. *Technologies*, *12*(8), 120. https://doi.org/10.3390/technologies12080120.

17. Chen, B., Colston, B., Boehnert, M., González-Rodríguez, J., Ruiz-Jiménez, J., Jaiswal, A. K., Jickells, S., et al. (2011). Determination of arsenic, mercury and barium in herbarium mount paper using dynamic ultrasound-assisted extraction prior to atomic fluorescence and absorption spectrometry. https://core.ac.uk/download/1645649.pdf (accessed on 29 May 2025).

18. Ciobanu, A. M., Baconi, D., Bălălău, C., Negrei, C., Stan, M., & Bârcă, M. (2015). Toxicological analysis of some drugs of abuse in biological samples. *Journal of Mind and Medical Sciences*, *2*(2), 108–127. https://doi.org/10.22543/2392-7674.1018.

19. Coopman, V., Blanckaert, P., Van Parys, G., Van Calenbergh, S., & Cordonnier, J. (2016). A case of acute intoxication due to combined use of fentanyl and 3,4-dichloro-N-[2-(dimethylamino)cyclohexyl]-N-methyl benzamide (U-47700). *Forensic Science International*, *266*, 68–72. https://doi.org/10.1016/j.forsciint.2016.05.001.

20. Crawford-Jakubiak, J. E., Alderman, E. M., Leventhal, J. M., Flaherty, E. G., Idzerda, S. M., Legano, L. A., Leventhal, J. M., et al. (2017). Care of the adolescent after an acute sexual assault. *Pediatrics*, *139*(5). https://doi.org/10.1542/peds.2016-4243.

21. Davis, J. R., Lane, H. W., & Stepaniak, P. C. (2025). Loss of signal: Aeromedical lessons learned from the STS-107 Columbia space shuttle mishap. Retrieved from: https://core.ac.uk/download/pdf/42730063.pdf (accessed on 29 May 2025).

22. Di Nunno, N., Esposito, M., Argo, A., Salerno, M., & Sessa, F. (2021). Pharmacogenetics and forensic toxicology: A new step towards a multidisciplinary approach. *Toxics*, *9*(11), 292. https://doi.org/10.3390/toxics9110292.

23. Dos Santos, B. P., Birk, L., Schwarz, P. K. N., Sebben, V. C., Sgaravatti, Â. M., de Gouveia, G. C., Silva Petry, A. U., de Menezes, F. P., Gonzaga, A. P., Schlickmann, P. F., Arbo, M. D., de Oliveira, T. F., & Eller, S. (2024). A validated dilute-and-shoot LC-MS-MS urine screening for the analysis of 95 illicit drugs and medicines: Insights from clinical and forensic Brazilian cases. *Journal*

of Analytical Toxicology, *48*(5), 314–331. https://doi.org/10.1093/jat/bkae005.

24. Duvall, N. (2017). "If experts differ, what are we to do in the matter?" The medico-legal investigation of gunshot wounds in a 1927 Scottish murder trial. *Social History of Medicine*, *30*(2), 367–388. https://doi.org/10.1093/shm/hkw066.
25. Fabricant, M. C., & Garrett, B. L. (2018). The myth of the reliability test. Retrieved from: https://core.ac.uk/download/213020569.pdf (accessed on 29 May 2025).
26. Faigman, D. L. (2008). Anecdotal forensics, phrenology, and other abject lessons from the history of science. Retrieved from: https://core.ac.uk/download/230095688.pdf.
27. Ferrara, L. (2018). The contribution of ethical reasoning skills in forensic science (Doctoral dissertation, Duquesne University). Retrieved from: https://dsc.duq.edu/etd/1426 (accessed on 29 May 2025).
28. Garrett, B. L., & Mitchell, G. (2018). The proficiency of experts. Retrieved from: https://core.ac.uk/download/213020407.pdf (accessed on 29 May 2025).
29. Goel, R., Kumar, D., & Arora, V. (2022). Forens(om)ic medicine: Omics in forensic medicine. *International Journal of Research in Medical Sciences*, *10*(2), 557–564. https://doi.org/10.18203/2320-6012.ijrms20220309.
30. Guijas, C., Montenegro-Burke, J. R., Domingo-Almenara, X., Palermo, A., Warth, B., Hermann, G., Koellensperger, G., et al. (2018). METLIN: A technology platform for identifying knowns and unknowns. *Analytical Chemistry*, *90*(6), 3156–3164. https://doi.org/10.1021/acs.analchem.7b04424.
31. Ho, K. C., Jentzen, J., Johnson, L. T., et al. (1994). Destructive hostility: The Jeffrey Dahmer case: A psychiatric and forensic study of a serial killer. Retrieved from: https://core.ac.uk/download/213059368.pdf (accessed on 29 May 2025).
32. Issa, S. Y. (2019). Forensic toxicology. Retrieved from: https://core.ac.uk/download/322440626.pdf (accessed on 29 May 2025).
33. Jannetto, P. J., Helander, A., Garg, U., Janis, G. C., Goldberger, B. A., & Ketha, H. (2018). The fentanyl epidemic and evolution of fentanyl analogs in the United States and the European Union. *Clinical Chemistry, 65*, 242–253. https://doi.org/10.1373/clinchem.2017.281626.
34. Kaushik, N., Pal, S. K., Sharma, A., Thakur, S., et al. (2017). Role of diatoms in diagnosis of death due to drowning: Case studies. https://core.ac.uk/download/483635548.pdf (accessed on 29 May 2025).
35. Kinoshita, H., Tanaka, N., Takakura, A., Jamal, M., Ito, A., Kumihashi, M., Kimura, S., et al. (2017). Simplified analysis of toxic gaseous substances in forensic practice: Experiences from Japan. Retrieved from: https://www.semanticscholar.org/paper/b17a9420da291c21a265b62866e5e05041ffd491 (accessed on 29 May 2025).
36. Kintz, P. (2018). Hair analysis in forensic toxicology: An updated review with a special focus on pitfalls. *Current Pharmaceutical Design, 23*. https://doi.org/10.2174/1381612823666170929155628.
37. Klingberg, J., Keen, B., Cawley, A., Pasin, D., & Fu, S. (2022). Developments in high-resolution mass spectrometric analyses of new psychoactive substances. *Archives of Toxicology, 96*, 949–967. https://doi.org/10.1007/s00204-022-03224-2.
38. Klinkner, M. (2008). Proving genocide? Forensic expertise and the ICTY. *Journal of International*

Criminal Justice, 6(3), 447–466. https://ssrn.com/abstract=1212077 (accessed on 29 May 2025).

39. Lechien, J. R., Chiesa-Estomba, C. M., Hans, S., Barillari, M. R., Jouffe, L., & Saussez, S. (2020). Loss of smell and taste in 2013 European patients with mild to moderate COVID-19. *Annals of Internal Medicine, 173*(9), 672–675. https://doi.org/10.7326/m20-2428.
40. Lowe, D. J., Torrance, H. J., Ireland, A. J., Bloeck, F., & Stevenson, R. (2017). SODAS: Surveillance of Drugs of Abuse Study. *European Journal of Emergency Medicine, 24*(2), 126–129. https://doi.org/10.1097/MEJ.0000000000000310.
41. Lynch, K. L. (2015). CLSI C62-A: A new standard for clinical mass spectrometry. *Clinical Chemistry, 62*, 24–29. https://doi.org/10.1373/clinchem.2015.238626.
42. Mannocchi, G., Pantano, F., Romolo, F. S., Tittarelli, R., et al. (2015). Recreational use, analysis and toxicity of tryptamines. https://core.ac.uk/download/54534388.pdf (accessed on 29 May 2025).
43. McCartney, C. (2011). The law-forensic science disciplinary divide: The Canadian experience.
44. Moreno, I. E. D. (2016). The role of miniaturized systems in analytical toxicology: New psychoactive substances. https://core.ac.uk/download/303998412.pdf (accessed on 29 May 2025).
45. Mores, C. M., Castro, M. B., & Melo, C. B. (2025). Forensic examinations in the investigations of crimes involving animals: A review. *Ciência Rural, 55*(3). https://doi.org/10.1590/0103-8478cr20240071.
46. Morgan, J. (2023). Wrongful convictions and claims of false or misleading forensic evidence. *Journal of Forensic Sciences, 68*, 908–961. https://doi.org/10.1111/1556-4029.15233.
47. Nodari, R., Arghittu, M., Bailo, P., Cattaneo, C., Creti, R., D'Aleo, F., Saegeman, V., et al. (2024). Forensic microbiology: When, where and how. *Microorganisms, 12*, 988. https://doi.org/10.3390/microorganisms12050988.
48. Parmar, P. (2023). The integration of artificial intelligence in the forensic medicine and its applications in medico-legal autopsy, forensic toxicology, and disaster victim identification. *International Journal of Forensic Sciences*. https://www.semanticscholar.org/paper/fc16f6a30cab5b4e85b76b323902ed9b047c2d0c (accessed on 29 May 2025).
49. Piraianu, A. I., Fulga, A., Mușat, C. L., Ciobotaru, O. R., Poalelungi, D. G., Stamate, E., Ciobotaru, O. C., et al. (2023). Enhancing the evidence with algorithms: How artificial intelligence is transforming forensic medicine. *Diagnostics, 13*, Article 2992. https://doi.org/10.3390/diagnostics13182992.
50. Poalelungi, D. G., Mușat, C. L., Fulga, A., Neagu, M., Neagu, A. I., Piraianu, A. I., & Fulga, I. (2023). Advancing patient care: How artificial intelligence is transforming healthcare. *Journal of Personalized Medicine, 13*(8), 1214. https://doi.org/10.3390/jpm13081214.
51. Reid, K. M., Suwalowska, H., Martin, L. J., & Heathfield, L. J. (2025). Ethical considerations in the routine identification of human remains in forensic mortuaries [Version 1; peer review: awaiting peer review]. *Welcome Open Research, 10*, 171. https://doi.org/10.12688/wellcomeopenres.23041.1.
52. Sanzyapova, R. R. (2025). The role of dentistry in forensic medicine: Identification of human

remains. *Patient-Oriented Medicine and Pharmacy*. https://www.semanticscholar.org/paper/d8db5ae62d74c13d619c3b0324e081b54abd3399 (accessed on 29 May 2025).

53. Saxena, S., & Deo, S. H. (2024). Implication of forensic science for private security. https://core.ac.uk/download/617189936.pdf (accessed on 29 May 2025).

54. Seywright, A., Torrance, H. J., Wylie, F. M., McKeown, D. A., Lowe, D. J., & Stevenson, R. (2016). Analysis and clinical findings of cases positive for the novel synthetic cannabinoid receptor agonist MDMB-CHMICA. *Clinical Toxicology, 54*(8), 632–637. https://doi.org/10.1080/15563650.2016.1186805.

55. Sh, J., Hugar, B., & Praveen, S. (2020). Determination of stature from index and ring finger lengths in South Indian population. *Journal of Forensic Medicine*, *14*(4), 795–799. Retrieved from: https://www.semanticscholar.org/paper/72c123b38b5775ba4623cc03bf7b5a76dc64b3db (accessed on 29 May 2025).

56. Singh, W. U., & Singh, K. P. (2023). The transformative role of artificial intelligence in forensic medicine and toxicology. *Journal of Medical Society, 37*, 101–102. https://doi.org/10.4103/jms.jms_54_24.

57. Speaker, P. J. (2017). FORESIGHT benchmark data 2015-2016. *Faculty & Staff Scholarship*, 1144. https://researchrepository.wvu.edu/faculty_publications/1144 (accessed on 29 May 2025).

58. Tai, S. S. C. (2018). *Chiral and Stable Isotope Analysis in Forensic Chemistry: Novel Psychoactive Substance Analysis* (Doctoral dissertation, University of Glasgow).

59. Tammi, T., & Viskari, I. (2021). *Report on Good Practices of Synthetic Opioid Preparedness, And Needs and Challenges in EU Member States: Deliverable D3.2*. https://core.ac.uk/download/591956267.pdf (accessed on 29 May 2025).

60. Teymourian, H., Parrilla, M., Sempionatto, J. R., Montiel, N. F., Barfidokht, A., Van Echelpoel, R., De Wael, K., et al. (2020). Wearable electrochemical sensors for the monitoring and screening of drugs. *ACS Sensors*, *5*(9), 2679–2700. https://doi.org/10.1021/acssensors.0c01318.

61. Vadysinghe, A., Edusooriya, D., Dayaratne, S. P., Manoratne, N. M. K., Abeysekara, Y., & Nissanka, P. W. A. D. P. M. (2017). Is the undergraduate forensic medicine teaching adequate to produce an expert medical witness? *Medico-Legal Journal of Sri Lanka*, *5*(1), 5. https://www.semanticscholar.org/paper/aeabce33a41a4da7a1b3ac45577f2f7b05916575 (accessed on 29 May 2025).

62. Vrees, R. (2017). Evaluation and management of female victims of sexual assault. *Obstetrical & Gynecological Survey, 72*, 39–53. https://doi.org/10.1097/ogx.0000000000000390.

63. Wille, S., Van Dijck, K., Van Assche, A., di Fazio, V., Ramiréz-Fernandéz, M. del M., Vanvooren, V., & Samyn, N. (2021). The interest of a systematic toxicological analysis combined with forensic advice to improve the judicial investigation and final judgment in drug facilitated sexual assault cases. *Pharmaceuticals, 14*. https://www.semanticscholar.org/paper/79c2d94ac127bf7dde45b85ed9fa5802fab11079 (accessed on 29 May 2025).

64. Wu, J., Luan, Y., Zhang, Q., Wang, F., & Rao, Y. (2024). Effects of dichloromethane, nitrate, and sulfhemoglobin-induced substances on carboxyhemoglobin detection: A comprehensive review. *Journal of Analytical Toxicology*. https://www.semanticscholar.org/paper/9a4148b9a9a47c9f29ba979851341f0c21f471e9 (accessed on 29 May 2025).

65. Zeppenfeld, K., Tfelt-Hansen, J., Riva, M., Winkel, B. G., Behr, E. R., Blom, N. A., Charron, P., et al. (2022). 2022 ESC guidelines for the management of patients with ventricular arrhythmias and the prevention of sudden cardiac death. *European Heart Journal, 43*, 3997–4126. https://doi.org/10.1093/eurheartj/ehac262.

DEATH AND ITS MEDICOLEGAL ASPECTS

4

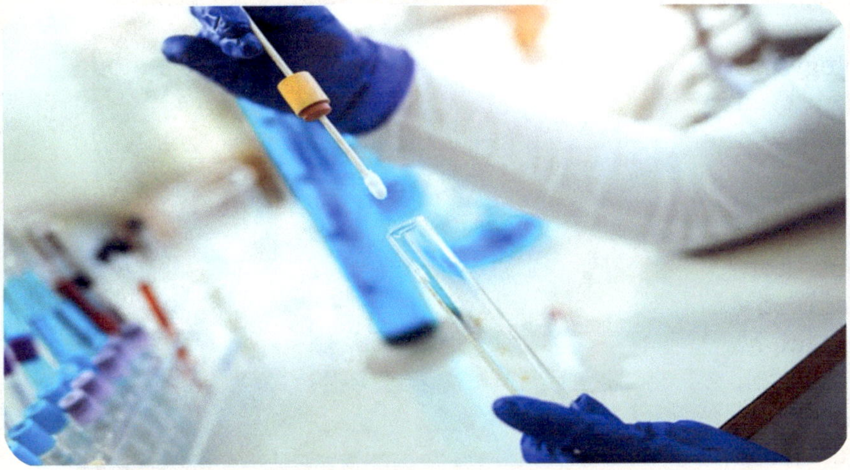

LEARNING OBJECTIVES

After studying this chapter, you will be able to:

1. Know the legal definitions and classifications of death;
2. Explain autopsy and its medicolegal importance;
3. Understand death investigation and the role of coroners;
4. Explain what happens in criminal law when someone dies.

Introduction

Death is much more than a personal loss because it usually leads to a range of legal and medical issues that reveal many things we might not notice. These days, the aftermath of death affects more than just people's emotions; it brings up many legal and ethical issues that touch public policies, medical care and investigations. When you dig into these medicolegal details, you often uncover pressing questions about informed consent, especially as new tech like AI keeps shifting how we work in medicine and investigate deaths (Poalelungi et al., 2023). In many cases, getting a grip on the moral ideas behind informed consent is crucial, because these principles lay the groundwork for research on human subjects, and they also help steer practices in forensic science (Budowle et al., 2023). All of these points together show the many aspects of death, where law, ethics and new technology come together and help prepare for further study.

Definition of Death in a Medical Context

It is still difficult in medicine to pinpoint when a person has died, because it involves ethical, legal and social issues. Instead of a single clear-cut moment, doctors often face a split: one moment when breathing and the heartbeat stop (what's sometimes called clinical death), versus when all brain activity permanently ends—each posing its own challenges in practice. The distinction is very important, since it affects organ transplants and the way legal death is defined in each place. Most of the time, new medical technology has made things more complicated, making it even harder to decide and raising questions about our legal systems.

Meanwhile, forensic anthropologists sometimes get into debates about how these distinctions affect things like ancestry estimation—which some critics say might even sustain racial biases—and overall, understanding what "death" means medically is key to untangling today's medicolegal issues (DiGangi et al., 2021; Rogers et al., 2020) .

Importance of Studying Medicolegal Aspects of Death

The medicolegal part of death matters a lot, not only because of the legal checks. In many cases, knowing what factors lead to a fatal outcome—take severe burn injuries with clear legal ties Dr. Ram et al. (2023) as an example—sheds light on why deaths occur, especially when injuries or violent acts are involved. With this kind of information, forensic investigations improve and healthcare teams can detect similar issues and risk factors involved in unexpected deaths. Studies that capture survivor experiences, for instance Thambithurai et al. (2024), remind us that including patient voices shapes more realistic care indicators. Ultimately, by diving into these details, both medical professionals and legal authorities can navigate ethical challenges, fine-tune policies, and work to ensure justice in unnatural death cases, thereby lifting the overall standard of societal care (Figure 4.1).

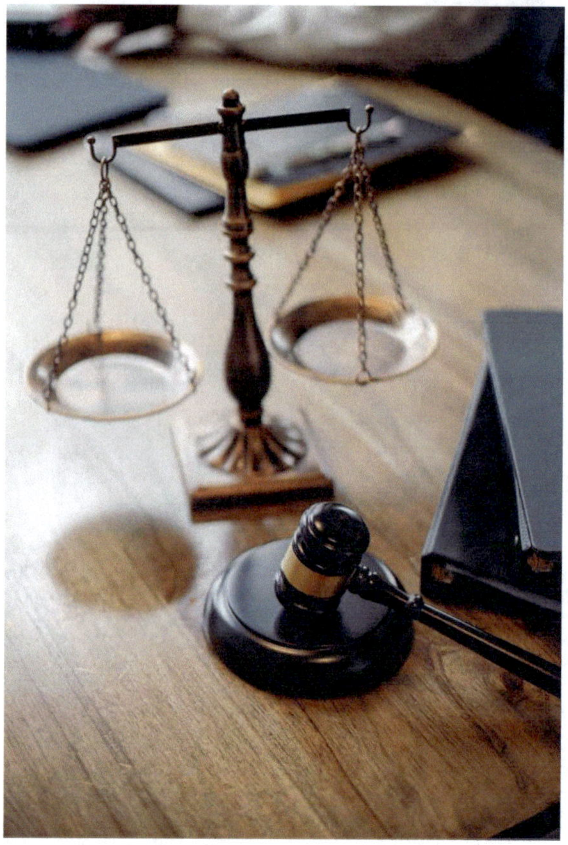

Figure 4.1. Medicolegal aspects of death.

Source: https://juriscentre.com/wp-content/uploads/2023/01/pexels-photo-5669619.jpeg?w=800.

Overview of the Relationship Between Medicine and Law

Medicine and law are often connected in surprising ways, mainly when matters about death and ethics arise. Over the years, people have updated their views on what causes death and this usually happens together with stricter laws. In 17th-century Rome, courts would ask medical experts to help decide if a woman's death was due to complications in childbirth and this led to many debates about what disease actually is. Many times, these disagreements indicated that doctors should care about legal issues since a medical decision could lead to major legal problems in malpractice or wrongful death cases. Nowadays, questions about consent and patient rights help keep the discussion between the two fields more detailed than it might appear at the beginning. To summarize, the close connection between medicine and law remains crucial for tackling not only tricky ethical problems but also for keeping legal accountability steady in healthcare (Renzi, 2010; Courson et al., 2014).

Historical Perspectives on Death and Legal Implications

Death has long sparked questions about the law and about culture. Experts say that how communities deal with death involves much more than just rules; it includes a variety of ethics, morals and government policies. In a lot of situations, our views on death are shaped by both religion and civic laws. For instance, how illnesses are recorded for legal purposes. Generally speaking, people dealing with serious health issues encounter different legal hurdles than those in better shape, as seen in the Maqasid Shariah principles aimed at protecting property and offspring (Anwar et al., 2024). The law's take on suicide, too, seems to have shifted over time; older views often favored strict punishment, but now there's more understanding and support (Wojnicz, 2024). All in all, the way death is handled in law reflects the influence of society's values on everyday rules and the sometimes complicated relationship between law and human life.

Relevance of the Topic in Contemporary Society

Death in the modern world is not straightforward because it involves matters that require various types of expertise, mainly where law and medicine meet. Because interpersonal violence is increasing and often affects the most vulnerable, forensic nurses play an even more important role. Having practical skills to identify victims and deal with legal matters, these nurses can affect patient outcomes and help us see violence differently. There's also a national online program for forensic training that's been boosting nurses' abilities in trauma-aware care and injury documentation, filling the gap many noted from their previous lack of forensic training (Brown et al., 2024). On top of that, figuring out whether remains are human or nonhuman in forensic anthropology calls for specialized training—something that, quite frankly, helps medical examiner offices work way better (Fourshee et al., 2022). In general such efforts help form a medicolegal system that can handle the complexities of real-life situations.

Methodology for Research and Analysis

Looking at death from a medicolegal perspective is not simple, because there are many details to consider and a good research and analysis approach is needed. Besides focusing only on statistics like mortality rates, researchers also pay attention to the special details that make each case different. For example, Sabirova et al. (2025) goes into how flow cytometry is used to track changes in cells after death, which ties back to the biological factors at play. In most cases, Mirashk et al. (2025) also points out that Design Science Research (DSR) can be pretty useful in building predictive models that mix numerical data with those qualitative nuances, thereby deepening our insight into medicolegal risk. Researchers who use mixed methods often discover different aspects of death which allows for more subtle ways to view their findings. To summarize, this kind of rigorous—if sometimes a bit messy—approach not only powers academic studies but also feeds into practical forensic science, continually nudging the field's evolving landscape (Figure 4.2).

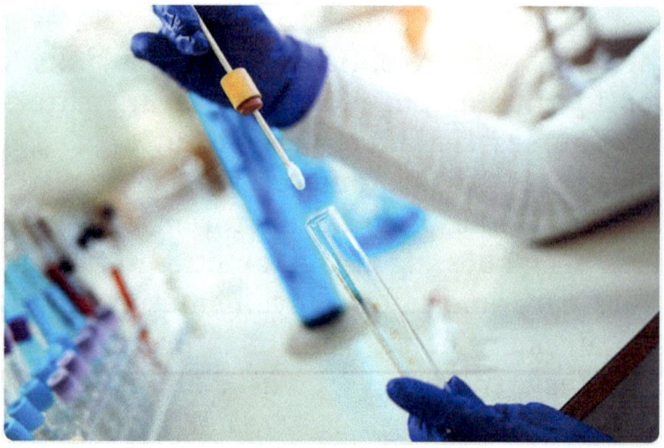

Figure 4.2. Examining death within a medicolegal framework isn't as straightforward as it might seem.

Source: https://i.imgur.com/L5buhy3.jpg.

4.1. Legal Definitions and Classifications of Death

Learning Outcome

1. Understand clinical death versus biological death;
2. Know legal death and its implications;
3. Explain the determination of death;
4. Pay attention to the medical team's role in determining when death occurs;
5. Learn variations in legal definitions across jurisdictions;
6. Explain what brain death is and how it is treated by law;
7. Identify implications of misclassification of death;
8. Learn case studies illustrating legal definitions;
9. Keep up with new trends in how death is understood in the law.

Death can be complicated and the many legal definitions just make things more confusing for people working in medicine and law. Now, people often discuss death in different stages: first is clinical death, when breathing and the heart stop and then biological death, when the brain stops functioning entirely, even the parts that manage basic tasks. This isn't only about technical details; it is very important, especially in malpractice cases, because the type of death can determine who is held liable and the way the case is managed. For example, if something goes wrong during surgery—say, a perioperative peripheral nerve injury (PNI)—it might blur the line between clinical and biological death, a nuance that pops up in talks about patient safety in anesthesia (Chui et al., 2018). Also, when you consider conditions like metabolic syndrome and their potential effects on thinking, it becomes clear that getting our legal definitions right is pretty important since these classifications sometimes tie into larger matters like disability claims and healthcare costs (Ricci et al., 2017).

4.1.1. Clinical Death Versus Biological Death

The details of death are not always straightforward like people might believe. People refer to clinical death and its biological equivalent as two different things and this difference usually leads to big legal and ethical consequences. Consider clinical death first: it happens when your heart stops and you stop breathing and luckily, medical help may be able to start your heart again. When cells are damaged beyond repair and all the important functions cease, this is known as biological death and the organs eventually fail. This isn't only about legal terms—these differences affect who gets an organ, how inheritances are distributed and what kinds of care are given at the end of life. A complete lack of brain activity is usually taken as a sign that the person is in an irreversible state which is considered a legal indicator of death. That clear, yet sometimes fuzzy, distinction creates many ethical and legal dilemmas for both the healthcare team and families; even a small mix-up can end up causing some pretty serious consequences in critical care situations (Gokaba et al., 2024; Xu et al., 2024) (Figure 4.3).

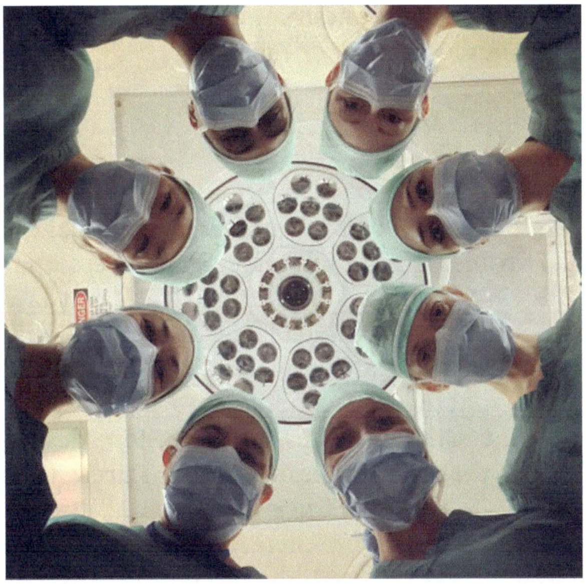

Figure 4.3. Clinical death versus biological death.

Source: https://study.com/cimages/multimages/16/clinical_death1466654726727194517.jpg.

4.1.2. Legal Death and its Implications

Death can be complicated and it takes more than one simple legal explanation, especially when medical issues are involved. What we consider to be a legal death changes over time and this usually leads to unexpected effects for doctors, families and society. Forensic investigators, who are essential in untangling these matters, often wrestle with mounting pressures at work; such stress, at times, dims their ability to dig into death cases effectively (Thorpe et al., 2024). How we determine a death as legal is now affected by social, political and mental well-being factors. Contemporary issues, like climate change and mass migration, toss extra layers into the ethical mix of forensic work, making legal death assessments even more complicated and increasing the load on professionals (Smith et al., 2024). For these reasons, investing in caring and flexible workplaces is essential for the well-being of medical staff and the stability of the medicolegal process which in turn helps society rethink its attitude toward death and its legal consequences.

4.1.3. Determination of Death: Criteria and Methods

Medicolegal work centers on determining death and it requires following standard steps instead of using a simple checklist. Experts check for signs such as a heart stopping or the brain not functioning at all and these signs often overlap. When cases are difficult, neuroimaging is used in addition to other tests to provide more details when the usual signs do not explain everything. Yet, in most cases, the fallout from a misstep can be serious; slight misreads or mishandling of forensic details might even lead to wrongful convictions (Morgan, 2023). Generally speaking, carefully following these established guidelines is seen as absolutely essential for keeping justice on track and for maintaining the public's trust in the medicolegal system (Poalelungi et al., 2023) (Figure 4.4).

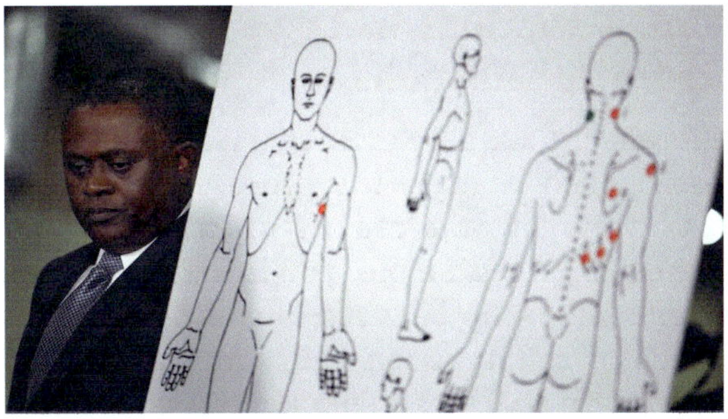

Figure 4.4. Determining death sits at the heart of medicolegal work—it's not a simple checklist but a matter where sticking to known steps counts.

Source: https://media.hswstatic.com/eyJidWNrZXQiOiJjb250ZW50Lmhzd3N0YXRpYy5jb20iLCJrZXkiOiJnaWZcL2F1dG9wc3ktbGlzdC5qcGciLCJlZGl0cyI6eyJyZXNpemUiOnsid2lkdGgiOjgyOH19fQ==.

4.1.4. The Role of Medical Professionals in Declaring Death

Declaring death is not just a usual part of the job—it involves more responsibilities than typical medical care. Providers in health care have to manage combining medical knowledge, legal rules and ethics, often trying to merge facts with the expectations of the community. For example, the Uniform Determination of Death Act is often used to set rules, but it also reminds everyone that being clear matters, as it helps families and medical staff when they need some legal protection when things go wrong. Recent events, especially during the COVID-19 crisis, have thrown these responsibilities into sharper relief, pushing healthcare workers to be extra transparent and build trust (Crowley et al., 2019; Nioi et al., 2021). Usually, these changes cause decisions that at first look like simple choices, but they end up affecting our entire legal system for medicine. In short, when doctors have to act fast, the results can change the course of science, law and ethics, even if the process is not always perfect.

4.1.5. Variations in Legal Definitions Across Jurisdictions

Different regions have their own ways of defining death which changes the process of medical-legal work and the results of investigations. In the U.S., for example, you'll find that some states tend to flip between labeling a case as a suicide or calling it self-injury mortality (SIM) (Rockett et al., 2022). This kind of change can result in incorrect data and less clear public health information, mainly for overdoses. Now, take a look at how postmortem examinations are handled in places like Italy and the U.S.—the legal approach there is largely a product of cultural tastes and slightly different regulatory rules (Moretti et al., 2021). In short, these inconsistencies make it difficult to standardize forensic practices and highlight the importance of more research and open talks which usually lead to improved understanding in the law and better outcomes.

4.1.6. The Concept of Brain Death and Its Legal Status

Brain death involves many medical, ethical and legal problems all at once. Medical professionals are trying to understand brain death, but laws are not keeping up which leads to problems with organ donation and family decisions. Brain death means that all brain activity is permanently gone and this is the usual definition, despite the fact that local customs and cultures differ. Sometimes, this murkiness leads to real clashes; think about cases involving pregnant women, where decisions end up weighing both the mother and her unborn child in ways that don't fit the usual rules (Gerber et al., 1966). As a result, the legal side of brain death stays hotly debated, pushing healthcare pros and legal experts into constant, sometimes uneasy chats to bridge the gap between modern medicine and society's values (Ocviyanti et al., 2021) (Figure 4.5).

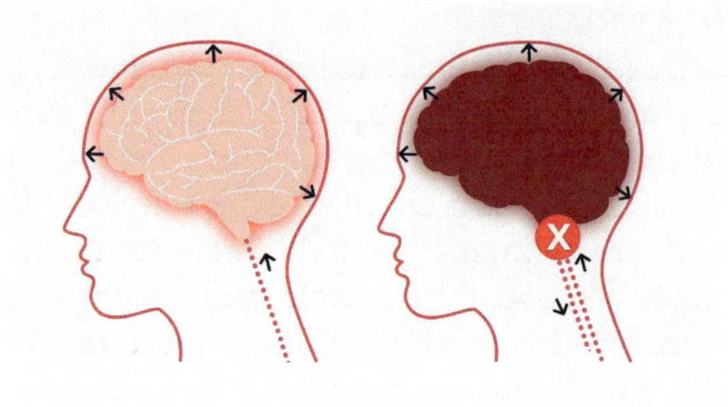

Figure 4.5. Brain death.

Source: https://chainedevie.org/sites/default/files/2021-06/blog-la-mort-cerebrale.jpg.

4.1.7. Implications of Misclassification of Death

Incorrectly classifying deaths creates confusion in medicolegal research, mainly when discussing suicide and poisoning. In most cases, research out of the United States shows that cases involving drug intoxication-related suicides often fly under the radar because there simply isn't enough psychological or psychiatric evidence, which in turn skews the numbers and messes with our overall efforts to keep track and prevent further tragedies (Caine et al., 2018). Such errors at times make us unsure about the real number of suicides which adds more difficulty to public health efforts. It's interesting to note that the drop we see in official suicide numbers from 1987–2000 might, in part, come from non-elderly suicides being lumped in with unintentional poisoning—a mix-up that only deepens the challenges faced by both national and regional epidemiological efforts (Leo et al., 2010). Basically, if we want data to be accurate and we want to design effective interventions, we cannot ignore these classification issues.

4.1.8. Case Studies Illustrating Legal Definitions

Once sudden cardiac death occurs, it causes many problems that make standard legal definitions no longer fit – especially after an autopsy takes place. It keeps being shown in case studies that SCD isn't just one problem; there are often hidden genetic factors involved in these sudden deaths, showing how complex the issue can be. For example, postmortem genetic testing has become a key approach in uncovering what went wrong – many experts now generally advise its use for families affected by these tragedies (Fellmann et al., 2019). It's interesting that research also finds gender differences, with women typically passing away later and more often due to non-ischaemic causes (Haukilahti et al., 2019), a detail that adds another twist to legal considerations. All of this encourages us to change our usual legal approaches and see SCD cases in a way that combines medical knowledge and legal investigation in a more flexible and human manner.

4.1.9. Future Trends in the Legal Understanding of Death

Societies evolve and our approach to death changes as well. Because ethics and technology keep changing, the laws about death are not constant and can change in surprising ways. Forensic examiners, for instance, now show up as crucial players in malpractice lawsuits; they dig into messy cases and, with a clear-cut approach, explain how medical practices line up with the outcomes we observe, ensuring that responsibility sticks while ethical standards remain front and center (Sobh et al., 2024).

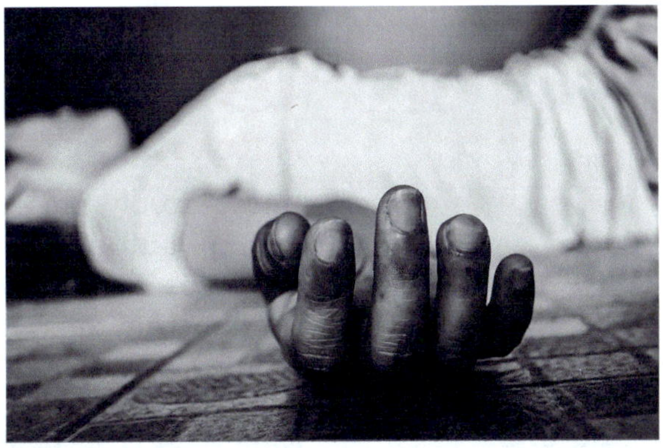

Figure 4.6. Societies change, and the way we handle issues like death shifts along with them.

Source: https://www.thestatesman.com/wp-content/uploads/2020/06/murder.jpg.

Suicide is also looked at from several social and economic angles. Studies that peek at regional differences in suicide rates point out how cultural factors and legal reactions mix together in interesting ways, hinting that local methods might someday shape broader legal changes (Wojnicz , 2024). To summarize, these trends suggest that a mix of perspectives—drawing from many different fields—is needed to truly grasp the future legal landscape of death, one that keeps pace with society's needs and the leaps made in medical science (Figure 4.6).

Test Your Knowledge

1. Define legal death.
2. What is the contrast between clinical death and biological death?
3. What does it mean to be brain dead and how is that legally established?

4.2. Autopsy and Its Medicolegal Importance

Learning Outcome

1. Understand the definition and purpose of an autopsy;
2. Explain types of autopsies;
3. Know the role of forensic pathologists;
4. Explain legal requirements for conducting autopsies;
5. Be able to interpret the results of an autopsy and their impact on legal proceedings;
6. Focus on ethical considerations in performing autopsies;
7. Find out how the findings from an autopsy influence investigations into crimes;
8. Identify public perception of autopsies and their necessity;
9. Discuss advances in autopsy techniques and technologies.

Figuring out the cause and circumstances of a death can be tough and usually requires us to examine the body. Often, when it's not obvious what caused or how someone died, a full postmortem exam is required instead of being optional. When a death is sudden or puzzling, an autopsy is sometimes needed to look for clues about any hidden health conditions. Nowadays, there's also the new twist of postmortem genetic testing, which, generally speaking, helps spotlight inherited conditions that might explain an untimely death in younger people; this insight often nudges families toward taking preventative measures (Fellmann et al., 2019). One can't overlook the old-school method of clinical-pathologic correlation—an approach with roots stretching back for centuries—that carefully maps out disease processes and, in doing so, reinforces the weight of autopsy findings in both medical and legal arenas (Williamson, 2019). In short, autopsies are a key and often overlooked part of today's medicolegal system because they supply important information for public health and legal decisions.

4.2.1. Definition and Purpose of an Autopsy

Unexpectedly, medicine and law come together during autopsies which have many more purposes than just finding out the cause of death. An autopsy is mainly about examining a body after death and this is often done by forensic pathologists to identify hidden health conditions. This work matters on several levels; generally speaking, it helps clarify individual tragedies like sudden cardiac death—where postmortem genetic testing, for example, can reveal underlying causes (Fellmann et al., 2019)—and it also plays a role in broader community health, especially during crises such as the COVID-19 pandemic when tracking disease spread becomes key (Moretti et al., 2021). In addition, autopsies add to the information used in big studies about public health which helps guide decisions and slowly advances medical knowledge. Naturally, having so many positives also raises ethical and practical issues which usually result in continuous discussion and joint efforts by those involved in autopsy education and practice. To summarize, this mix of methodical investigation and ethical debate shows just how intertwined and dynamic the worlds of medicine and law are (Figure 4.7).

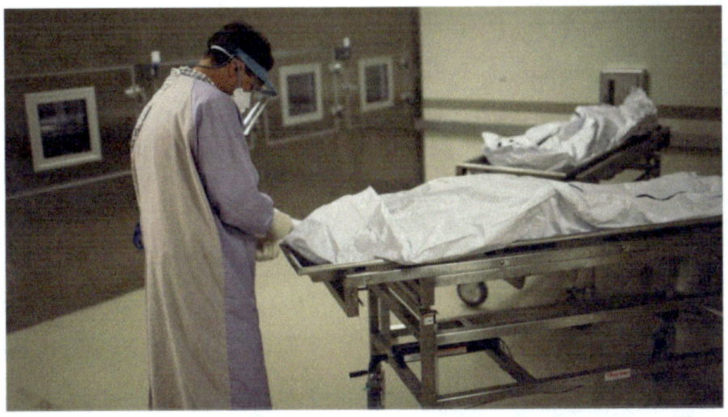

Figure 4.7. Medicine and law unexpectedly meet in the practice of autopsies, which do way more than just pinpoint why someone died.

Source: https://blog.ipleaders.in/wp-content/uploads/2020/10/new-mexico-forensics2_wide-d98e7e8e45d88133e8d5e581350769ad80cdb363.jpg.

4.2.2. Types of Autopsies: Clinical Versus Forensic

Death in medicolegal cases can create many unclear issues. Autopsies performed in hospitals are used to discover the cause of death and examine disease patterns which improves medical knowledge and patient care. Forensic autopsies are mainly concerned with legal issues and they are usually done when a death is sudden, unexpected or appears suspicious, to collect information for a criminal case. Most of the time, this difference influences consent and ethics, especially if the family of the deceased is not fully aware of the risks involved in a postmortem examination. In most cases, sticking to the principles of respect, beneficence, and justice is key, so that everyone involved is properly informed about what the autopsy process means—this is even more important when identifying missing persons through familial links and forensic genetic genealogy (Budowle et al., 2023; Nowinski et al., 2022).

4.2.3. The Role of Forensic Pathologists

There are often complications between death and the law and forensic pathologists are called when things don't make sense. They investigate cases when something doesn't feel right or looks suspicious—trying to solve puzzles that are not easy to understand. Running an autopsy helps learn the reason for someone's death and also helps identify public health issues, especially when a new illness like COVID19 appears. They also testify in court, where they explain their medical findings and how they relate to the legal arguments, usually helping the case. The pandemic has, in a way, shouted out that our old autopsy guidelines just won't cut it anymore—forcing these specialists to continually adapt to unpredictable challenges, all while trying to support both legal proceedings and community health goals (Kim et al., 2020) (Figure 4.8).

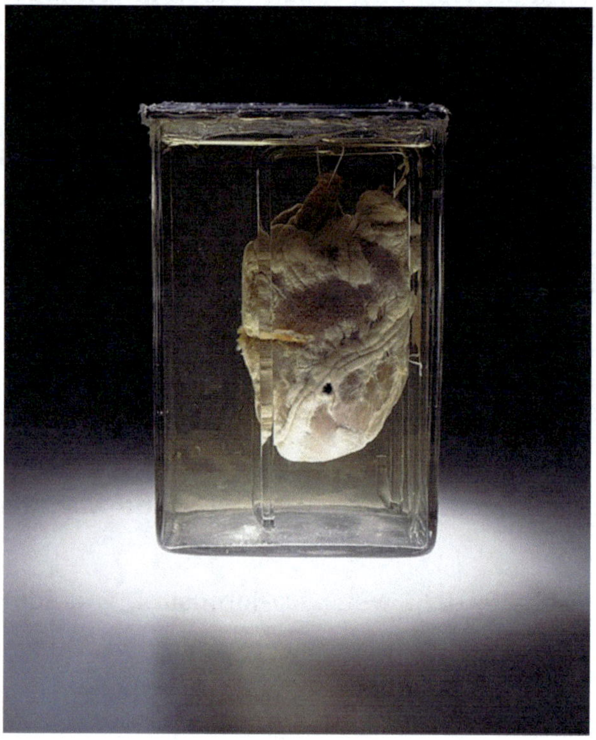

Figure 4.8. The role of forensic pathologists.

Source: https://en.wikipedia.org/wiki/File:Forensic_medicine_heart.jpg.

4.2.4. Legal Requirements for Conducting Autopsies

There are many legal rules that must guide every step of an autopsy. These rules not only make sure the investigation is clear, but also help look after the rights of those who have passed and their families. Normally, the law sets out when an autopsy should be done, using the way someone died, the events surrounding it and local rules as factors. When working with the rules, forensic experts often have to weigh the technical aspects against moral issues, mainly when dealing with marginalized communities. Many forensic anthropologists and similar professionals are wedded to finding better, fairer practices; there's a growing push to be more inclusive, even when it comes to recognizing a range of gender identities during death investigations, as noted in recent studies (Adams et al., 2023; Nasnodkar et al., 2023). Such a change in viewpoint usually impacts both the way procedures are done and the way society views death in general.

4.2.5. Autopsy Findings and their Implications in Legal Cases

Most of the time, looking into a death means carefully examining autopsy results which often play a key role in shaping legal outcomes. For example, spotting bacteria like Escherichia coli during postmortem tests can point to problems such as symmetrical peripheral gangrene or even a psoas abscess, gently nudging the case toward claims of medical negligence or wrongful death (Sangita et al., 2025).

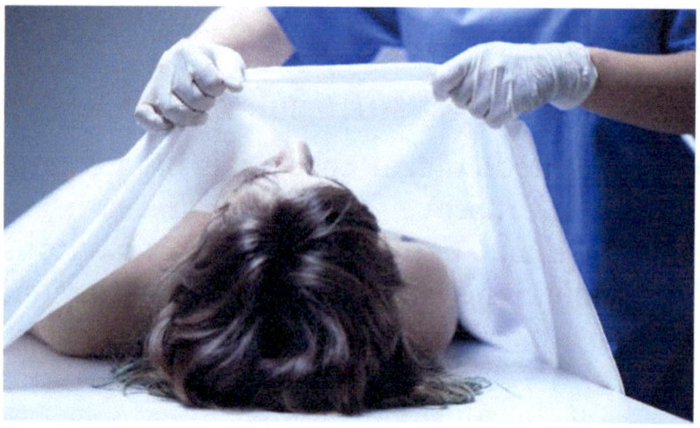

Figure 4.9. Autopsy findings and their implications in legal cases.

Source: https://www.livelaw.in/h-upload/2020/10/19/750x450_383059-post-mortem.jpg.

It's not only about what's inside the body—the hard part can be telling if the fractures happened before or after the person died which helps reveal more about the injury and the cause and manner of death. Odd as it may seem, the texture and appearance of broken bones often throw in some valuable forensic clues, subtly influencing interpretations about what occurred (Moirangthem et al., 2024). To summarize, these autopsy clues stretch far beyond mere medical observations; they weave into the legal fabric of the case, showing just how intertwined forensic insights are with courtroom debates (Figure 4.9).

4.2.6. Ethical Considerations in Performing Autopsies

There are many times when cultural beliefs and medical practices do not agree and this can make autopsies very complicated. Take Kerala, for instance—despite high literacy rates, many people still seem uneasy about the whole idea, usually pointing to their religious beliefs and a nagging worry over possible disfigurement (Babu et al., 2025). In most cases, these doubts help us see that showing cultural sensitivity when dealing with ethics matters is very important; if we fail to do this, people may doubt the law and the legal system. When studying violent deaths in Senegal, it becomes clear that forensic science and law enforcement need to know the local social and legal situation for autopsies to be accurate. In short, ethical practices should put clear informed consent and some straightforward education first, so folks can better understand how autopsies actually help serve both public health and legal goals (Oumar et al., 2024).

4.2.7. The Impact of Autopsy Results on Criminal Investigations

The results of an autopsy are very important in crime investigations, even though they may be overlooked sometimes. They do not only report the details of the death; they also notice and reveal clues about suspicious deaths such as blunt force trauma or poisoning. A thorough review of the body can sometimes suggest that something suspicious occurred which can change the course of the case.

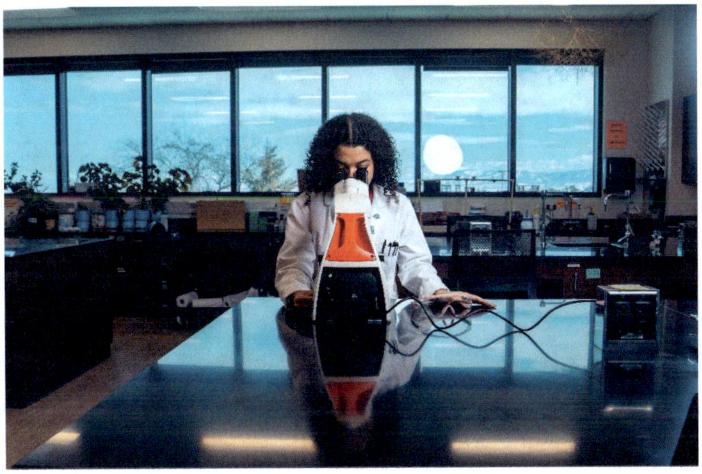

Figure 4.10. Autopsy findings matter—a lot—in crime investigations, even if it's easy to overlook just how crucial they are.

Source: https://erau.edu/-/media/images/university/hub-spoke/images-for-development/20240209-makenzi-patterson-09474-full.jpg?as=0&hash=FA163059592E8592C6DD87BB4C85C758.

In many cases, the information gleaned doesn't stop at explaining a death; it can also reveal insights into underlying disease processes, occasionally linking seemingly isolated cases into a broader outbreak—consider how, during the recent pandemic, forensic pathologists' observations proved generally indispensable (Moretti et al., 2021). Ultimately, this kind of knowledge shapes law enforcement strategies while reinforcing the legal system's backbone, underscoring the need for thorough medicolegal practices in our ongoing quest for justice (Nioi et al., 2021) (Figure 4.10).

4.2.8. Public Perception of Autopsies and Their Necessity

Autopsies can cause a variety of reactions whenever death is brought up. Many people discuss if it is right to examine a body after someone dies, considering our cultural beliefs. Although many agree that these practices help medicine and find out the true cause of death, some are still concerned about showing disrespect to the body or going against deeply held beliefs. Take consent and respectful treatment for example – these issues echo past lapses in medical oversight (J et al., 2024). In many Islamic contexts, the debate still smolders as folks try to tie scientific exploration with genuine reverence for those who have passed on (Aziz et al., 2023). To summarize, what people think about autopsies is shaped by a messy mix of ethics, tradition, and medical needs, calling for more open chats and better understanding (Figure 4.11).

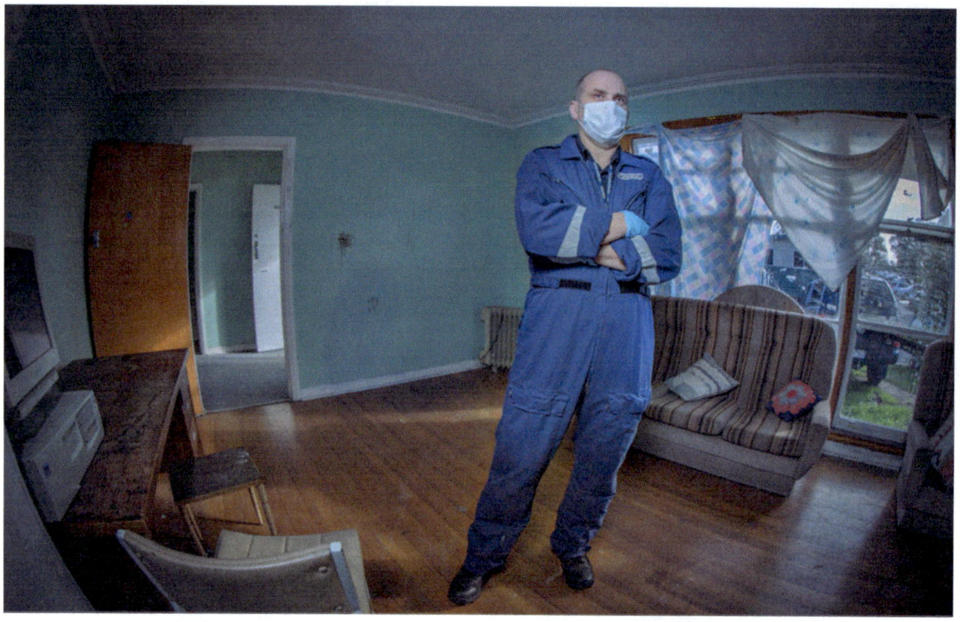

Figure 4.11. Many people admit that such practices push medicine forward and help pin down accurate causes of death, yet worries linger about disrespecting the body's sanctity or stepping on deeply held personal beliefs.

Source: https://live-production.wcms.abc-cdn.net.au/53176455b40f6ae5613e45f911801a64?src.

4.2.9. Advances in Autopsy Techniques and Technologies

Forensic science has advanced, affecting the way autopsies are done and making it simpler to find out the cause of death. Now, digital histopathology and 3-D imaging are common – they allow experts to examine the body's interior without making big incisions and with great detail. It allows for less physical effort by the doctor while still uncovering a lot about the patient's health; this is a smart way to learn more. It is important to mention that experts in forensics such as forensic pathologists and scientists, often team up to improve how postmortem analysis is done. Also, dealing with tricky metabolic problems – think disorders linked to metabolic dysfunction-associated steatohepatitis – shows that, in most cases, personalizing assessments in forensic work is becoming more and more necessary (Abrol, 2024). To summarize, these improvements not only raise the bar for forensic evaluations but also help build a broader picture of death and all its complicated aspects (Lonardo et al., 2024).

Test Your Knowledge

1. What is an autopsy?
2. Differentiate between clinical and medico-legal autopsy.
3. What is the minimum requirement for a medico-legal autopsy?

4.3. Death Investigation and the Role of Coroners

Learning Outcome

1. Explain the overview of the death investigation process;
2. Understand the role and responsibilities of a coroner;
3. Know the differences between coroners and medical examiners;
4. Examine the role of coroners in investigating deaths;
5. Identify challenges faced by coroners in their duties;
6. Know the importance of death certificates;
7. Learn case studies of notable death investigations;
8. Look at the effects of death investigations on the health of the public;
9. Explain future developments in death investigation practices.

The number of unanticipated death investigations has been increasing and this has made coroners responsible for more important duties. They are responsible for understanding the causes and circumstances of death which helps both law and public health. Because of the COVID-19 crisis, the usual way autopsies were performed had to be changed to protect staff. Forensic pathologists, grappling with these unexpected challenges, often offer key insights into disease workings that, in turn, help track outbreaks and trends (Murphy, 2023). As laws are updated, the rules for their work are also modified which means they must stay informed about informed consent and patient safety. In most cases, these steady improvements let the medicolegal field evolve to meet legal and ethical demands while still keeping death investigations as thorough as possible (Murphy, 2023).

4.3.1. Overview of the Death Investigation Process

Medicolegal death investigations are more involved than they appear and what the public thinks is significant. Even though Kerala has a high literacy rate, its traditional views about death are still present. Research shows that roughly 92% of people know about medicolegal autopsies; still, many get mixed up about what they're actually for, and cultural or even religious doubts mean that acceptance isn't complete (Babu et al., 2025). On a related note, studies on professional training reveal that even veterinarians can be caught off guard when dealing with death, hinting at a broader flaw in educational focus across several fields (Alves et al., 2024). In most cases, ramping up public awareness alongside improved training in death investigations seems pretty vital to secure truly informed consent and gain wider societal acceptance (Figure 4.12).

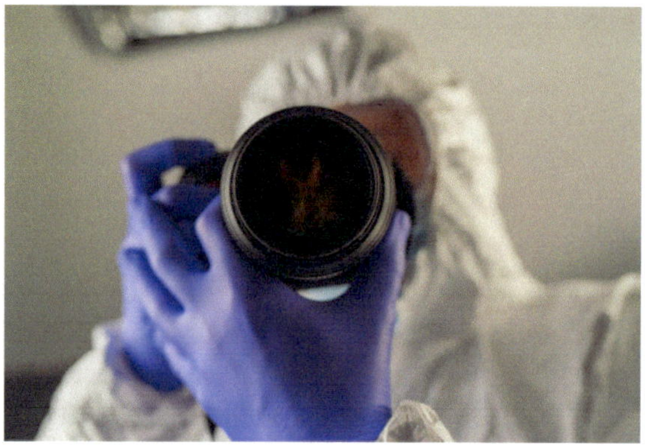

Figure 4.12. Death investigations in medicolegal cases aren't just dry procedures—they're intricate affairs where public opinion matters.

Source: https://ncjtc-static.fvtc.edu/images/training/TR00005771_20171212091837.jpg.

4.3.2. The Role and Responsibilities of a Coroner

Investigating deaths that seem unusual places the coroner in the middle of linking medicine and law. They usually look into the circumstances, collect evidence, conduct autopsies when appropriate and help families understand the process of working with the law. The variety of tasks in this job which is greater than most people realize, can result in confusion about medicolegal autopsies. For example, a study in Kerala showed that while many folks appreciate the value of these procedures, around 6% still have doubts based on cultural views (Babu et al., 2025). In cases that get tricky, such as with neurological conditions like temporal lobe epilepsy—which can muddle legal responsibility as well as forensic checks—the coroner's work becomes even more key (Noé López-Amador et al., 2024). In short, as well as meeting legal duties, coroners help us learn more about death and its effects.

4.3.3. Differences Between Coroners and Medical Examiners

Death investigations can be messy. The difference between coroners and medical examiners is sometimes not easy to notice. Most coroners are chosen by the people and come from different walks of life and they might not have the medical training some believe they should have—this can result in mixed findings.

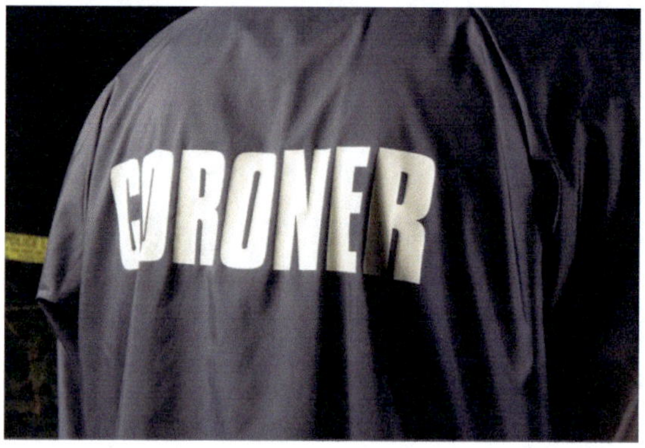

Figure 4.13. Coroners are usually picked by voters and come from all sorts of backgrounds, and they often don't have the medical schooling that some expect—this can make their results a bit uneven.

Source: https://cdn.route-fifty.com/media/img/cd/2021/10/28/iStock_184980512/860x394.jpg.

Unlike coroners, medical examiners are usually licensed doctors who have chosen to focus on forensic pathology; they rely on autopsies and other steps to determine how someone died. Because they have strong medical knowledge, they can handle complex cases, but coroners must rely on local rules that change from place to place. Generally speaking, these differences point to why a more standardized approach to death investigations is needed, as the current system has some clear gaps that affect both the service and the safety of medicolegal death investigators (Vicks et al., 2019). Knowing the background of these professionals is key when you're trying to tell human remains apart from nonhuman ones, which matters to the quality of forensic analysis (Fourshee et al., 2022) (Figure 4.13).

4.3.4. Legal Authority of Coroners in Death Investigations

Investigating deaths depends a lot on coroners—they explain the cause of death and also suggest how each case is related to public health. They are allowed to perform autopsies, collect evidence and issue death certificates; these things can affect the outcome of trials and help form new laws. Look at the challenges during the COVID-19 pandemic (Moretti et al., 2021): coroners had to wrestle with strict rules meant to control infection, which made routine postmortem exams unexpectedly tricky. It appears that having flexible policies helps them do their work and keep everyone safe. When you turn your attention to ancestry estimation in forensic anthropology, it's clear that new methods must wrangle with a messy mix of ethics and legal rules—challenges that all too often hit marginalized communities the hardest (DiGangi et al., 2021).

4.3.5. Challenges Faced by Coroners in Their Duties

The many duties that coroners have to handle make their job in medicolegal investigations very complicated. There have been more complicated death cases lately, mainly because of a rise in suicides and drug-related deaths. COVID-19, for instance, seems to have deepened these challenges by ramping up social isolation and straining mental health among vulnerable folks—factors coroners now must weigh in their evaluations (Gaddis et al., 2024). Because it is hard to tell suicides apart from other fatalities, data collection is affected which can change our view of mortality trends. To summarize, this situation generally points to the need for broader training and more uniform procedures so that coroners can better navigate the ever-changing landscape of death, with clear impacts on public health and safety (Rockett et al., 2021) (Figure 4.14).

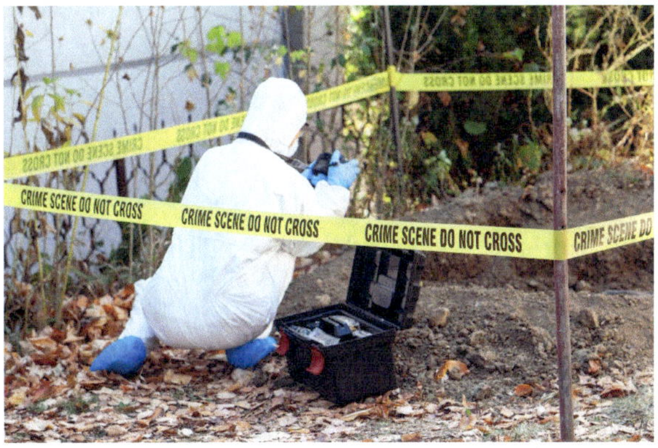

Figure 4.14. Coroners juggle a maze of duties that make their work in medicolegal investigations far from straightforward.

Source: https://www.openaccessgovernment.org/wp-content/uploads/2021/09/dreamstime_xl_220627441-scaled.jpg.

4.3.6. The Importance of Death Certificates

When medicine and law meet, especially on matters as sensitive as mortality, good record-keeping is very important. Death certificates are not only legal papers; they also hold a lot of public health information. They give the person's identity, the cause of death and the events leading up to it which can guide both public health and police investigations. A lot of the time, if these documents are not accurate, you could get a wrong idea about how diseases are spreading or how mortality rates are changing. Take, for instance, debates over ancestry estimation in forensic anthropology, which have stirred up concerns about racial bias in medicolegal realms (DiGangi et al., 2021). Research on obstructive sleep apnea and its link to increased accident risk also shows that proper paperwork is key to crafting clear clinical guidelines and safety standards (Bonsignore et al., 2020) (Figure 4.15).

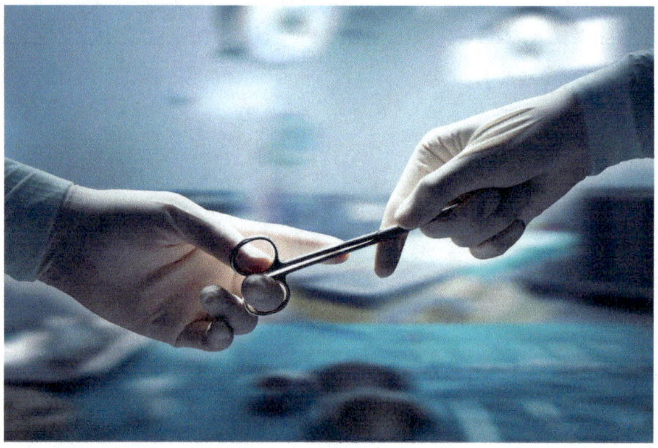

Figure 4.15. Death certificates aren't merely legal forms; they serve as rich sources of public health details.

Source: https://media.npr.org/assets/img/2016/05/03/doctor-failure_custom-b39c26855ae37f87ed227682d106bfdb743d9e0a.jpg?s=1100&c=50&f=jpeg.

4.3.7. Case Studies of Notable Death Investigations

Death investigations are full of unexpected problems and this is often shown by studying real cases that highlight the key tasks of medicolegal death investigators. When you dig into these cases, it becomes pretty clear that not having solid rules and a consistent training system frequently puts a dent in how investigations are handled, as noted in recent reviews of current practices (Vicks et al., 2019). In most cases, the heavy emotional load and stress that investigators deal with only add more hurdles to their everyday work, sometimes nudging them toward burnout—which then messes with their overall performance and job satisfaction (Thorpe et al., 2024). In general, handling these issues is key for the progress of medicolegal practices; it highlights the importance of proper oversight and strong support systems that look after investigators which leads to better and more reliable death investigations. In short such an approach helps the field develop and respond to society's need to know more about the consequences of these tragedies.

4.3.8. The Impact of Death Investigations on Public Health

Both death investigations and public health help society in ways that may not be noticed at first. Looking into why people die – often by probing events like sudden heart stoppages (SCD) – gives us vital data that, in many cases, inform public health actions and even steers genetic counseling (Fellmann et al., 2019).

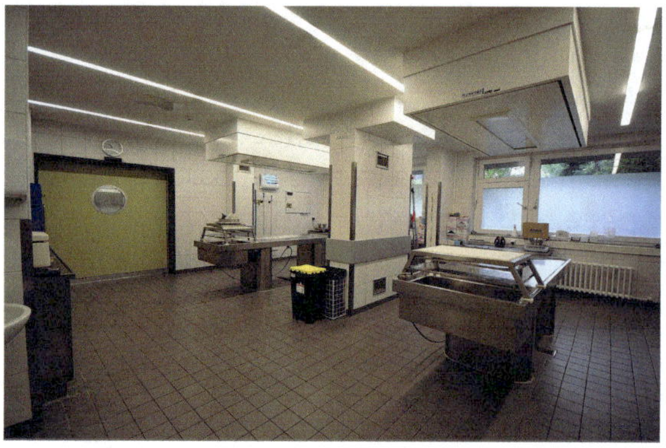

Figure 4.16. Death investigations and public health shape society's well-being in ways that aren't always immediately obvious.

Source: By Ralf Roletschek (talk) - Infos über Fahrräder auf fahrradmonteur.de - Own work, FAL, https://commons.wikimedia.org/w/index.php?curid=22886399.

It's also evident that a lot of medical students don't get enough nutrition training, which points to an urgent need for better education in this area to help prevent health problems at both the personal and community levels (Crowley et al., 2019). Using results from autopsies that suggest important epidemiological points and encouraging specialists to cooperate, helps health officials design interventions that improve the results. In general, these investigations not only shine light on the underlying causes of death but also lay the groundwork for sound public health policy and a more responsive healthcare system (Figure 4.16).

4.3.9. Future Developments in Death Investigation Practices

The fast development of technology is causing changes in the way death investigations are handled. Forensic analysis and AI are now assisting with hard cases which makes it easier to find out who did what and why. Across different regions, guidelines (often kicked off by various medical groups) end up stirring a kind of casual consistency that nobody expected. Take the Royal College of Obstetricians and Gynaecologists; they've long backed the notion that sticking to evidence-based clinical practices can subtly steer medicolegal protocols (Murphy, 2023). Then there's the idea that throwing nutrition basics into medical training might, in many instances, boost new doctors' knack for recognizing health factors tied to a death (Crowley et al., 2019). When all these pieces are put together, sometimes in unexpected ways, we can see a clearer approach forming which may help improve health outcomes and make forensic law more reliable.

Test Your Knowledge

1. What is the main responsibility of a coroner in an investigation of a death?
2. How are coroners and medical examiners different from each other?

4.4. Medicolegal Implications of Death in Criminal Law

Learning Outcome

1. Understand homicide and its legal definitions;
2. Describe the part that forensic evidence plays in solving homicide cases.
3. Pay attention to the idea of manslaughter and the differences it has from other crimes.
4. Understand what the law says about assisted death and euthanasia.
5. Study how death influences civil liability cases.
6. Examine the functions of expert witnesses in matters of death.
7. Learn high-profile cases that shaped death-related laws;
8. Find out where mental health definitions of death meet the legal definitions.
9. Keep up with new changes in death and criminal law.

Medicolegal death investigators are important in separating criminal law from cases that end in death. They are at the center of investigating and carefully recording deaths, mainly those that seem suspicious or might be crimes. In most cases, the fact that there isn't any firm regulation and no mandatory accreditation (Vicks et al., 2019) creates a whole host of problems that end up muddling the investigation process. Plus, heavy workloads and the constant push from the organization often wear investigators down, which can mean they sometimes struggle to keep up both accuracy and genuine compassion (Thorpe et al., 2024).

All in all, this combination of problems indicates that a more uniform system of training and support is required in medicolegal work; this helps investigators and maintains the trust and reliability of our justice system, making sure each case receives proper attention, even if it is not always perfect.

4.4.1. Homicide and its Legal Definitions

There are many legal meanings to homicide and these can vary a lot depending on the place. Because forensic experts use these legal lines to guide their investigations, how they are drawn is very important. A case may be charged as murder or manslaughter based on whether the intent or guilt is seen differently which affects the court verdict and the actions taken at the scene. In most cases, recent work shows that medicolegal death investigators are key to working through these tangled definitions, although their field still lacks standardized training and clear guidelines (Vicks et al., 2019). Look at serial murder cases, as some FBI studies point out (Holland et al., 2015)—understanding these legal nuances becomes absolutely essential for practitioners trying to do justice and improve their investigations. To summarize, the way legal definitions mix with medicolegal practices paints the picture of how homicide probes are shaped (Figure 4.17).

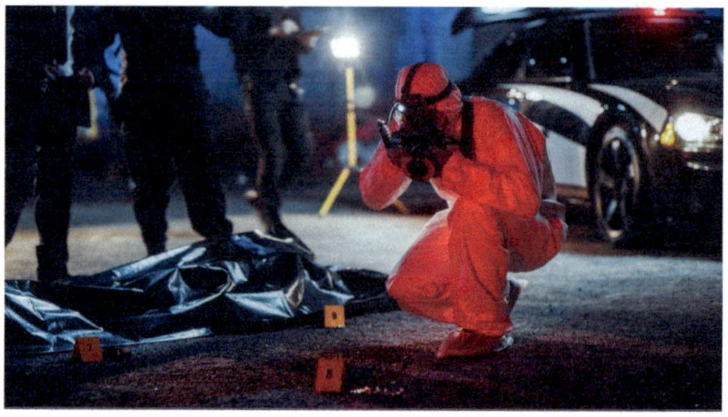

Figure 4.17. Homicide.

Source: https://legalcareerpath.com/wp-content/uploads/2024/04/iStock-1481901859.jpg.

4.4.2. The Role of Forensic Evidence in Homicide Cases

Homicide investigations are messy, with a lot happening and forensic evidence is the key point. Forensic anthropology and genetic testing are used by science to learn about the victim and what happened in the time leading up to their death. Sometimes, checking out skeletal remains reveals ancestral hints that can nail an identification down, although some experts have raised concerns over racial bias in these techniques (DiGangi et al., 2021). Then again, breakthroughs in genetic testing have proven to be a big deal, especially when a sudden cardiac death happens; in most cases, pinpointing a genetic predisposition can shed light on hidden causes, which in turn shifts the medicolegal narrative a bit (Fellmann et al., 2019). In short, mixing together all these pieces of forensic evidence doesn't just help crack a case—it also reminds us that ethical issues are always in the mix, demanding a balance of firm science and genuine care in the quest for justice (Figure 4.18).

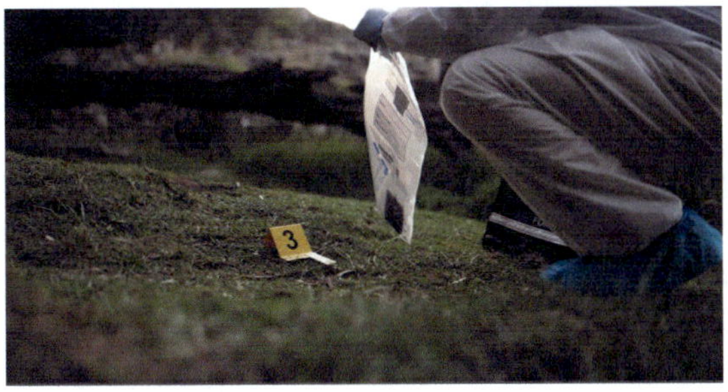

Figure 4.18. The Role of forensic evidence in homicide cases.

Source: https://www.aerlawgroup.com/wp-content/uploads/2024/09/The-Role-of-Forensic-Evidence-in-Murder-Trials.jpg.

4.4.3. The Concept of Manslaughter and its Distinctions

It is very important to understand the differences between manslaughter, since this is often considered when law and medicine look at cases of death. A lot of people think that manslaughter is less serious than homicide and it is often divided into two types that can be hard to define. Sometimes manslaughter is called voluntary manslaughter, referring to an action done with intent, but not premeditated, while involuntary manslaughter usually happens by accident, because of carelessness or recklessness. Usually, this difference greatly influences who is held legally responsible and what the consequences are. At the same time, debates on euthanasia, offering a fresh yet complex lens on death, tend to mix these ideas—tapping into evolving views on personal freedom and the right to a dignified end (Halina Pérez Álvarez et al., 2021; Simonović, 2024). Such discussions, emphasizing a fairer treatment in legal outlooks, reflect a gradual shift towards more compassionate approaches in dealing with matters of life and death (Figure 4.19).

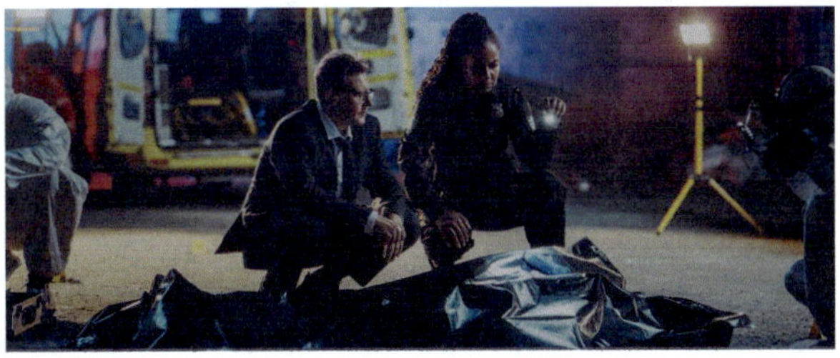

Figure 4.19. Manslaughter.

Source: https://www.agpllp.ca/wp-content/uploads/2024/09/manslaughter-cases.webp.

4.4.4. Legal Consequences of Assisted Death and Euthanasia

The topic of assisted death is always ongoing. There are many differences in laws from one place to another which makes us ask what people should have. In America, around 56,000 people are sentenced to life without parole and most of them live through long periods of distress in prison. The argument over letting prisoners choose euthanasia raises questions about our moral beliefs and laws—is a dignified death something everyone should have or do laws differ from one country to another? Here, the laws on euthanasia often clash with people's basic rights such as the right to life, freedom of choice and being protected from cruelty. In most cases, the absence of one shared international legal standard only makes the inequalities worse and complicates the safety nets that should protect citizens (Long et al., 2024; Michałkiewicz-Kądziela et al., 2023).

4.4.5. The Impact of Death on Civil Liability Cases

Death and civil liability often interact in ways that cause many legal challenges for society. If a person dies because of someone else's mistake, tort law becomes especially important by figuring out who is at fault and trying to bring balance to the situation for those affected. Civil liability is a way to address wrongs; families are usually able to seek damages to help with emotional pain, loss of companionship and financial problems. Over the centuries, as medical know-how improved, forensic methods evolved too, which only underscores just how critical an accurate cause-of-death determination is in these cases (Fatović-Ferenčić et al., 2010). The way we define liability can change and this is clear from past rulings that draw a difference between events that require legal action and those that are just unfortunate accidents. Generally speaking, the way death factors into civil liability not only shapes individual legal battles but also mirrors wider social ideas about who bears responsibility and what ethical behavior should look like (Wecht et al., 2000).

4.4.6. The Role of Expert Witnesses in Death-related Cases

Sorting through the confusing details in death cases depends a lot on expert witnesses. Forensic pathologists and other similar pros often step in to help sort out the difference between stillbirths and live births (Krywanczyk et al., 2024)—a distinction that can end up having huge, sometimes unexpected, legal knock-on effects for both families and healthcare providers. Since practices differ from one place to another, it is usually very important to have an expert on the ground to ensure investigations are clear and reliable. The autopsy, a process that digs into the core details of how and why someone died, adds a lot to the legal conversation (Narayankar et al., 2024)—it's one of those steps that makes the whole investigation feel more solid. Drawing on many solid science and hard-earned clinical know-how, these experts not only back up the legal system but also help make sense of the tangled issues surrounding death, even if the topic remains as complex as ever (Figure 4.20).

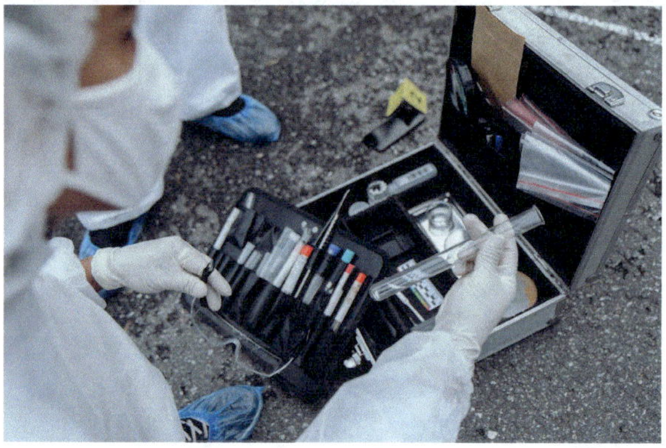

Figure 4.20. Expert witnesses are key players in sorting out the messy details that pop up when we try to figure out what happened in death cases.

Source: https://www.all-about-forensic-science.com/images/the-role-of-forensic-evidence-in-criminal-defense-cases.png.

4.4.7. High-profile Cases That Shaped Death-related Laws

Famous cases can lead to changes in laws concerning death in the medical legal field. Sometimes a major case captures the public's interest and also results in tougher guidelines for forensic science, particularly in the area of human remains. Take isotope analysis for instance—it's one of those techniques that shows, generally speaking, how fresh scientific ideas can slip into legal cases; it helps authorities figure out where unidentified remains might have come from, boosting both the accuracy and speed of investigations (Bartelink et al., 2019). Most of the time, important court decisions show that it is important to consider what patients think about end-of-life care. Getting various opinions together and including patients is now very important for dealing with complex healthcare challenges. All of this clearly points to a need for laws that stay nimble, adapting as medical ethics and patient rights evolve (McGoon et al., 2018).

4.4.8. The Intersection of Mental Health and Legal Definitions of Death

Discussions on what is death become complicated when mental health becomes involved. Society sometimes considers that mental health issues can change how we view the importance of life. For infanticide cases, the reason behind the act becomes very important in legal discussions. The strict rules in some mental health places such as forcing people to stay, can make people ask if patients are considered mentally "done" even if they are physically alive. Because it's not always clear if someone is dead or alive, this area leads to many legal arguments that make us reconsider how mental health is linked to death. At the end of the day, all this blur underlines the need for comprehensive mental health policies to tackle these deep challenges (Belayneh et al., 2025).

4.4.9. Future Legal Trends Regarding Death and Criminal Law

There are new connections between medicine and law and soon standard rules for medicolegal investigations may be used more often. Right now, many death investigators in this field haven't earned their proper accreditation—a gap repeatedly pointed out in the literature (Vicks et al., 2019)—and this shortcoming tends to throw a wrench into smooth service delivery. Most of the time, new legal structures will prefer simple training and basic rules to ensure that death investigations are more reliable. Burnout, too, is starting to stand out; the heavy stress these professionals face often chips away at their job satisfaction, and that situation might just spur lawmakers to tweak workplace conditions and boost support structures (Thorpe et al., 2024). In short, these changes are designed to make investigations more effective and also look after the people who do most of the work.

Test Your Knowledge

1. Define homicidal death with one example.
2. How is a postmortem examination important in solving crimes?
3. How does the time since a person's death affect criminal law?

Summary

Death and the medical and legal aspects of it bring up many issues that are not always easy to group together. Many studies tell us that medicolegal death investigators (MDIs) are right in the middle of handling tricky cases—often wrestling with problems like inconsistent training and shaky accreditation standards. Research generally shows that while MDIs seem pretty sure about what they do, the lack of uniform rules can sometimes put both their effectiveness and safety at risk (Vicks et al., 2019). Burnout also looms large here, a sign of the real psychological strain this line of work can impose, and it hints that better organizational support might help boost morale and resilience among these professionals (Thorpe et al., 2024). Facing these challenges is not only another layer of bureaucracy; it is a significant step toward making sure death investigations are carried out with the highest level of professionalism which is good for both the public and the people involved.

It's not just that we die—it leads to many questions and problems in both law and medicine. Knowing when a person has died is closely related to ethical issues and these issues usually guide clinical practice and affect laws concerning life support. Traumatic brain injuries (TBI) only add to these murky end-of-life debates, generally prompting the call for simple, clear protocols to assist doctors during challenging moments. Having patients, families and healthcare professionals involved adds a human aspect, so the process of making decisions together feels less like a machine. To summarize, this discussion points toward a framework built on fairness and shared responsibility—a model that, in many instances, balances the practicalities of death with promoting sustainability and the overall well-being of everyone involved (Philippe Bégin et al., 2020; Pinchi et al., 2017).

KEY TERMS FROM THIS CHAPTER

Accreditation	Accuracy	Civil liability
Compassion	Criminal law	Euthanasia
Genetic predisposition	Genetic testing	Homicide
Investigators	Mental health	Organization
Penalties	Racial bias	Regulation

Short Answer Questions

1. What is the legal significance of certifying death?
2. Who has the authority to declare someone legally dead?
3. Define suspicious death.
4. What distinguishes natural death from unnatural death in terms of the law?
5. What is the legal term presumption of death?
6. In what ways is a death certificate used in legal and administrative situations?
7. List two examples of medico-legal cases of death.
8. Mention two important organs commonly examined during an autopsy.
9. What types of deaths are typically investigated by coroners?

Critical Thinking Questions

1. The minimum duration of continuous absence after which a person is presumed legally dead (in many jurisdictions) is:

a. 3 years
b. 5 years
c. 7 years
d. 10 years

2. Which of these is not a way that death is categorized in forensic medicine?

a. Natural
b. Suicidal
c. Suspicious
d. Homicidal

3. When someone is considered brain dead, it is legally the same as death for these cases:

a. Asphyxia
b. Organ transplantation
c. Drowning
d. Electrocution

4. For which deaths should the police be informed and does a medico-legal autopsy need to be performed?

a. Death due to terminal cancer
b. Death in ICU under a doctor's care
c. Death during surgery
d. Death by suspected poisoning

5. The first visible sign of death is usually:

a. Coldness of body

b. Rigor mortis
c. Cessation of respiration
d. Loss of skin elasticity

Answers to Critical Thinking Questions

1. (c); 2. (c); 3. (c); 4. (d); 5. (c)

References

1. Abouelkeir, R., Ali, A. A., Abdelsatar, M. F., Rashed, L. A., & Alsaeed, S. A. (2022). Application of the methylated markers (spectrin beta and DEAD-box protein) for definitive differentiation between fresh and aged semen by evaluating their role in identifying semen from mixed body fluids. *International Journal of Medical Toxicology and Forensic Medicine, 12*(4), 386. https://doi.org/10.32598/ijmtfm.v12i4.38615.
2. Abrol, V. (2024). *Forensic Science: Revealing the Clues*. IntechOpen eBooks. https://doi.org/10.5772/intechopen.1003870.
3. Adamec, V., Köbölová, K., Pavlíková, S., et al. (2019). Current approaches of occupational and safety health management in work environments containing nanoparticles. *Transactions of the VSB–Technical University of Ostrava Safety Engineering Series, XIV*(2). https://core.ac.uk/download/287648860.pdf (accessed on 29 May 2025).
4. Adeola, H. A., Van Wyk, J. C., Arowolo, A. T., & Khumalo, N. P. (2018). Human hair as a testing substrate in the era of precision medicine: Potential role of 'omics-based approaches. *IntechOpen*. https://doi.org/10.5772/intechopen.77215.
5. Advisory Council on the Misuse of Drugs. (2011). Consideration of the novel psychoactive substances ('legal highs'). https://core.ac.uk/download/1643031.pdf (accessed on 29 May 2025).
6. Ahmed, Y. A., Ali, S., & Ghallab, A. (2018). Hair histology as a tool for forensic identification of some domestic animal species. *EXCLI Journal, 17*, 663–670. https://doi.org/10.17179/excli2018-1478.
7. Balhareth, A. A. S., Jamesh, M., Zabarah, G. A., Almotlaq, M. M., Alabaaltahin, M. A. M., Al Jaarah, A. H., Aldawsari, A. G., Almastaneer, K. A. M., Alyami, S. M., & Al Yami, A. S. H. (2024). The role of forensic medicine in modern criminal justice: A review of current practices and innovations. *Journal of Eco Humanism, 3*(7), 2699–2707. https://doi.org/10.62754/joe.v3i7.4669.
8. Basso, C., Aguilera, B., Banner, J., Cohle, S., d'Amati, G., de Gouveia, R. H., di Gioia, C., Fabre, A., Gallagher, P. J., Leone, O., Lucena, J., Mitrofanova, L., Molina, P., Parsons, S., Rizzo, S., Sheppard, M. N., Mier, M. P. S., Kim Suvarna, S., Thiene, G., van der Wal, A., & Association for European Cardiovascular Pathology. (2017). Guidelines for autopsy investigation of sudden cardiac death: 2017 update from the Association for European Cardiovascular Pathology. *Virchows Archiv, 471*(6), 691–705. https://doi.org/10.1007/s00428-017-2221-0.
9. Bhoyar, L., Mehar, P., & Chavali, K. (2024). An overview of DNA degradation and its implications

in forensic caseworks. *Egyptian Journal of Forensic Sciences, 14*. https://doi.org/10.1186/s41935-024-00389-y.

10. Boriwala, A., & Hankare, M. (2024). Literature review about forensic toxicology and poisoning. *Journal of Ayurveda and Integrated Medical Sciences*, *9*(4), 176–183. https://jaims.in/jaims/article/view/3079 (accessed on 29 May 2025).
11. Boronat Ena, M. del M., Cowan, D., & Abbate, V. (2021). Ambient ionization mass spectrometry applied to new psychoactive substance analysis. *Mass Spectrometry Reviews, 42*, 3–34. https://doi.org/10.1002/mas.21695.
12. Buzdar, Z. A., Murad, T., Shabbir, S., Ahmed, A., Soomro, T. A., & Masood, R. (2024). Estimating age on the autopsy table: A postmortem study of forensic investigations. *Journal of Saidu Medical College, Swat*. https://www.semanticscholar.org/paper/fde681bc296472e9b38d3a4bc9801e2195d2b32b (accessed on 29 May 2025).
13. Capiau, S., Stove, C., & Velghe, S. (2016). Opening the toolbox of alternative sampling strategies in clinical routine: A key role for (LC-)MS/MS. Retrieved from: https://core.ac.uk/download/84043363.pdf (accessed on 29 May 2025).
14. Casparsen, C. (2024). The role of toxicology in forensic investigations. *International Journal of Forensic Medicine*, *6*(1), 31–33.
15. Caudill, D. S. (2009). Arsenic and old chemistry: Images of mad alchemists, experts attacking experts, and the crisis in forensic science. Retrieved from: https://core.ac.uk/download/229258057.pdf (accessed on 29 May 2025).
16. Chango, X., Flor-Unda, O., Gil-Jiménez, P., & Gómez-Moreno, H. (2024). Technology in forensic sciences: Innovation and precision. *Technologies*, *12*(8), 120. https://doi.org/10.3390/technologies12080120.
17. Chen, B., Colston, B., Boehnert, M., González-Rodríguez, J., Ruiz-Jiménez, J., Jaiswal, A. K., Jickells, S., et al. (2011). Determination of arsenic, mercury and barium in herbarium mount paper using dynamic ultrasound-assisted extraction prior to atomic fluorescence and absorption spectrometry. https://core.ac.uk/download/1645649.pdf (accessed on 29 May 2025).
18. Ciobanu, A. M., Baconi, D., Bălălău, C., Negrei, C., Stan, M., & Bârcă, M. (2015). Toxicological analysis of some drugs of abuse in biological samples. *Journal of Mind and Medical Sciences*, *2*(2), 108–127. https://doi.org/10.22543/2392-7674.1018.
19. Coopman, V., Blanckaert, P., Van Parys, G., Van Calenbergh, S., & Cordonnier, J. (2016). A case of acute intoxication due to combined use of fentanyl and 3,4-dichloro-N-[2-(dimethylamino)cyclohexyl]-N-methyl benzamide (U-47700). *Forensic Science International*, *266*, 68–72. https://doi.org/10.1016/j.forsciint.2016.05.001.
20. Crawford-Jakubiak, J. E., Alderman, E. M., Leventhal, J. M., Flaherty, E. G., Idzerda, S. M., Legano, L. A., Leventhal, J. M., et al. (2017). Care of the adolescent after an acute sexual assault. *Pediatrics*, *139*(5). https://doi.org/10.1542/peds.2016-4243.
21. Davis, J. R., Lane, H. W., & Stepaniak, P. C. (2025). Loss of signal: Aeromedical lessons learned from the STS-107 Columbia space shuttle mishap. Retrieved from: https://core.ac.uk/download/pdf/42730063.pdf (accessed on 29 May 2025).
22. Di Nunno, N., Esposito, M., Argo, A., Salerno, M., & Sessa, F. (2021). Pharmacogenetics and

forensic toxicology: A new step towards a multidisciplinary approach. *Toxics, 9*(11), 292. https://doi.org/10.3390/toxics9110292.

23. Dos Santos, B. P., Birk, L., Schwarz, P. K. N., Sebben, V. C., Sgaravatti, Â. M., de Gouveia, G. C., Silva Petry, A. U., de Menezes, F. P., Gonzaga, A. P., Schlickmann, P. F., Arbo, M. D., de Oliveira, T. F., & Eller, S. (2024). A validated dilute-and-shoot LC-MS-MS urine screening for the analysis of 95 illicit drugs and medicines: Insights from clinical and forensic Brazilian cases. *Journal of Analytical Toxicology, 48*(5), 314–331. https://doi.org/10.1093/jat/bkae005.
24. Duvall, N. (2017). "If experts differ, what are we to do in the matter?" The medico-legal investigation of gunshot wounds in a 1927 Scottish murder trial. *Social History of Medicine, 30*(2), 367–388. https://doi.org/10.1093/shm/hkw066.
25. Fabricant, M. C., & Garrett, B. L. (2018). The myth of the reliability test. Retrieved from: https://core.ac.uk/download/213020569.pdf (accessed on 29 May 2025).
26. Faigman, D. L. (2008). Anecdotal forensics, phrenology, and other abject lessons from the history of science. Retrieved from: https://core.ac.uk/download/230095688.pdf.
27. Ferrara, L. (2018). The contribution of ethical reasoning skills in forensic science (Doctoral dissertation, Duquesne University). Retrieved from: https://dsc.duq.edu/etd/1426 (accessed on 29 May 2025).
28. Garrett, B. L., & Mitchell, G. (2018). The proficiency of experts. Retrieved from: https://core.ac.uk/download/213020407.pdf (accessed on 29 May 2025).
29. Goel, R., Kumar, D., & Arora, V. (2022). Forens(om)ic medicine: Omics in forensic medicine. *International Journal of Research in Medical Sciences, 10*(2), 557–564. https://doi.org/10.18203/2320-6012.ijrms20220309.
30. Guijas, C., Montenegro-Burke, J. R., Domingo-Almenara, X., Palermo, A., Warth, B., Hermann, G., Koellensperger, G., et al. (2018). METLIN: A technology platform for identifying knowns and unknowns. *Analytical Chemistry, 90*(6), 3156–3164. https://doi.org/10.1021/acs.analchem.7b04424.
31. Ho, K. C., Jentzen, J., Johnson, L. T., et al. (1994). Destructive hostility: The Jeffrey Dahmer case: A psychiatric and forensic study of a serial killer. Retrieved from: https://core.ac.uk/download/213059368.pdf (accessed on 29 May 2025).
32. Issa, S. Y. (2019). Forensic toxicology. Retrieved from: https://core.ac.uk/download/322440626.pdf (accessed on 29 May 2025).
33. Jannetto, P. J., Helander, A., Garg, U., Janis, G. C., Goldberger, B. A., & Ketha, H. (2018). The fentanyl epidemic and evolution of fentanyl analogs in the United States and the European Union. *Clinical Chemistry, 65*, 242–253. https://doi.org/10.1373/clinchem.2017.281626.
34. Kaushik, N., Pal, S. K., Sharma, A., Thakur, S., et al. (2017). Role of diatoms in diagnosis of death due to drowning: Case studies. https://core.ac.uk/download/483635548.pdf (accessed on 29 May 2025).
35. Kinoshita, H., Tanaka, N., Takakura, A., Jamal, M., Ito, A., Kumihashi, M., Kimura, S., et al. (2017). Simplified analysis of toxic gaseous substances in forensic practice: Experiences from Japan. Retrieved from: https://www.semanticscholar.org/paper/b17a9420da291c21a265b62866e5e05041ffd491 (accessed on 29 May 2025).
36. Kintz, P. (2018). Hair analysis in forensic toxicology: An updated review with a special focus

on pitfalls. *Current Pharmaceutical Design, 23*. https://doi.org/10.2174/1381612823666170929155628.

37. Klingberg, J., Keen, B., Cawley, A., Pasin, D., & Fu, S. (2022). Developments in high-resolution mass spectrometric analyses of new psychoactive substances. *Archives of Toxicology, 96*, 949–967. https://doi.org/10.1007/s00204-022-03224-2.

38. Klinkner, M. (2008). Proving genocide? Forensic expertise and the ICTY. *Journal of International Criminal Justice, 6*(3), 447–466. https://ssrn.com/abstract=1212077 (accessed on 29 May 2025).

39. Lechien, J. R., Chiesa-Estomba, C. M., Hans, S., Barillari, M. R., Jouffe, L., & Saussez, S. (2020). Loss of smell and taste in 2013 European patients with mild to moderate COVID-19. *Annals of Internal Medicine, 173*(9), 672–675. https://doi.org/10.7326/m20-2428.

40. Lowe, D. J., Torrance, H. J., Ireland, A. J., Bloeck, F., & Stevenson, R. (2017). SODAS: Surveillance of Drugs of Abuse Study. *European Journal of Emergency Medicine, 24*(2), 126–129. https://doi.org/10.1097/MEJ.0000000000000310.

41. Lynch, K. L. (2015). CLSI C62-A: A new standard for clinical mass spectrometry. *Clinical Chemistry, 62*, 24–29. https://doi.org/10.1373/clinchem.2015.238626.

42. Mannocchi, G., Pantano, F., Romolo, F. S., Tittarelli, R., et al. (2015). Recreational use, analysis and toxicity of tryptamines. https://core.ac.uk/download/54534388.pdf (accessed on 29 May 2025).

43. McCartney, C. (2011). The law-forensic science disciplinary divide: The Canadian experience.

44. Moreno, I. E. D. (2016). The role of miniaturized systems in analytical toxicology: New psychoactive substances. https://core.ac.uk/download/303998412.pdf (accessed on 29 May 2025).

45. Mores, C. M., Castro, M. B., & Melo, C. B. (2025). Forensic examinations in the investigations of crimes involving animals: A review. *Ciência Rural, 55*(3). https://doi.org/10.1590/0103-8478cr20240071.

46. Morgan, J. (2023). Wrongful convictions and claims of false or misleading forensic evidence. *Journal of Forensic Sciences, 68*, 908–961. https://doi.org/10.1111/1556-4029.15233.

47. Nodari, R., Arghittu, M., Bailo, P., Cattaneo, C., Creti, R., D'Aleo, F., Saegeman, V., et al. (2024). Forensic microbiology: When, where and how. *Microorganisms, 12*, 988. https://doi.org/10.3390/microorganisms12050988.

48. Parmar, P. (2023). The integration of artificial intelligence in the forensic medicine and its applications in medico-legal autopsy, forensic toxicology, and disaster victim identification. *International Journal of Forensic Sciences*. https://www.semanticscholar.org/paper/fc16f6a30cab5b4e85b76b323902ed9b047c2d0c (accessed on 29 May 2025).

49. Piraianu, A. I., Fulga, A., Mușat, C. L., Ciobotaru, O. R., Poalelungi, D. G., Stamate, E., Ciobotaru, O. C., et al. (2023). Enhancing the evidence with algorithms: How artificial intelligence is transforming forensic medicine. *Diagnostics, 13*, Article 2992. https://doi.org/10.3390/diagnostics13182992.

50. Poalelungi, D. G., Mușat, C. L., Fulga, A., Neagu, M., Neagu, A. I., Piraianu, A. I., & Fulga, I. (2023). Advancing patient care: How artificial intelligence is transforming healthcare. *Journal of Personalized Medicine, 13*(8), 1214. https://doi.org/10.3390/jpm13081214.

51. Reid, K. M., Suwalowska, H., Martin, L. J., & Heathfield, L. J. (2025). Ethical considerations in the routine identification of human remains in forensic mortuaries [Version 1; peer review: awaiting peer review]. *Welcome Open Research, 10*, 171. https://doi.org/10.12688/wellcomeopenres.23041.1.

52. Sanzyapova, R. R. (2025). The role of dentistry in forensic medicine: Identification of human remains. *Patient-Oriented Medicine and Pharmacy*. https://www.semanticscholar.org/paper/d8db5ae62d74c13d619c3b0324e081b54abd3399 (accessed on 29 May 2025).

53. Saxena, S., & Deo, S. H. (2024). Implication of forensic science for private security. https://core.ac.uk/download/617189936.pdf (accessed on 29 May 2025).

54. Seywright, A., Torrance, H. J., Wylie, F. M., McKeown, D. A., Lowe, D. J., & Stevenson, R. (2016). Analysis and clinical findings of cases positive for the novel synthetic cannabinoid receptor agonist MDMB-CHMICA. *Clinical Toxicology, 54*(8), 632–637. https://doi.org/10.1080/15563650.2016.1186805.

55. Sh, J., Hugar, B., & Praveen, S. (2020). Determination of stature from index and ring finger lengths in South Indian population. *Journal of Forensic Medicine, 14*(4), 795–799. Retrieved from: https://www.semanticscholar.org/paper/72c123b38b5775ba4623cc03bf7b5a76dc64b3db (accessed on 29 May 2025).

56. Singh, W. U., & Singh, K. P. (2023). The transformative role of artificial intelligence in forensic medicine and toxicology. *Journal of Medical Society, 37*, 101–102. https://doi.org/10.4103/jms.jms_54_24.

57. Speaker, P. J. (2017). FORESIGHT benchmark data 2015-2016. *Faculty & Staff Scholarship*, 1144. https://researchrepository.wvu.edu/faculty_publications/1144 (accessed on 29 May 2025).

58. Tai, S. S. C. (2018). *Chiral and Stable Isotope Analysis in Forensic Chemistry: Novel Psychoactive Substance Analysis* (Doctoral dissertation, University of Glasgow).

59. Tammi, T., & Viskari, I. (2021). *Report on Good Practices of Synthetic Opioid Preparedness, And Needs and Challenges in EU Member States: Deliverable D3.2*. https://core.ac.uk/download/591956267.pdf (accessed on 29 May 2025).

60. Teymourian, H., Parrilla, M., Sempionatto, J. R., Montiel, N. F., Barfidokht, A., Van Echelpoel, R., De Wael, K., et al. (2020). Wearable electrochemical sensors for the monitoring and screening of drugs. *ACS Sensors, 5*(9), 2679–2700. https://doi.org/10.1021/acssensors.0c01318.

61. Vadysinghe, A., Edusooriya, D., Dayaratne, S. P., Manoratne, N. M. K., Abeysekara, Y., & Nissanka, P. W. A. D. P. M. (2017). Is the undergraduate forensic medicine teaching adequate to produce an expert medical witness? *Medico-Legal Journal of Sri Lanka, 5*(1), 5. https://www.semanticscholar.org/paper/aeabce33a41a4da7a1b3ac45577f2f7b05916575 (accessed on 29 May 2025).

62. Vrees, R. (2017). Evaluation and management of female victims of sexual assault. *Obstetrical & Gynecological Survey, 72*, 39–53. https://doi.org/10.1097/ogx.0000000000000390.

63. Wille, S., Van Dijck, K., Van Assche, A., di Fazio, V., Ramiréz-Fernandéz, M. del M., Vanvooren, V., & Samyn, N. (2021). The interest of a systematic toxicological analysis combined with forensic advice to improve the judicial investigation and final judgment in drug facilitated sexual assault cases. *Pharmaceuticals, 14*. https://www.semanticscholar.org/paper/79c2d94ac127bf7dde45b85ed9fa5802fab11079 (accessed on 29 May 2025).

64. Wu, J., Luan, Y., Zhang, Q., Wang, F., & Rao, Y. (2024). Effects of dichloromethane, nitrate, and sulfhemoglobin-induced substances on carboxyhemoglobin detection: A comprehensive review. *Journal of Analytical Toxicology*. https://www.semanticscholar.org/paper/9a4148b9a9a47c9f29ba979851341f0c21f471e9 (accessed on 29 May 2025).

65. Zeppenfeld, K., Tfelt-Hansen, J., Riva, M., Winkel, B. G., Behr, E. R., Blom, N. A., Charron, P., et al. (2022). 2022 ESC guidelines for the management of patients with ventricular arrhythmias and the prevention of sudden cardiac death. *European Heart Journal, 43*, 3997–4126. https://doi.org/10.1093/eurheartj/ehac262.

POSTMORTEM CHANGES

5

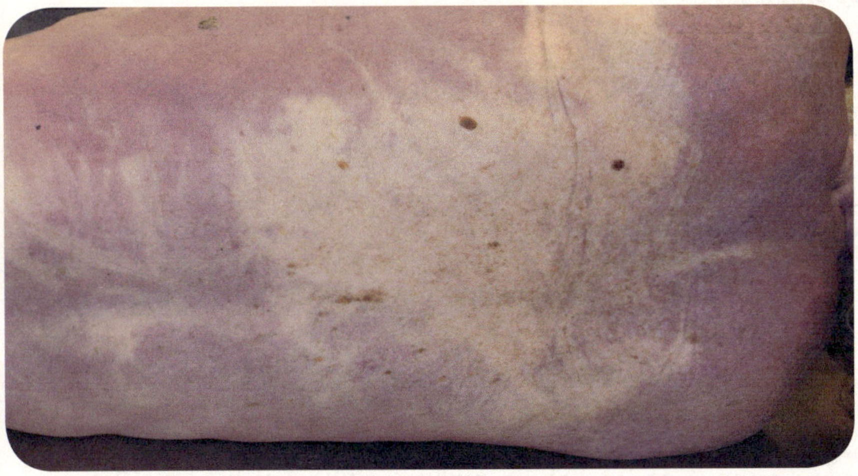

LEARNING OBJECTIVES

After studying this chapter, you will be able to:

1. Explain types of postmortem changes;
2. Identify factors influencing postmortem changes;
3. Discuss forensic applications of postmortem changes;
4. Learn case studies and real-world applications.

Introduction

Looking at what happens after someone dies helps us learn about many natural and forensic changes. Changes in the body after death such as decay and altered metabolism, give hints about the whole decay process, sometimes in interesting ways. In most cases, even something as unexpected as how licorice is processed can tell us a lot; recent studies show that small tweaks in old, traditional methods may alter the quality and concentration of bioactive compounds, which then impact medicinal formulas (Sun et al., 2024). Then there's the issue of brain energy use in Alzheimer's disease: research indicates that postmortem pH fluctuations can hint at underlying neural activity and might even tie in with typical evaluations such as Braak staging (Hagihara et al., 2024). All in all, these findings increase our understanding of what happens after death and also help move forward progress in both medical and forensic science.

Definition of Postmortem Changes

After someone dies, the body experiences changes that you may not have predicted. It's not just one neat process either—first, the body cools down (that's usually called algor mortis), then the muscles get stiff (what we call rigor mortis), and after a while blood begins to settle in the lower parts, leading to discoloration known as livor mortis. The body slowly loses heat; muscle contractions occur due to chemical changes and blood remaining in the body creates visible marks. Overall such changes are useful in forensic investigations, as they can suggest the time and manner of death. Researchers have even ventured beyond traditional methods—sometimes employing ideas like checking the iris after death (Sansola et al., 2015)—to open up new ways of identifying people. Additionally, looking into complications from anesthesia during surgery, in most cases, can make figuring out the exact cause of death a pretty tangled puzzle (Argo et al., 2019) (Figure 5.1).

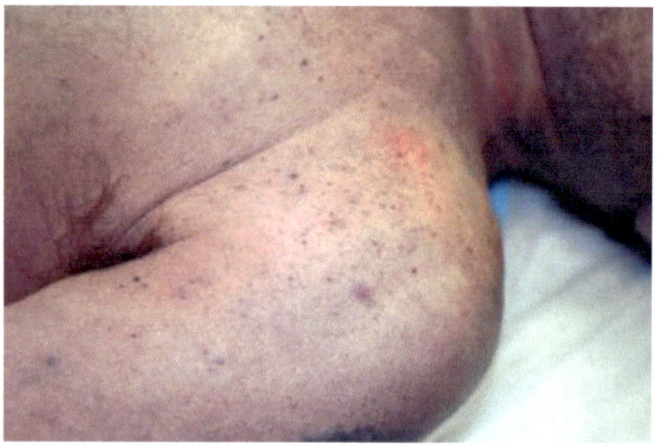

Figure 5.1. Postmortem changes.

Source: https://img.medscapestatic.com/pi/meds/ckb/49/9649tn.jpg.

Importance of Studying Postmortem Changes

The study of body decomposition is important in real-life forensic investigations. Figuring out the details of decomposition can sometimes suggest when the death took place and what happened before it which investigators use to solve real cases. There's also a curious twist with tiny microbes; research suggests these organisms sometimes stick around unaltered for long periods, which might connect objects at a scene to a particular individual (Kodama et al., 2018). In cases of missing persons, such insights become even more important—experts at the Forensic Unit of the International Committee of the Red Cross, for example, point out that mixing various investigative methods helps improve the search and identification process (Puerto et al., 2021). In short, studying postmortem changes helps develop forensic techniques and also serves real-world purposes.

Historical Context of Postmortem Examination

The ways postmortem practices were carried out in the 19th century tell us a lot about the society and culture of that era. At this time, dissection was becoming very popular, especially in cities like New York and this often led to people stealing bodies from graves in ways that were not ethical. Resurrectionists, who often went after society's more vulnerable folks, stirred up a host of ethical debates about how we treat those who have passed on (Novak et al., 2014). At that time, photographs of the dead were taken, as seen in Stanley Burns' work which reflects how society wanted to remember people. Photos of the deceased weren't just morbid images—they were staged, frequently featuring clothing that trailed the latest fashion trends, meant to convey respect and a final touch of dignity (Aldridge et al., 2008). For the most part, these traditions broke the links between death, memories and social identity and their effects are still felt today.

Overview of the Types of Body Changes

Once someone dies, their body changes in a way that usually indicates how much time has passed.

After death, muscles contract and become stiff which is called rigor mortis and this usually begins a few hours in. As time passes, blood pools in the lower parts of the body, leaving skin discoloration and showing the position of the body at the time of death. The body's temperature decreases as well which is called algor mortis and how quickly it cools depends on the environment. Forensic experts use these overlapping signs as a natural clock to find out how long ago the person died. Newer techniques, like shear wave elastography (SWE), have started measuring how organ stiffness shifts, adding a fresh twist to forensic investigations (Kara et al., 2024; Taskent et al., 2025). Although it may look simple, these little, related signs highlight the complexity of what happens after death.

Relevance to Forensic Science

Forensic work turns on knowing what happens after death. Hair, for example, can be surprisingly revealing – researchers have gone on to build animal hair databases based on detailed studies, like one done on domestic animals in Upper Egypt (Ahmed et al., 2018). RNA decay, which you might think is just technical mumbo-jumbo, now shows promise in clocking the time since death; in most cases, tracking its gradual fading in tissues offers a fresh angle that can actually beat out methods relying only on DNA (Young et al., 2011). It has been observed that using several types of biological markers can help find the deceased's identity and set the order of events. In most cases, the understanding from hair and RNA supports each other, each providing some details, but the picture can look a little messy sometimes. By combining what is seen daily with technical information, the accuracy of solving crimes improves.

Significance in Legal Investigations

It is very important to understand how bodies change after death in legal investigations—this helps create timelines and identify people. The way evidence is evaluated can change the outcome of a case and influence how the public views our legal system. Updating our methods by embracing new tech for gathering and analyzing evidence is pretty important, if not vital, to keep judicial proceedings both fair and efficient (Turysbek et al., 2024). Radiocarbon analysis is also very important because it helps forensic anthropologists estimate dates of birth and death which is key to confirming identity in legal matters. A range of case studies has shown over and over how radiocarbon dating ties into the criminal justice system—demonstrating how it can narrow down candidate lists while offering insights that are useful in both archaeological and medico-legal contexts (Bertrand et al., 2024) (Figure 5.2).

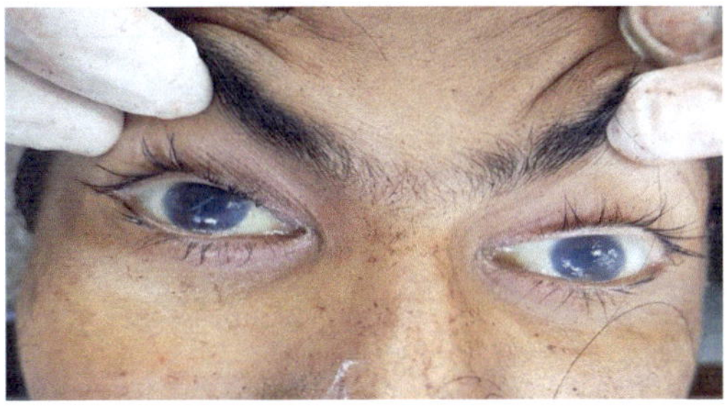

Figure 5.2. Grasping how bodies change after death is crucial in legal investigations—it helps set up timelines and figure out identities in ways that matter.

Source: https://media.springernature.com/lw685/springer-static/image/chp%3A10.1007%2F978-981-99-1377-0_7/MediaObjects/505341_1_En_7_Fig4_HTML.jpg.

Ethical Considerations in Postmortem Studies

Ethical issues that arise from postmortem studies are difficult to define and handle. When human remains are studied by bioarcheology, it leads to difficult questions about respecting the dead and how their families feel. In most cases, researchers today have to deal with the mistakes of the past such as how skeletons were collected, as seen at the University of Louisville. Institutions, meanwhile, sometimes drift into a kind of structural indifference that can even lead to harm against marginalized groups (Zuckerman et al., 2024); this unthinking approach has compelled a rethink of how remains are used in research. Balancing scientific curiosity with the deep cultural respect for the dead turns into a real challenge, particularly when community histories remain patchy because of earlier ethical oversights (Appenzeller et al., 2015). In short, being more thoughtful and caring is usually necessary for us to make improvements in ethical practices.

5.1. Types of Postmortem Changes

Learning Outcome

1. Know the definition and process of rigor mortis;
2. Explain the characteristics and significance of livor mortis;
3. Define algor mortis;
4. Describe stages and factors of decomposition;
5. Discuss autolysis;
6. Understand putrefaction;
7. Learn the conditions and outcomes of mummification;
8. Focus on skeletonization;
9. Know adipocere formation.

Examining the process after death helps us understand the changes in the body that happen when life ends which is useful for solving mysteries and for medical research. Rigor mortis, decomposition and autolysis are changes that help the body break down after death. Usually, new molecular profiling methods let researchers take a closer, more detailed look at postmortem brain tissue, uncovering specific molecular traits in different cell types that matter a lot in conditions such as Alzheimer's and Parkinson's (Mätlik et al., 2025). There are also new technologies that can tell apart tumor tissue from regular brain tissue after death which could lead to improved surgery and a clearer view of brain pathology, as gliomas have different electrical impedance from normal tissue . All these unusual shifts, when put together, help develop better diagnostic tests and even new treatments (Mätlik et al., 2025).

5.1.1. Rigor Mortis: Definition and Process

Forensic teams usually check what occurs in the body right after death and one obvious sign is that muscles stiffen. Rigor mortis occurs because the body has little ATP which causes actin and myosin to bind, making the muscles stiff. Rigor mortis usually starts two to six hours after death, but the temperature and health of the person before they died can make the timing different.

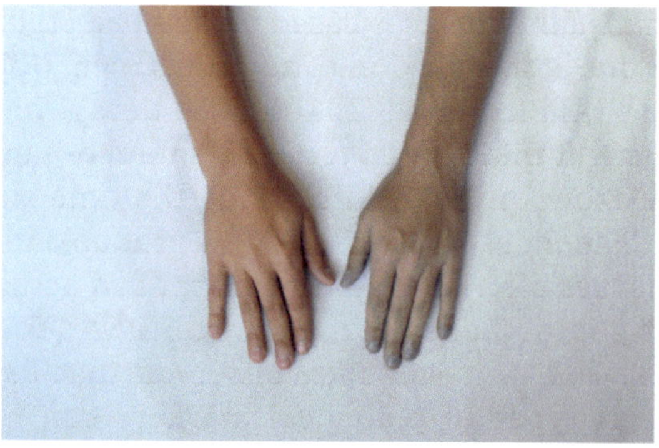

Figure 5.3. Rigor mortis.

Source: https://lh3.googleusercontent.com/proxy/2WyeeTdPj5tmEwISz6DvUb3V0qUBHIK61OhfPB92NNWNI_3W-gTDXbjstPfQ5XOQqfgiTDIgJDPYSIPxhupMpNgwqpOvrgPBtQmD2LEgft7TxvEOq04B1M1SQwu1xj1EOlxk6pi6ioQykEheoQ.

When the muscles firm, investigators can use this to create a rough timeline to find out when the person likely passed away. In many cases, experts mix this info with other decay signs—like shifts in temperature and the local environment—to fine-tune their guess at the postmortem interval, ultimately giving more weight to their overall forensic findings (Bautista et al., 2015; Reisdorf et al., 2018) (Figure 5.3).

5.1.2. Livor Mortis: Characteristics and Significance

Postmortem changes often tell us a lot about the circumstances surrounding the death and livor mortis is a good example. After death, the blood begins to flow and gathers in areas that are not normally pulled down by gravity and this change usually happens within a few hours which helps forensic teams estimate the time of death. The color you notice which is usually reddish-purple, may not be the same every time, as it can depend on things like room temperature or the circumstances of death. Sometimes, like in cases of sodium nitrite poisoning, the usual hue may twist into a brownish or greyish tint, a change that tends to muddy the waters when decomposition is well underway (Chang et al., 2025). Recent studies generally point out that these subtle patterns in livor mortis serve as important hints during investigations, helping to piece together the nuances and timings of an event (Henrikson et al., 2018) (Figure 5.4).

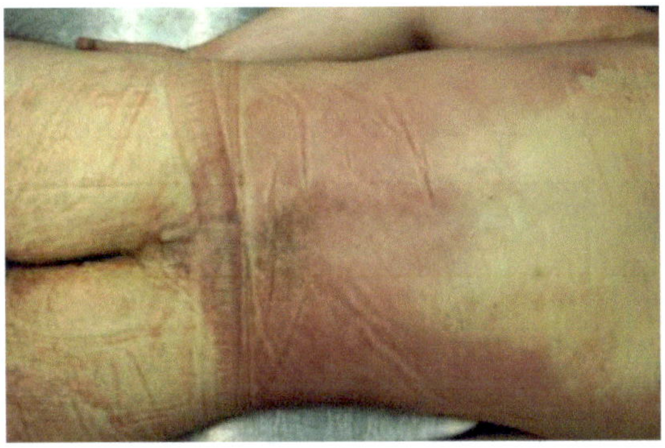

Figure 5.4. Livor mortis.

Source: https://www.researchgate.net/publication/363411227/figure/fig1/AS:11431281083689217@1662731524865/Livor-mortis-or-lividity-on-the-posterior-aspect-of-the-body-3.jpg.

5.1.3. Algor Mortis: Cooling of the Body

When someone dies, their body cools down which forensic experts use to help estimate the time of death. The rate of cooling varies a lot; it depends on how warm the air is and if the person was wearing clothes. Researchers, generally speaking, have found that models such as the MARS model do a pretty good job of mapping these heat drops, showing different cooling patterns over various postmortem periods as recorded in controlled environments (Eliyani et al., 2017). On top of that, nailing down the postmortem interval (PMI) is tricky because natural body differences and other outside influences come into play (Bautista et al., 2015). To summarize, wrapping your head around algor mortis not only helps crack cases but also gives us a deeper look at the body's subtle changes after death (Figure 5.5).

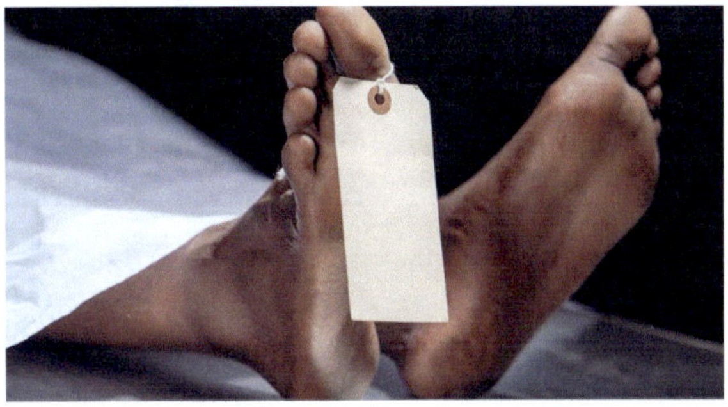

Figure 5.5. Algor mortis.

Source: https://simplyforensic.com/wp-content/uploads/2021/08/Dead-rep-d_d-jpg.webp.

5.1.4. Decomposition: Stages and Factors

It is very important in forensics to know how the body decomposes, especially when trying to estimate the time since death. The process doesn't follow a neat, one-step plan—it kicks off with early changes like the body cooling (algor mortis), stiffening (rigor mortis) and blood settling, before finally shifting into putrefaction.

Many factors, including weather, body size and details of the death, seem to play a role in these stages. Generally speaking, research shows that a heavier carcass can decompose faster, which means we need more detailed studies to sort out these differences (Ikpa et al., 2025). Shifts in the tiny microbial world during decay also come into play when estimating how long a body might have been submerged, as seen in the changes in bacterial diversity and numbers at various steps (Wallace et al., 2021). All these details blend to create a multilayered, although sometimes untidy, view of decomposition that is still very important for both forensic analysis and legal cases.

5.1.5. Autolysis: Cellular Breakdown

When life ends, the cells in the body suddenly stop being organized and start breaking apart in strange ways. Right away, autolysis takes over—internal enzymes start to break down the structures that kept the cells intact.

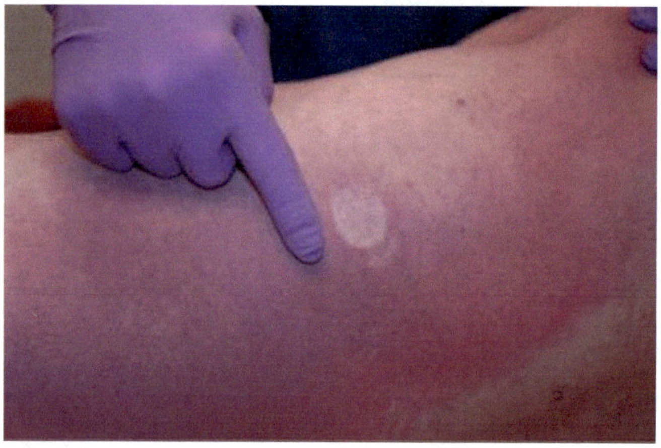

Figure 5.6. Autolysis.

Source: https://img.medscapestatic.com/pi/meds/ckb/56/9656tn.jpg.

In a way, this self-destruction makes it easier for microbes to do the important job of decomposition. Generally speaking, as autolysis carries on, the tissue's chemical signature also shifts; you can often spot a boost in nitrogen isotopes in the fluids produced, a change that contrasts with the original makeup of the tissue (Keenan et al., 2019). This change also means that decay becomes less about a cell breaking down on its own and more about microbes outside the cell playing a big role. Interestingly, programmed cell death (PCD) plays a somewhat similar role by managing how cells disassemble, yet its effects in multicellular organisms are even more tangled and complex (Daneva et al., 2016). To summarize, getting a handle on autolysis sheds light on the many intricate ways our tissues start to fall apart once life has gone (Figure 5.6).

5.1.6. Putrefaction: Microbial Activity

Putrefaction demonstrates that microbes are important for decomposing human bodies. After death, the body goes through various changes and bacteria grow rapidly, using many chemical processes to break down the body's organic parts—this can cause some mess. This active microbial crowd not only speeds up decay but also shifts its own makeup over time, with those changes often serving as subtle clues for estimating how long it's been since death (Dowell-Curby et al., 2017). These organisms usually grow best in certain areas which are shaped by the soil, insects and even the skin traces there. Plus, even though molecules like glycans have been observed hanging around in tissue samples from centuries past, which, in most cases, deepens our grasp of both forensic methods and the natural processes surrounding decomposition (Dowell-Curby et al., 2017) (Figure 5.7).

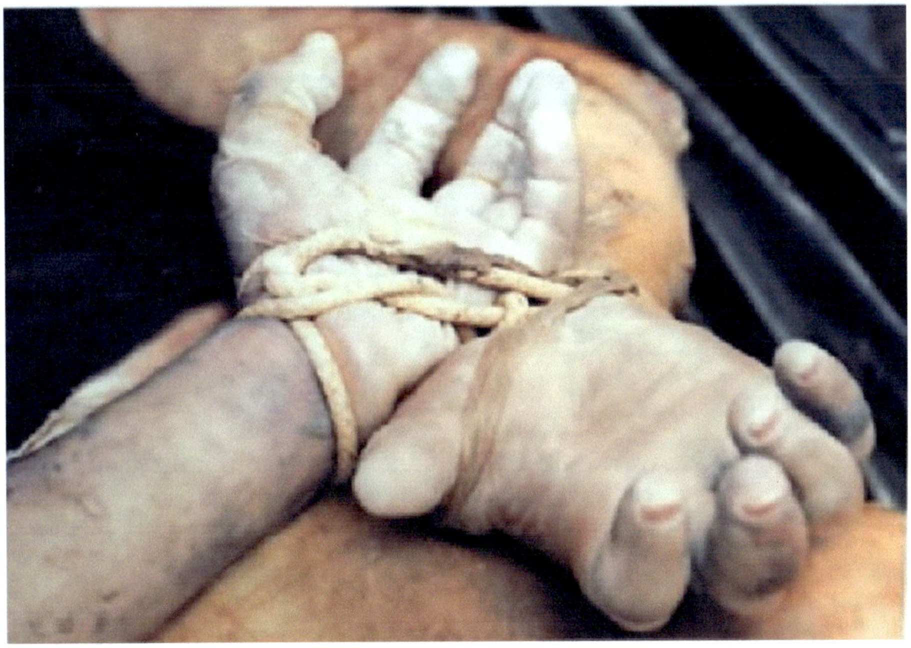

Figure 5.7. Putrefaction shows how microbes end up being critical in breaking down human remains.

Source: By Tampa Police Department - YouTube: https://www.youtube.com/watch?v=uYn5HDCBChk – View/save archived versions on archive.org and archive.today, Public Domain, https://commons.wikimedia.org/w/index.php?curid=36500079.

5.1.7. Mummification: Conditions and Outcomes

The outcome after death is affected by the specific conditions in the area where the body lies. As an example, mummification can happen which means the body's soft tissues remain longer than they should have. You commonly notice this in very hot and dry places; the combination of high heat and low moisture causes the body to dehydrate rapidly which slows down the action of germs and enzymes that would break down the tissues. Mummified remains can reveal small details about how people lived and what happened at the time of their death and they can also suggest the general conditions of the environment. Learning how mummification works might be very useful for forensic experts who try to reconstruct a timeline of decomposition. Sure, approaches such as scoring a body's features or tracking subtle changes in decay can be tricky, yet they open up promising avenues for deepening our grasp of these unusual preservation processes (Mee, 2020; Pittner et al., 2020) (Figure 5.8).

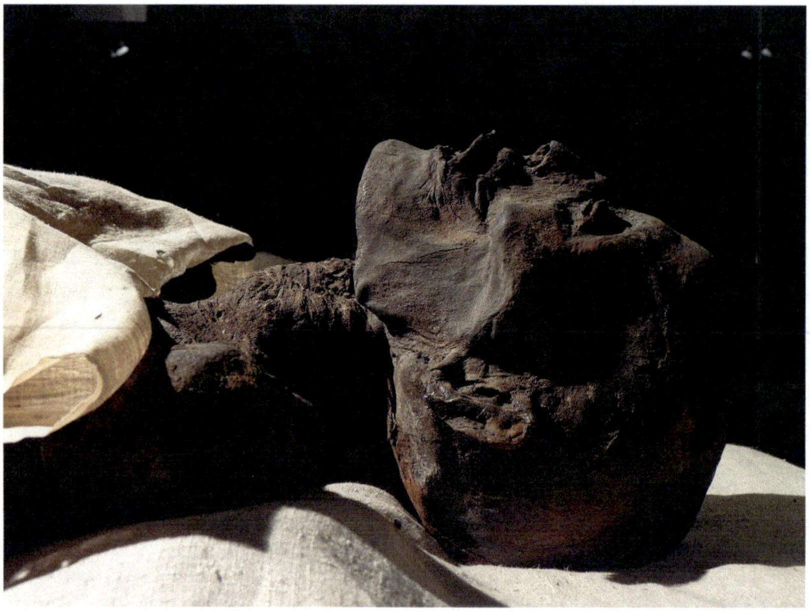

Figure 5.8. Mummification.

Source: By Alyssa Bivins - Own work, CC BY-SA 4.0, https://commons.wikimedia.org/w/index.php?curid=52559243.

5.1.8. Skeletonization: Timeline and Factors

A body gradually breaks down into its skeleton as decay happens, influenced by many different factors in the environment and the body. In forensic work, getting a good grip on these factors is pretty key, especially when you're trying to nail down the minimum postmortem interval (mPMI). Take, for instance, when a body is covered with cloth or plastic; this can reduce exposure to the air and prevent insects from reaching the body which are major factors in soft tissue breakdown. One study Joseph et al. (2017) looked at pig heads hidden away in hard-shell cases and fabric suitcases, and, generally speaking, noted that these heads had insects showing up much later compared to uncased controls, effectively stretching out the timeline for skeletonization. Temperature and moisture, by the way, are just as important, with small shifts sometimes speeding things up or, in most cases, slowing them down (Dautartas et al., 2009). All of these elements must be carefully watched over when trying to understand what happened in a forensic scene.

5.1.9. Adipocere Formation: Process and Implications

Soft tissues may alter in a strange way after death which is known as adipocere. Fats are broken down by hydrolysis and then, surprisingly, they form a waxy, soap-like layer that appears to outline the body. You normally discover adipocere when a body is in an oxygen-poor environment such as in water or deep underground, since this tends to slow down the whole decay process. Research shows that this transformation can be important in forensic work, yet its degree tends to depend on things like ambient temperature and the type of material surrounding the remains (Adlam et al., 2014). In some studies, deeper burial or certain aquatic conditions noticeably change how fast decomposition and adipocere formation occur, subtly pointing to a close link between environmental settings and how well the remains hold together (Westling et al., 2012). To summarize, understanding these changes is pretty key for estimating time since death and keeping crucial evidence intact (Figure 5.9).

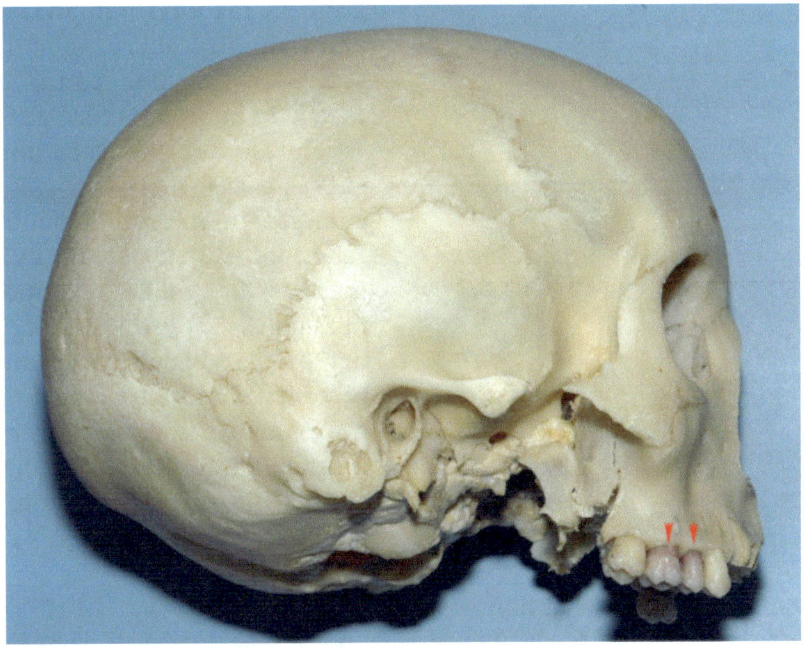

Figure 5.9. Adipocere formation.

Source: https://ars.els-cdn.com/content/image/3-s2.0-B9780128037591000096-f09-46-9780128037591.jpg.

Test Your Knowledge

1. What are postmortem changes?
2. What is algor mortis?
3. What is livor mortis (postmortem lividity)?

5.2. Factors Influencing Postmortem Changes

Learning Outcome

1. Identify environmental conditions such as temperature and humidity;
2. Know body composition;
3. Identify the cause of death;
4. Perform estimation methods of time since death;
5. Study how clothing and coverings can change the process of decomposition;
6. Explain the presence of insects;
7. Determine if the body was found inside or outside;
8. Focus on trauma and injuries;
9. Describe microbial flora's role in decomposition.

It is very important to understand what happens after a person dies in forensic work. There are many factors involved, like body size, the way someone dies and the environment which influence how fast a body decomposes.

Research generally shows that larger or heavier bodies tend to experience early changes differently – think of the cooling of the body (algor mortis), muscle stiffening (rigor mortis), and blood settling (livor mortis) – as earlier studies Ikpa et al. (2025) have pointed out. How samples are obtained matters a lot; blood components can be altered by changes in time. In one systematic look at natural compounds in blood after death, scientists uncovered noticeable fluctuations in metabolite levels during roughly the first 48 hours—a reminder, in most cases, that time is a crucial factor (Steuer et al., 2024).

All these details, put together, show that understanding postmortem changes requires looking at a number of different aspects at once.

5.2.1. Environmental Conditions: Temperature and Humidity

The kind of postmortem changes seen depends a lot on the environment such as temperature and humidity. Microbes and enzymes are more active in warmer conditions which causes decay to happen more rapidly. For example, when the temperature dips from +10°C to −10°C, decay rates can shift noticeably due to changes in microbial behavior and chemical reactions (Rörup et al., 2024). Humidity also matters; high moisture helps preserve biological molecules, but low humidity causes materials to dry quickly which can change the state of the remains. Generally speaking, getting a grip on these factors is key for forensic work since they influence how fast decay happens and help in estimating the postmortem interval (Wang et al., 2024) (Figure 5.10).

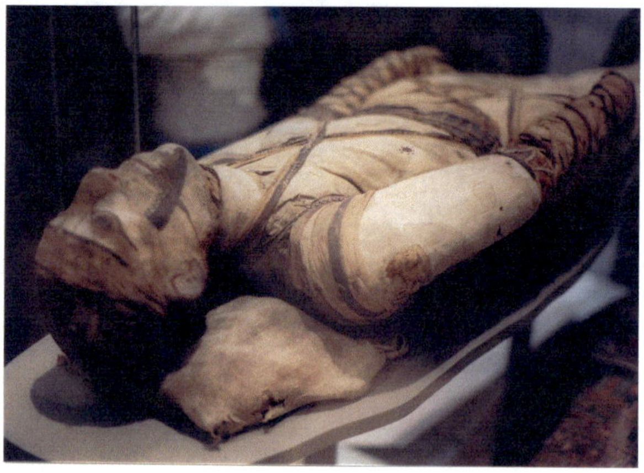

Figure 5.10. Postmortem changes hinge a lot on environmental conditions—temperature and humidity play unexpected roles.

Source: CC BY-SA 3.0, https://commons.wikimedia.org/w/index.php?curid=15047.

5.2.2. Body Composition: Fat and Muscle Content

The way a body is made up, plus what happens after death, can teach us about the slow breakdown of tissues. How much fat a body has compared to muscle is very important because it affects how the body deals with outside conditions and natural aging. When fat content is high, you might see an uptick in lipid oxidation; a pattern that, for instance, shows up in meat where a drop in both taste and nutrition happens as rancid compounds form (Amaral et al., 2018). Muscle tissues, on the other hand, deal with their own kind of complexity: enzymes known as matrix metalloproteinases (MMPs) help dismantle the supportive structures outside cells. In many cases, if the activity of these MMPs goes a bit off, the degradation speeds up, echoing patterns we often associate with certain diseases (Cabral-Pacheco et al., 2020). To summarize, checking a body's makeup isn't just about understanding changes after death—it also hints at broader issues of tissue degeneration in healthy and diseased states alike (Figure 5.11).

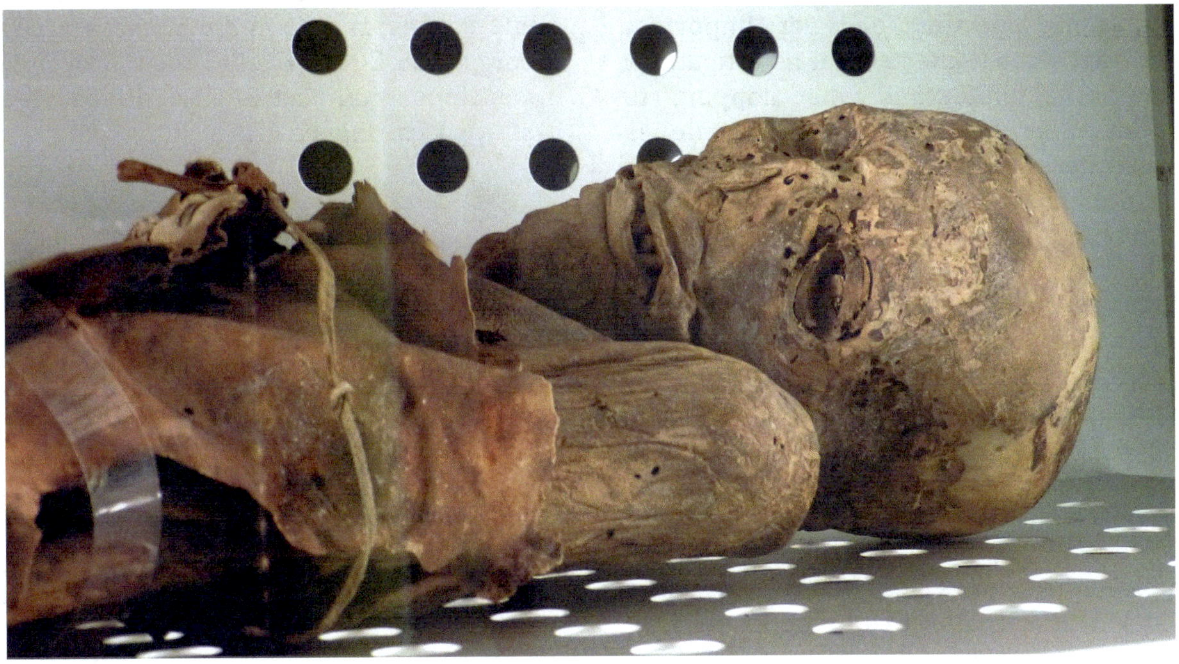

Figure 5.11. Body composition and what happens after death often go hand in hand, offering a window into how tissues slowly break down.

Source: By Wolfgang Sauber - Own work, CC BY-SA 3.0, https://commons.wikimedia.org/w/index.php?curid=31575361.

5.2.3. Cause of Death: Natural Versus Unnatural

It is not always easy to understand why a person has died, especially when you need to tell between natural and unnatural causes. Studies usually indicate that the majority of child deaths are caused by things like abuse or neglect, not by normal accidents. One investigation spanning various trauma centers found that roughly 9.7% of pediatric deaths were linked to trauma and about 10.3% to neglect; still, most cases ended up being accidental, which is particularly disconcerting for preschool-aged kids (Wagensveld et al., 2020). That's why it's very important to do proper post-mortem examinations in cases where the cause is not clear, so we can correctly identify unnatural deaths. In most cases, new techniques such as minimally invasive autopsies (MIA) have been introduced as promising diagnostic alternatives that might help reveal hidden factors behind these deaths (Wagensveld et al., 2020). Bringing together innovative and traditional methods could play a big role in lowering the number of unnatural deaths that are not noticed in different populations.

5.2.4. Time Since Death: Estimation Methods

The time since a person died is very important in forensics, since it affects legal investigations and helps us understand what happens to the body after death. Different techniques are tried here, sometimes just by looking at physical signs and at other times by relying on advanced imaging. Take, for instance, some recent research that generally points to postmortem computed tomography (PMCT) as a useful tool for spotting radiomic details in the brain's lateral ventricles. These marks, when run through statistical models, seem to connect with the PMI, spotlighting things like median Hounsfield Units and even the surface area of the ventricles (Bergamin et al., 2024). Also, a closer look at organs—kidneys being a prime example—often shows clear microscopic shifts that kick in shortly after death; the intensity of these changes usually appears to match both the surrounding temperature and the elapsed time (Bhawnani et al., 2017). All these methods together help us see the timeline after death in more detail.

5.2.5. Clothing and Coverings: Effects on Decomposition

The type of clothing and coverings on a body can change its decomposition which forensic experts consider when calculating PMI. Little pockets in everyday fabrics can influence the temperature and moisture around a body which can usually influence the growth of microbes and the rate of decay. What's interesting is that some materials can keep insects away or change how the body deals with the outdoors which might delay or alter the usual stages of decomposition. Under certain conditions, you might even find adipocere—a kind of waxy substance coming from fat tissue—making PMI estimates even trickier and obscuring details of soft tissues (Fields et al., 2023). In general, paying attention to these special ways of decay such as those affected by clothing, is very important. This nuanced understanding proves vitally important for law enforcement when they piece together crime scenes and compare witness accounts (Georgy et al., 2017). Overall, the role of clothing in decomposition isn't as straightforward as it first appears (Figure 5.12).

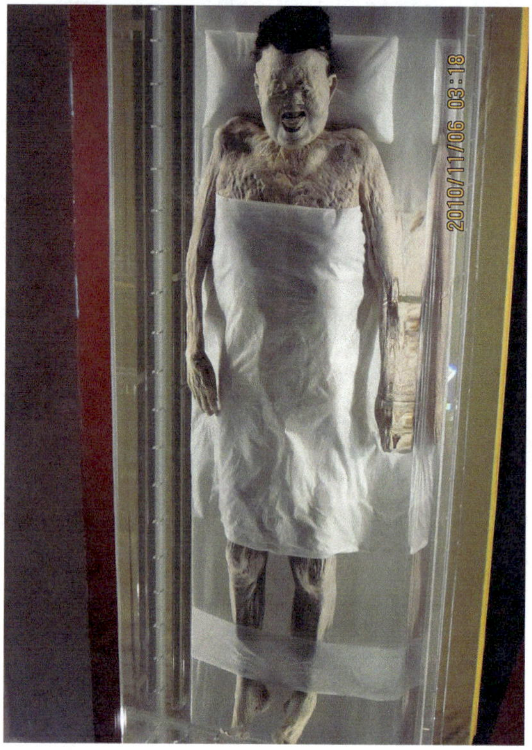

Figure 5.12. Clothing and coverings often change how human remains break down, a factor that forensic experts take into account when estimating the so-called post-mortem interval (PMI).

Source: By Huangdan2060 - Own work, Public Domain, https://commons.wikimedia.org/w/index.php?curid=19674578.

5.2.6. Presence of Insects: Entomological Studies

Although insect studies may seem unusual at the start, they give valuable information about the events after death. To find out how long since death, experts often observe bugs and their life cycles which, in most cases, helps them estimate the PMI. If a body is hidden such as in a suitcase, its decomposition will be different from what happens to a body left out in the open. Take this: while typical remains attract blowflies almost immediately, insect activity may be delayed in a concealed setting, which muddles the PMI guesswork (Jädt et al., 2024). New molecular techniques, in most cases, add to the picture by boosting data accuracy and letting scientists tweak how they collect and analyze insect evidence (Jawad et al., 2019). All in all, these developments make sure that almost every aspect of PMI is considered—even when some details are missed sometimes in an unpredictable way.

5.2.7. Location of the Body: Indoor Versus Outdoor

What happens to a body depends a lot on where it is after death. When a body is inside, there is often less temperature change and fewer scavengers which appears to slow the decay process. On the outside, things become much more unpredictable; weather changes, humidity and sun or wind all work together to break down the skin faster. More than temperature, sudden changes, moisture and being exposed to the outside are important for decomposition.

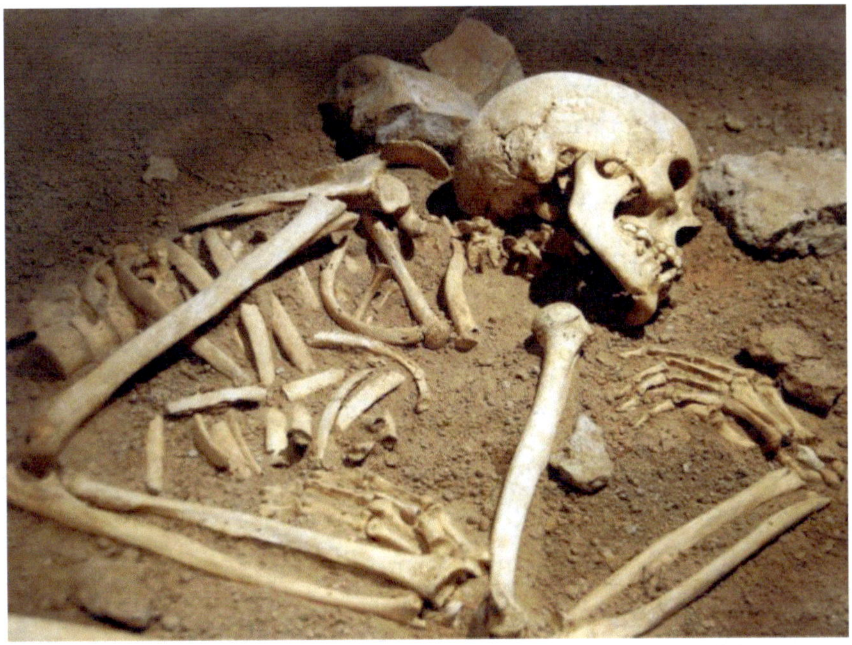

Figure 5.13. A body's surroundings have a big say in how it breaks down after death.

Source: https://media.post.rvohealth.io/wp-content/uploads/sites/3/2020/01/326356_2200-732x549.jpg.

When looking at many forensic cases, it is clear that the location of the remains, whether open or inside, affects the way they decay and the insects involved which makes the location key to understanding how and when the remains were affected. Lately, omics techniques, for instance, have been hinting that environmental factors complicate postmortem analysis even further, reminding us that careful forensic checks are needed in a variety of settings (Jädt et al., 2024; Procopio et al., 2024) (Figure 5.13).

5.2.8. Trauma and Injuries: Impact on Changes

Many times, trauma leads to lasting changes in the brain and this needs further investigation. In contact sports, repeated head impacts can quietly build up over time, sometimes nudging toward chronic issues like Chronic Traumatic Encephalopathy (CTE), even when that first concussion seems pretty minor. A hit to the head may not seem serious at the time, but its effects can appear gradually over the years as memory problems or changes in mood which can be difficult to understand. Studies have even picked up small, telling signs—biomarkers like miR-21 and GFAP observed during postmortem checks (Sage et al., 2018)—which oddly enough serve as clues mapping the long, winding journey from injury to brain decline. To summarize, this knotty link between early brain trauma and later changes underscores, in most cases, why we need more careful research to unravel these injury mechanisms and put together better safeguards for those at risk (Pinchi et al., 2018).

5.2.9. Microbial Flora: Role in Decomposition

Decomposition is not as simple as it looks; it is mostly the result of many microbes breaking down the tissues after someone has passed away. When the usual gut bacteria decline, other microbes, with and without oxygen, move in and help the body get rid of nutrients by new methods. Research shows, generally speaking, that these microbial shifts follow certain patterns; surprisingly, groups like Lactobacillus, Dubosiella, and Enterococcus often jump out as useful signposts for estimating time since death (Liu et al., 2021). Some scientists have even started testing advanced machine learning ideas to predict these intervals by looking closely at the mix of microbes—a method that not only deepens our grasp of host–microbe interactions but also hints at fresh approaches in forensic science and personalized medicine (Marcos-Zambrano et al., 2021). To summarize, these findings remind us how these tiny organisms, despite their imperfections and occasional quirks, play an essential role in the natural recycling process (Figure 5.14).

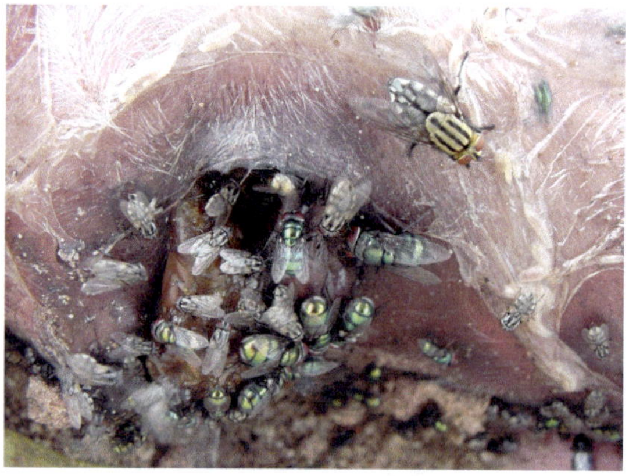

Figure 5.14. Decomposition isn't as straightforward as it might first appear—it's largely driven by many microbes that get to work breaking down tissues after death.

Source: https://media.australian.museum/media/dd/images/Some_image.width-1600.7a33905.jpg.

Test Your Knowledge

1. List the primary factors that influence postmortem changes.
2. Does the temperature around a body change the speed of postmortem changes?

5.3. Forensic Applications of Postmortem Changes

Learning Outcome

1. Estimating the time of death;
2. Identifying the cause of death;
3. Know legal implications;
4. Explain the role in homicide investigations;
5. Learn use in mass disaster scenarios;
6. Focus on collaboration with forensic entomologists: benefits;
7. Discuss technological advancements such as imaging and analysis;
8. Focus on ethical considerations in forensic practices;
9. Describe training and education for forensic professionals.

Knowing about what happens after death can tell us both the date and the sequence of events leading up to it. Checking chemical shifts in eye fluids, for example, can be a solid way to gauge the PMI; a study on domestic pigs even showed clear swings in sodium, potassium, and glucose levels over time (Pali et al., 2024). Things like humidity can disrupt autolysis which makes it harder to estimate the time of death. One line of research looked at how various humidity settings affect organs such as the liver and pancreas, revealing some distinct autolytic signs that help us better grasp postmortem processes (Pali et al., 2024). In general, these discoveries improve the way forensics is done and help make sure the causes of unexpected animal deaths are correctly understood which often matters greatly for justice and animal welfare.

5.3.1. Estimating Time of Death: Methods and Accuracy

The moment a person is considered dead is an intersection between what is needed in practice and what is discovered by science in forensic medicine. Investigators mix a range of methods, from tracking muscle stiffening (rigor mortis) and the settling of blood (livor mortis) to noting changes in eye clarity, to hint at how much time has passed—a process that, in most cases, has its ups and downs. Research points out that checking potassium levels in the gel-like substance of the eye, the vitreous humor, can sometimes deliver a surprisingly accurate estimate compared to traditional physical assessments (Hindawy et al., 2019) . The findings generally show a strong tie between these measures and the postmortem interval, with potassium levels often emerging as the most trustworthy marker (Romano et al., 2017). Mixing several approaches seems to sharpen the overall accuracy of time-of-death estimates—a move many experts consider vital for keeping forensic investigations on track (Figure 5.15).

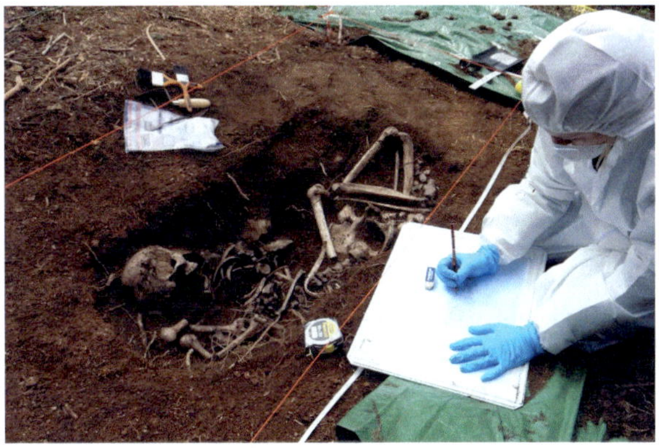

Figure 5.15. Determining exactly when a person has died sits at a crossroads between practical needs and scientific inquiry in forensic medicine.

Source: https://ugc.futurelearn.com/uploads/images/14/86/1486ad87-ebdf-4143-99b8-a1c2b73b6a30.jpg.

5.3.2. Identifying Cause of Death: Implications for Investigations

Forensic investigators must determine the cause of death because it guides legal actions and public health policies. In most situations, experts look at physical signs and chemical signals found at the scene after death which can help explain the circumstances. Recent progress in postmortem biochemistry has brought in new markers that can fine-tune the diagnostic process, especially in puzzling scenarios like hypothermia where the usual visual inspections and microscope work sometimes leave us wanting clear answers (Rousseau et al., 2018). It's also becoming clear that looking into inherited conditions, particularly in sudden cardiac arrest cases, can open up avenues for family screening and preventative tactics that reverberate through community heart health (Abrams et al., 2021). In short, nailing down the exact cause of death isn't merely about fulfilling a legal requirement—it carries real consequences that touch families directly and influence broader public health strategies (Figure 5.16).

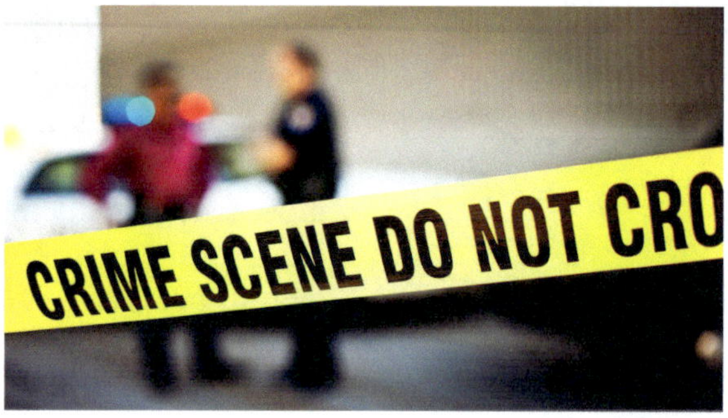

Figure 5.16. Determining why someone passed away is a key step in forensic work.

Source: https://media.hswstatic.com/eyJidWNrZXQiOiJjb250ZW50Lmhzd3N0YXRpYy5j-b20iLCJrZXkiOiJnaWZcL2NzaS1sZWFkLmpwZyIsImVkaXRzIjp7InJlc2l6ZSI6eyJ3aWR0aCI6IjEy-MDAifX19.

5.3.3. Legal Implications: Evidence in Court

The analysis done after a death has important legal consequences for what evidence can be used in court. For example, it is very important to know exactly what happened before, during and after a death, since these details can change the outcome of the case. The information obtained from examining a body usually helps to determine the sequence of events and possible causes which can guide how a criminal investigation and trial are handled. A quick glance back into history shows that practices like dissecting human remains once looked on with deep religious disfavor, have slowly become an indispensable part of both medical study and legal scrutiny, revealing just how vital anatomical insight is when courts weigh evidence (Ghosh, 2015). Also, recognizing behavioral factors—especially those seen in adolescents—drives home the point that understanding social and psychological elements is key in these investigations (Casey, 2014).

5.3.4. Role in Homicide Investigations: Case Studies

Often, clues found after death are important for solving a homicide. Rigor mortis, livor mortis and putrefaction can easily tell us when the person died and what was happening at that time. Experts say that knowing the rate of these changes can help them determine if the person died inside or outside and sometimes it indicates a struggle beforehand. In most cases, when international experts talk about genetic factors in sudden deaths, they point to how useful genetic testing can be in tricky homicide cases, especially when hereditary issues are suspected (Fellmann et al., 2019). Also, mixing insights about behavior and the scene itself shows that investigators often need to mix methods from different fields (Caine, 2013). All of these clues, coming together in a sometimes oddly natural way, boost the clarity and precision in solving cases (Figure 5.17).

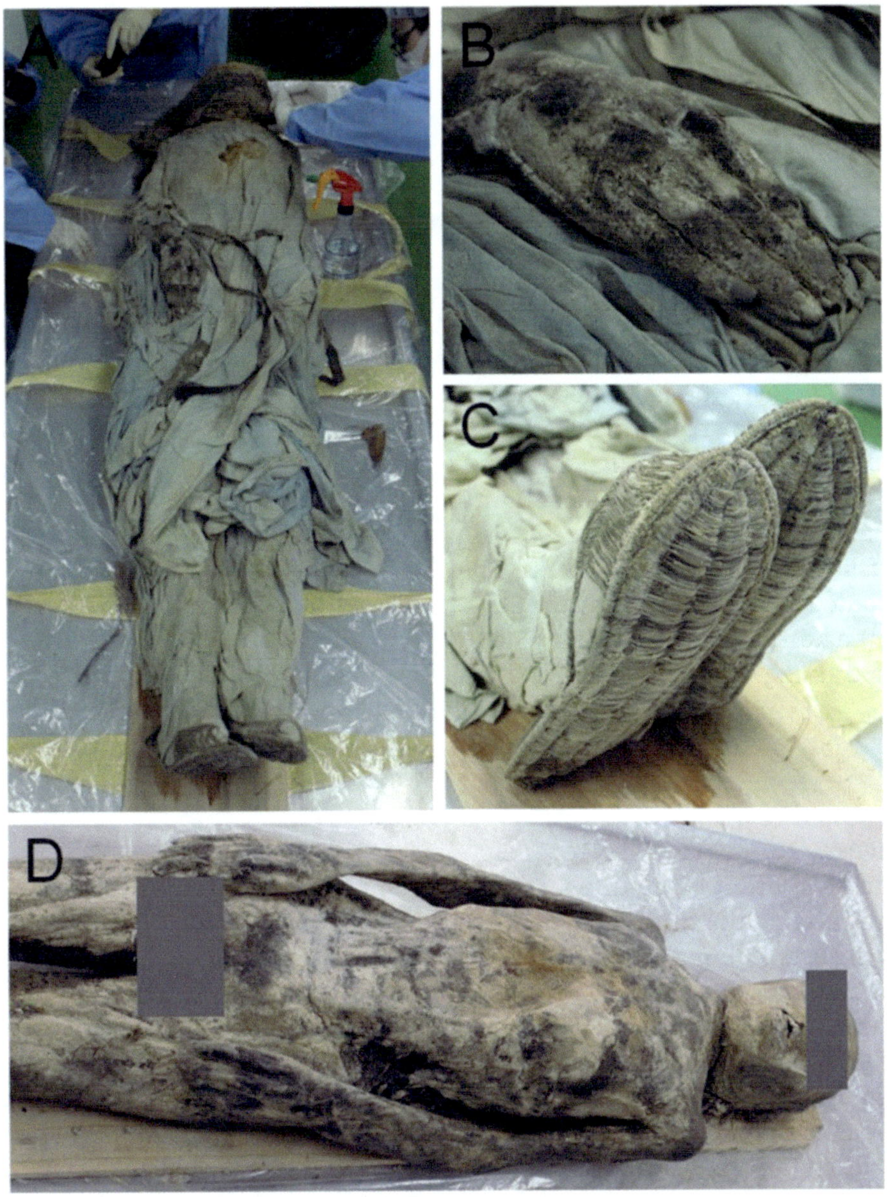

Figure 5.17. Postmortem clues can often be the key to understanding a homicide.

Source: By Kim Y, Lee I, Jung G, Kim M, Oh C, Yoo D, Lee W, Lee E, Cha S, Shin D - Image file from Kim Y, Lee I, Jung G, Kim M, Oh C, Yoo D, Lee W, Lee E, Cha S, Shin D (2014). "Radiological Diagnosis of Congenital Diaphragmatic Hernia in 17th Century Korean Mummy." PLOS ONE. DOI:10.1371/journal.pone.0099779. PMID 24988465. PMC: 4079512., CC BY 4.0, https://commons.wikimedia.org/w/index.php?curid=34839946.

5.3.5. Use in Mass Disaster Scenarios: Challenges and Techniques

After disasters affect a large number of people, handling the remains is a tough job that requires better solutions. As bodies break down naturally, parts like lower limbs and feet might end up scattered, making it harder to pinpoint who they belonged to while also drawing public curiosity and exposing some of the blind spots in current forensic research (Barrett et al., 2014). The large number of deaths can overload local and national services which leads to many experts, including dental hygienists, being called in to help. Sure, there aren't many training programs for these folks, but research generally suggests that multimedia-based education may boost how well they learn and even stir more interest in dealing with mass fatality scenarios (Bruhn et al., 2015). You could say that after such events, the job is to untangle the mess and deal with a lack of proper training.

5.3.6. Collaboration with Forensic Entomologists: Benefits

Postmortem investigations rely on forensic entomology which can often bring unexpected help, mainly in estimating the time since death. Looking at how insects colonize a body gives experts a kind of timeline that can prove crucial for law enforcement (Parsons et al., 2009). Joining forces with entomologists, investigators look at data from the area to see how different environmental factors impact decay. Take, for example, research out in west central Montana; it generally shows that decomposition can unfold in ways that differ a lot from what happens in other climates, reinforcing the idea that each region plays its own role (Parsons et al., 2009). Occasionally, using new techniques such as listening to carrion insects, can lead to better ways of tracking species which in turn improves PMI predictions. To summarize, mixing forensic science with the study of insects doesn't just boost the investigative process but also deepens our overall grasp of postmortem changes in varied ecological settings (Figure 5.18).

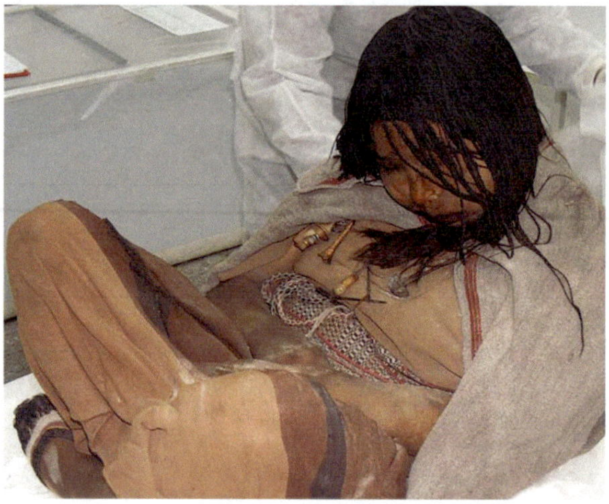

Figure 5.18. Forensic entomology comes into its own in postmortem investigations, often providing unexpected benefits.

Source: By grooverpedro - https://www.flickr.com/photos/116565391@N02/12336665294/, CC BY 2.0, https://commons.wikimedia.org/w/index.php?curid=31011225.

5.3.7. Technological Advancements: Imaging and Analysis

Advances in imaging have helped us understand postmortem cases better and find out who the person was and what happened to them. Take virtopsy, for example—it uses MSCT and MRI to give us a non-invasive glimpse inside a body, revealing details about inner structures and autopsy lesions that generally hold up against traditional methods (Zakaria et al., 2012). Iris recognition is also stepping into the spotlight, showing an 80% match rate in early tests even if it sometimes fumbles with a 20% false reject rate (Sansola et al., 2015). Most of the time, using these tools allows investigators to check forensic evidence more quickly and accurately, mainly when dealing with sudden or violent deaths. In short, it's obvious that forensic science and modern imaging and recognition technologies have developed together.

5.3.8. Ethical Considerations in Forensic Practices

There is often a connection between ethics and forensic work, mainly in cases involving the dead. Genetic testing after death—say, when sudden cardiac death is in play—can unearth valuable clues about why someone passed, and in most cases, it even tips off families about possible inherited risks; yet, it also brings up prickly issues of consent and privacy (Fellmann et al., 2019). After someone passes away, testing their DNA can put us in situations with many ethical questions that are hard to avoid. In the meantime, as forensic anthropology pushes ahead with newer ways of estimating age—mixing histological techniques with tech integrations—the questions about how we treat remains become more pressing than ever (Ubelaker et al., 2019). Most experts are now collaborating across different fields and using public money which helps advance science and earns people's confidence in the forensic process.

5.3.9. Training and Education for Forensic Professionals

Because forensic science has advanced, we now need a strong training system for people working in the field, especially to learn about the small changes that occur after death. Now, because forensic anthropology is so specialized, it is necessary to make sure there are clear qualification standards and a complete range of training for most cases. The push for clearer rules appears to relate to discussions about what experts should do—since their results can have a big effect on people. Some experts argue that getting involved with professional groups helps keep those ethical rules in check, sort of reducing risks when people work outside one's area of expertise (Passalacqua et al., 2021). And then there's the issue of cognitive biases sneaking into decision-making, making it crucial for forensic pathologists to undergo rigorous training that shows them how to spot and counter these biases so their conclusions stay both fair and well-informed (Dror et al., 2021). To summarize, a well-built educational framework is key to nurturing both skill and integrity in forensic practice (Figure 5.19).

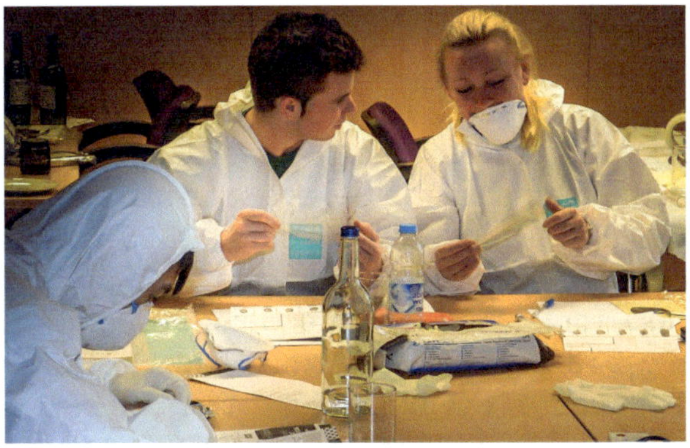

Figure 5.19. Training and education for forensic professionals.

Source: https://theforensicinstitute.com/uploads/images/singleimages/csetrio.jpg.

Test Your Knowledge

1. Why is documenting injuries crucial in homicide investigations?
2. How is time of death estimated in homicide cases?

5.4. Case Studies and Real-World Applications

Learning Outcome

1. Explain famous historical cases;
2. Learn some modern forensic cases;
3. Study the effects of postmortem changes on the possibility of wrongful convictions;
4. Give attention to how postmortem changes are used in solving cold cases;
5. Learn cross-disciplinary studies of anthropology and forensic science;
6. Learn international perspectives;
7. Discuss the role of postmortem changes in exhumations;
8. Learn case studies involving mass graves;
9. Identify future directions in forensic research.

Because of new technologies, forensic science is now exploring fresh ways to examine and recognize bodies after they die. Recently, a few case studies using iris scans—even in postmortem scenarios—have shown around an 80% match rate (Sansola et al., 2015), which generally points to a promising edge in using these tools. At the same time, research on how bodies break down has been exploring the impact of environmental factors; in several controlled experiments, however, the standard scales for decomposition alone haven't quite hit statistically solid ground (Santos et al., 2019). Most of the time such mixed results lead investigators to combine advanced biometric tools with careful checks done on-site. By using both strategies, the chances of correctly identifying the remains are increased and it also helps forensic pathology deal better with the sometimes-difficult tasks of medicolegal investigations.

5.4.1. Famous Historical Cases: Analysis of Postmortem Changes

Analyzing cases from history where things happen after death can reveal new facts about biology and forensic techniques. Louis XVI is a good example; his decay was affected by both the environment and the way he was buried. It's interesting that these changes after death can tell us about the decay process and possibly suggest what happened just before the person died. Forensic science has advanced a lot recently, using tissue studies and bug evidence to reconstruct crime scenes and this has helped real investigations. It could be argued that these studies are useful, as they help us relate what happened in the past to what happens today in forensics. In many instances, this mix of biology and investigation helps us trace evolutionary tweaks via genetic analysis (Haroche, 2013; Jónsson et al., 2014). All in all, small findings after death help us rethink both the natural events and the history of what happened.

5.4.2. Modern Forensic Cases: Lessons Learned

Important cases are leading forensic science to explore new areas which can result in both great successes and some surprising mistakes. Tracking the after-death changes in each case can be messy and their effects are often seen in the legal process. Upgrading technology has usually made the process of analysis more reliable, but discussions about handling human remains are still lively. I've noticed that Europe's rules on body donation are in a constant state of flux, with regular updates aiming to iron out ethical wrinkles (Brenner et al., 2023). In another corner, cybersecurity studies digging into past breaches make it clear that mixing old mistakes with new strategies is key to warding off future issues (Singla et al., 2023). All of this points out that forensic practices are always forced to adapt when science and ethics meet. In a way, it's a reminder that progress in this field is never a straight line but a series of unpredictable turns (Figure 5.20).

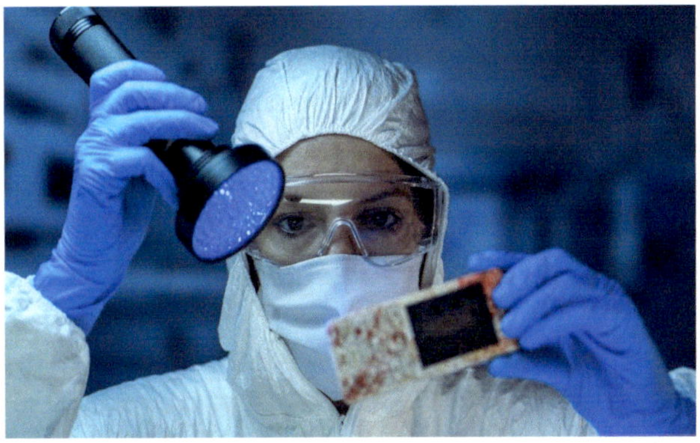

Figure 5.20. High-profile cases keep pushing forensic science into new territories, sparking sharp successes and some unexpected blunders.

Source: https://akm-img-a-in.tosshub.com/indiatoday/images/story/202503/forensic-scientist-at-work-063220120-16x9_0.jpg?VersionId=5eHKxdhBzCMMNin782aohqXIyd1FpCWW.

5.4.3. Impact of Postmortem Changes on Wrongful Convictions

When postmortem changes occur, it makes legal cases very difficult, mainly when wrongful convictions are possible. When the body starts to fail, DNA starts to lose its structure which can cause chaos quickly. Temperature swings, humidity, and even everyday pollutants can trigger processes like hydrolysis and oxidation – which, in many instances, leave DNA samples too damaged for proper forensic work (Bhoyar et al., 2024). Not only does this issue make it hard to estimate when the person died; it can also mess up the investigation and cause misunderstandings in the evidence. It is true that next-generation sequencing can sometimes recover bits of degraded DNA, but depend too much on these tools and you may become overconfident in results that can be wrong. In most cases, these ongoing changes remind us that evidence needs careful and continuous re-examination, especially in the delicate context of wrongful conviction cases (Sandhi et al., 2023).

5.4.4. Use of Postmortem Changes in Cold Cases

Looking at what happens after someone dies is now important in reopening cold cases, especially if the usual methods fail. They can show us the last moments of the deceased, the setting at the time and the condition of the body. In fact, writing down biochemical findings—researchers have shown that glucose and electrolytes can be important signs—is also very important. At times, using histological techniques lets forensic experts spot tiny signals of trauma or disease that earlier reviews might have simply skipped over (Mangin et al., 2018). New work in sifting through postmortem brain tissue has shown that axons often stick together pretty well, opening the door for ultrastructural checks related to potential neurodevelopmental quirks (Liu et al., 2014). All of these bits of info do more than back up forensic work; they add another layer that helps us piece together the deceased's medical and mental history (Figure 5.21).

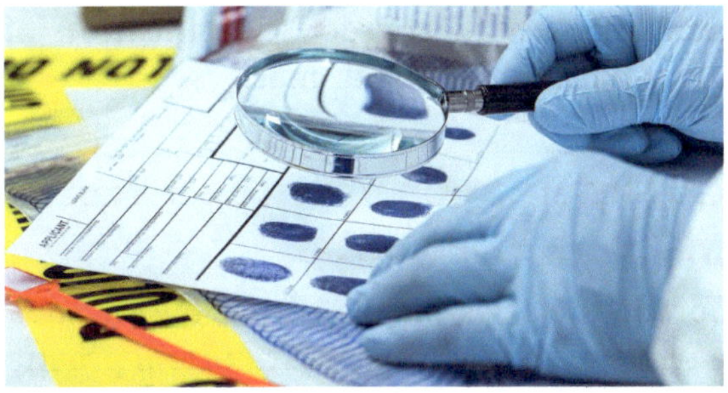

Figure 5.21. Examining the changes that kick in after death has become a key part of reopening cold cases, especially when the usual methods just don't seem to work.

Source: https://images.deccanherald.com/deccanherald%2F2024-01%2Fe2aa2be0-06ca-40f0-9fab-b403479f8dda%2FiStock_838277822.jpg?rect=0%2C30%2C1254%2C658&w=1200&ar=40%3A21&auto=format%2Ccompress&ogImage=true&mode=crop.

5.4.5. Cross-disciplinary Studies: Anthropology and Forensic Science

Anthropology and forensic science work together in surprising ways to show us how things change after a person dies and how society and identity are connected. In many violent cases, forensic anthropologists are involved and this has made it obvious that considering gender identity is not just a secondary concern. In most cases, people are now recognizing the reality of lived gender experience—especially for transgender and gender diverse (TGD) individuals—which presses forensic methods to confront some deep-seated, systemic anti-trans biases (Adams et al., 2023). Sometimes, when experts are handling disaster victim identification (DVI) operations, the obstacles they face remind us that working across different disciplines and being culturally sensitive—particularly in international scenarios—is pretty much a must (Adamovic et al., 2023). Through combining knowledge from several fields, anthropologists and forensic scientists can create approaches that are less rigid but more detailed and just which helps with correct identification and dealing with wider social matters.

5.4.6. International Perspectives: Variations in Practices

Different societies manage what follows death in a wide variety of ways. Postmortem practices differ widely around the world because of cultural traditions, laws and healthcare trends. In some places, traditional rituals about the community's spiritual well-being are important, but in other places things are handled in a formal, controlled way. In general, some people prefer to bury the body right away, as a sign of respect, but other cultures allow for more time to observe the body if forensic or scientific work is needed. Because of this mix of old traditions and modern methods, there are often problems about consent and the proper handling of human remains. Because global communication is always sharing ideas, it can lead to the mixing of different traditions into new forms. To summarize, these evolving trends mean that organizations must stay nimble and rethink how they safeguard information as cultural and professional viewpoints keep shifting (Bakir et al., 2023).

5.4.7. Role of Postmortem Changes in Exhumations

Looking at how a body changes after death matters, especially when the cause of death is still unknown after a long time. As a body starts to break down, it produces signs that experts can use, sometimes in unexpected manners, to discover what happened. Research generally shows that how quickly a body decomposes can hinge on things like how deep it's buried or the local weather and soil conditions (Adlam et al., 2014), so the clues aren't always straightforward. In cases where exhumation takes place after a long interval, toxicology becomes even trickier; altered drug levels might muddy the waters when trying to pinpoint a cause of death, especially with substances such as pharmaceuticals or pesticides (Albano et al., 2023). Recognizing these shifts not only shapes the course of the forensic exam, but also drives home the idea that time plays a huge role in what evidence we can actually recover (Figure 5.22).

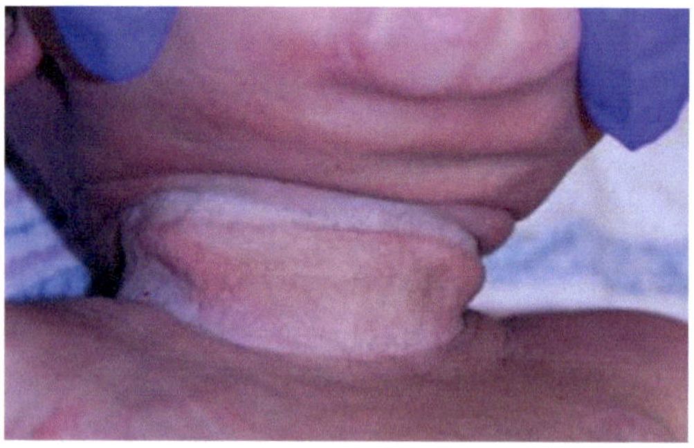

Figure 5.22. Role of postmortem changes in exhumations.

Source: https://img.medscapestatic.com/pi/meds/ckb/84/9684tn.jpg.

5.4.8. Case Studies Involving Mass Graves: Challenges Faced

Investigating mass graves is very difficult, as it is hard to link the remains to previous records and the process of justice and remembering becomes unclear. In Chile, for example, the aftermath of enforced disappearances during the Pinochet's regime shows how messy it can get—mixing skeletal clues with old records often leads to mix-ups because methods are not always sharp and past traumas can obscure what happened (Quinn et al., 2014). At the U.S.-Mexico border, the humanitarian crisis going on shows that structural violence is a real problem and it even affects how the remains of people are handled after their deaths. Various dying conditions trigger taphonomic shifts that mess with accurate identification, resulting in sometimes unmarked graves that, in most cases, leave families without the closure they desperately seek (Kaplan et al., 2024).

5.4.9. Future Directions in Forensic Research

Forensic research has changed and now combines new imaging techniques with a closer examination of structural violence which creates new opportunities in postmortem studies. Autopsies have long been the reliable go-to, but postmortem magnetic resonance imaging (PMMR) is emerging as a less intrusive option that, generally speaking, could boost how accurately diagnoses are made while easing ethical worries—especially in difficult cases like perinatal and childhood losses (Arthurs et al., 2017). Studies looking at migrant communities even hint that structural violence leaves its mark on biological clues and can steer the postmortem process in unexpected directions (Kaplan et al., 2024). All these changes, in many respects, suggest that various fields are being merged; they help improve forensic methods and also give some justice and respect to the deceased and their families.

Test Your Knowledge

1. What is an exhumation in a forensic context?
2. What postmortem changes are commonly observed in exhumed bodies?

Summary

Finding the PMI can be very challenging in forensic investigations. Researchers are noticing that both changes in protein levels and the makeup of microbes can give important hints. For instance, HMGB1 in the blood tends to hit its peak roughly 48 hours after death, while the muscle tissue—shown by a drop in desmin staining—gradually reveals signs of cellular breakdown (Albloshi, 2024). It's also interesting that the mouth's microbial community often changes in unpredictable ways, influenced by factors like temperature and humidity, which in most cases can help hint at how much time has passed (Langit et al., 2024). All things considered, pairing biomarker signs with changes in microbes seems to help forensic experts better estimate PMI and learn new things about postmortem changes.

A look at what happens after death shows us how a body gradually slows down and may start to break apart. People discuss many changes that happen to a body after death such as rigor mortis and algor mortis which occur at unexpected times and give useful details for forensic investigations. Usually, the appearance of rigor mortis can give an idea of when someone died and the activity of decaying microbes points out that where and how the body is kept can affect its condition. You might also notice that brain inflammation—seen in conditions such as Alzheimer's disease—makes it necessary to check postmortem brain tissues for any hidden markers (Kinney et al., 2018). Plus, shortages in healthcare resources, especially during messy times like the COVID-19 crisis, have shifted how postmortem exams are handled across the world (Rubin et al., 2020).

KEY TERMS FROM THIS CHAPTER

- Chemical reactions
- Data accuracy
- Decomposition
- Different decay patterns
- Enzymes
- Lipid oxidation
- Livor mortis
- Matrix metalloproteinases
- Minimally invasive autopsies
- Omics techniques
- Postmortem computed tomography (PMCT)
- Postmortem interval (PMI)
- Rigor mortis
- Scavengers
- Surface area
- Temperature
- Trauma centers

Short Answer Questions

1. When does rigor mortis usually start after a person has died?
2. What is putrefaction?
3. What are the early postmortem changes?
4. Name two signs of late postmortem changes.
5. How does body weight influence postmortem changes?
6. How does clothing affect the rate of changes that happen after death?
7. Describe how the environment affects the way decomposition happens.
8. What is the effect of humidity on postmortem changes?

Critical Thinking Questions

1. Rigor mortis refers to:
   a. Cooling of the body after death
   b. Stiffening of muscles after death
   c. Discoloration of skin due to blood pooling
   d. Decomposition of soft tissues

2. Postmortem lividity (livor mortis) is first noticed in:
   a. Hands and feet
   b. Face
   c. Dependent parts of the body
   d. Abdomen

3. Which of the following is the earliest postmortem change?
   a. Rigor mortis
   b. Putrefaction
   c. Livor mortis
   d. Algor mortis

4. Which alteration after death helps to find out the position of the body?
   a. Rigor mortis
   b. Algor mortis
   c. Livor mortis
   d. Putrefaction

5. Which factor does not influence rigor mortis?
   a. Age of the deceased
   b. Temperature of surroundings

c. Gender of the deceased
d. Cause of death

Answers to Critical Thinking Questions

1. (b); 2. (c); 3. (d); 4. (c); 5. (c)

References

1. Abad Santos, J. (2019). Decomposition of pig carcasses at varying room temperature. https://core.ac.uk/download/228080080.pdf (accessed on 29 May 2025).
2. Abu Bakar @ Zakaria, M. Z., Ibrahim, A. O., & Mustapha, M. N. (2012). Applicability of virtuosi in veterinary practice: A short review. https://core.ac.uk/download/42992189.pdf (accessed on 29 May 2025).
3. Adamovic, N., Howes, L. M., White, R., & Julian, R. (2023). Understanding the challenges of disaster victim identification: Perspectives of Australian forensic practitioners. *Forensic Sciences Research, 8*, 107–115. https://doi.org/10.1093/fsr/owad020.
4. Adlam, A. L. R., Arnold, J., Bachmann, L., Baraybar, J. P., Burns, C., Carter, D. O., et al. (2014). A preliminary examination of differential decomposition patterns in mass graves. https://core.ac.uk/download/1441337.pdf (accessed on 29 May 2025).
5. Ahmed, Y. A., Ali, S., & Ghallab, A. (2018). Hair histology as a tool for forensic identification of some domestic animal species. http://arxiv.org/abs/1807.02668 (accessed on 29 May 2025).
6. Albano, G. D., Zerbo, S., La Spina, C., Midiri, M., Guadagnino, D., D'Anna, T., Buscemi, R., & Argo, A. (2023). Toxicological analysis in tissues following exhumation more than two years after death (948 days): A forensic perspective in a fatal case. *Toxics, 11*(6), 485. https://doi.org/10.3390/toxics11060485.
7. Albloshi, A. M. K. (2024). Postmortem interval estimation of time since death: Impact of non-histone binding proteins, immunohistochemical, and histopathological changes *in vivo*. *Journal of Medicine and Life, 17*, 897–902. https://www.semanticscholar.org/paper/043ca6f62c25cf0cfa25f85329a630542c4db1f1 (accessed on 29 May 2025).
8. Aldridge, R. J. (2008). Dress in the United States of America as depicted in postmortem photographs, 1840–1900. https://core.ac.uk/download/217397902.pdf.
9. Amaral, A. B., da Silva, M. V., & Lannes, S. C. S. (2018). Lipid oxidation in meat: Mechanisms and protective factors–a review. *Food Science and Technology, 38*, 1–15. https://doi.org/10.1590/fst.32518.
10. An, H. J., Bereuter, T. L., Dimapasoc, L., Garrido, F., et al. (2014). Glycosylated proteins preserved over millennia: N-glycan analysis of Tyrolean Iceman, Scythian Princess and Warrior. *Scientific Reports, 4*, 4963. https://core.ac.uk/download/323070031.pdf.
11. Appenzeller, O., Bromage, T., Khairat, R., Nerlich, A., & Rühli, F. (2015). Bioarcheology: Medicine, biology, and forensic sciences. *BioMed Research International, 2015*. https://www.semanticscholar.org/paper/e5e554195963822215198544 2dfe00dfaeb67431 (accessed on 29 May 2025).
12. Argo, A., Buscemi, R., Karch, S. B., Lanzarone, A., Roccuzzo, R., & Zerbo, S. (2019).

Perioperative and anesthetic deaths: Toxicological and medico legal aspects. https://core.ac.uk/download/224993621.pdf (accessed on 29 May 2025).

13. Arjun, B. S., Alekya, B., Hari, R. S., V. V., Mahadevan, A., & Pandya, H. (2022). Electromechanical characterization of human brain tissues: A potential biomarker for tumor delineation. *IEEE Transactions on Biomedical Engineering, 69*, 3484–3493. https://www.semanticscholar.org/paper/b37705bdc1075cc2fbf441b29212223c04a82134 (accessed on 29 May 2025).

14. Arthurs, O. J., Hutchinson, J. C., & Sebire, N. J. (2017). Current issues in postmortem imaging of perinatal and forensic childhood deaths. https://core.ac.uk/download/79553300.pdf (accessed on 29 May 2025).

15. Bakir, R., & Marvik, V. (2023). Information security culture: An investigation into the impact of a large-scale cyberattack. https://core.ac.uk/download/577835881.pdf (accessed on 29 May 2025).

16. Barrett, J., Bidmos, M. A., Bilge, A., British Broadcasting Corporation, et al. (2014). The foot in forensic human identification–A review. https://core.ac.uk/download/30660095.pdf (accessed on 29 May 2025).

17. Bautista, R. (2015). Survey of biological factors affecting the determination of the postmortem interval. https://core.ac.uk/download/236084552.pdf (accessed on 29 May 2025).

18. Bergamin, E., Boldrini, L., De Vita, V., et al. (2024). Exploring radiomic features of lateral cerebral ventricles in postmortem CT for postmortem interval estimation. https://core.ac.uk/download/638780623.pdf (accessed on 29 May 2025).

19. Bertrand, B., Clauzel, T., Richardin, P., Bécart, A., Morbidelli, P., Hédouin, V., & Marques, C. (2024). Application and implications of radiocarbon dating in forensic case work: When medico-legal significance meets archaeological relevance. *Forensic Sciences Research, 9*. https://www.semanticscholar.org/paper/f71993cf5ce191e912a2544c0785fd34c10cccce (accessed on 29 May 2025).

20. Bhawnani, D., Goyal, M., & Thakur, R. (2017). A study on estimation of time since death after histological examination of kidney. https://core.ac.uk/download/543137047.pdf (accessed on 29 May 2025).

21. Bhoyar, L., Mehar, P., & Chavali, K. (2024). An overview of DNA degradation and its implications in forensic caseworks. *Egyptian Journal of Forensic Sciences, 14*. https://doi.org/10.1186/s41935-024-00389-y.

22. Brenner, E., Bleys, R. L. A. W., De, R., Catereniuc, I., Chirculescu, A. R. M., Destrieux, C., Eppler, E., et al. (2023). The legal and ethical framework governing body donation in Europe–2nd update on current practice. *Annals of Anatomy–Anatomischer Anzeiger, 252*, 152195. https://doi.org/10.1016/j.aanat.2023.152195.

23. Bruhn, A. M., Diawara, N., Newcomb, T. L., et al. (2015). Performance of dental hygiene students in mass fatality training and radiographic imaging of dental remains. https://core.ac.uk/download/217287010.pdf (accessed on 29 May 2025).

24. Cabral-Pacheco, G. A., Garza-Veloz, I., Castruita-De la Rosa, C., Ramirez-Acuña, J. M., Perez-Romero, B. A., Guerrero-Rodriguez, J. F., Martínez-Avila, N., et al. (2020). The roles of matrix metalloproteinases and their inhibitors in human diseases. *International Journal of Molecular Sciences, 21*, 9739. https://doi.org/10.3390/ijms21249739.

25. Caine, E. D. (2013). Forging an agenda for suicide prevention in the United States. *American Journal of Public Health, 103*, 822–829. https://doi.org/10.2105/ajph.2012.301078.

26. Casey, B. J. (2014). Beyond simple models of self-control to circuit-based accounts of adolescent behavior. *Annual Review of Psychology, 66*, 295–319. https://doi.org/10.1146/annurev-psych-010814-015156.

27. Chang, S., Jeon, S., Han, H. J., Kim, D. G., Hwang, S., & Kim, H. (2025). Suicidal cases involving sodium nitrite: Focus on crime scene and investigation. *Korean Journal of Legal Medicine*. https://www.semanticscholar.org/paper/a18d0e0b764299e0fb91107a77c4c4696f0ac2e1 (accessed on 29 May 2025).

28. Daneva, A., Gao, Z., Van Durme, M., & Nowack, M. K. (2016). Functions and regulation of programmed cell death in plant development. *Annual Review of Cell and Developmental Biology, 32*, 441–468. https://doi.org/10.1146/annurev-cellbio-111315-124915.

29. Dautartas, A. M. (2009). The effect of various coverings on the rate of human decomposition. https://core.ac.uk/download/268805448.pdf (accessed on 29 May 2025).

30. Donovan Adams, S. H., Blatt, T. M., Flaherty, J. D., Isa, M. I., Michael, A., & Smith, A. C. (2023). Shifting the forensic anthropological paradigm to incorporate the transgender and gender diverse community. *Humans, 3*, 142–165. https://doi.org/10.3390/humans3030013.

31. Dowell-Curby, J. (2017). A review of the microbiome associated with human decomposition. https://core.ac.uk/download/141488869.pdf (accessed on 29 May 2025).

32. Dror, I. E., Melinek, J., Arden, J. L., Kukucka, J., Hawkins, S., Carter, J., & Atherton, D. S. (2021). Cognitive bias in forensic pathology decisions. *Journal of Forensic Sciences, 66*, 1751–1757. https://doi.org/10.1111/1556-4029.14697.

33. Eliyani, H., Ma'ruf, A., Rantam, F. A., et al. (2017). Postmortem interval estimation time from algometric temperature of rats expressed by MARS model approach. https://core.ac.uk/download/417402230.pdf (accessed on 29 May 2025).

34. Fellmann, F., van El, C., Charron, P., Michaud, K., Howard, H., Boers, S. N., Clarke, A., et al. (2019). European recommendations integrating genetic testing into multidisciplinary management of sudden cardiac death. *European Journal of Human Genetics, 27*, 1763–1773. https://doi.org/10.1038/s41431-019-0445-y.

35. Fields, E. (2023). Postmortem interval estimation within the context of adipocere formation. https://core.ac.uk/download/599632011.pdf (accessed on 29 May 2025).

36. Georgy, J., & Petersen, C. (2017). The effect of suitcase concealment on the insect colonization: A pilot study in Western Australia. https://core.ac.uk/download/85259609.pdf (accessed on 29 May 2025).

37. Ghosh, S. K. (2015). Human cadaveric dissection: A historical account from ancient Greece to the modern era. *Anatomy & Cell Biology, 48*, 153–153. https://doi.org/10.5115/acb.2015.48.3.153.

38. Gorgeva, E., Hoogewerff, J., Robertson, J., et al. (2023). The potential of bioacoustics for surveying carrion insects. https://core.ac.uk/download/597770538.pdf (accessed on 29 May 2025).

39. Hagihara, H., & Miyakawa, T. (2024). Decreased brain pH correlated with progression of Alzheimer disease neuropathology: A systematic review and meta-analyses of postmortem studies. *International Journal of Neuropsychopharmacology, 27*. https://www.semanticscholar.

org/paper/49fdfa9d7ff6e67716fd0dab145cc64a85352f93 (accessed on 29 May 2025).

40. Haroche, S. (2013). Nobel lecture: Controlling photons in a box and exploring the quantum to classical boundary. *Reviews of Modern Physics, 85*, 1083–1102. https://doi.org/10.1103/revmodphys.85.1083.

41. Henrikson, Z. A., Vermette, C., Schwean-Lardner, K., & Crowe, T. (2018). Effects of cold exposure on physiology, meat quality, and behavior of turkey hens and toms crated at transport density. *Poultry Science, 97*, 347–357. https://www.semanticscholar.org/paper/fe4eb10629c3f0883f70282a108f65381515aa63 (accessed on 29 May 2025).

42. Hindawy, R. F., El Sawaf, H., Ramsis, M., Hussein, A., Adly, N., & Abdelkader, A. (2019). Vitreous potassium concentration as a predictor of postmortem interval in severe burn deaths at Alexandreia mortuary. *The Egyptian Journal of Forensic Sciences and Applied Toxicology*. https://www.semanticscholar.org/paper/8ff0e7f9d0c48c26258c04c4a651c238231fd610 (accessed on 29 May 2025).

43. Ikpa, J. O., Umana, U. E., Timbuak, J. A., & Tanko, M. (2025). Comparative study of early postmortem changes in Sus scrofa domestica models in the Savannah Region of Cross River State, Nigeria. Dutse *Journal of Pure and Applied Sciences*. https://www.semanticscholar.org/paper/35100c910d80e041367f4043e21913cc67806e51 (accessed on 29 May 2025).

44. Jawad, M., Khalid, M., Mona, S., et al. (2019). *Forensic Entomology: A Comprehensive Review*. https://core.ac.uk/download/268082179.pdf (accessed on 29 May 2025).

45. Jónsson, H., Schubert, M., Seguin-Orlando, A., Ginolhac, A., Petersen, L., Fumagalli, M., Albrechtsen, A., et al. (2014). Speciation with gene flow in equids despite extensive chromosomal plasticity. *Proceedings of the National Academy of Sciences, 111*, 18655–18660. https://doi.org/10.1073/pnas.1412627111.

46. Joseph, S., Reinecke, G., & Dadour, I. (2016). Suitcase concealment: An interdisciplinary analysis of the taphonomy processes and their effect on PMI estimation.

47. Kaplan, M. A., & Znachko, C. (2024). A spectrum of violence: The intersection of antemortem and postmortem embodiment in migrant death investigation at the U.S. Mexico border. *Human Biology Open Access Pre-Prints, 217*. https://digitalcommons.wayne.edu/humbiol_preprints/217 (accessed on 29 May 2025).

48. Kara, F., & Kantarci, K. (2024). Understanding proton magnetic resonance spectroscopy neurochemical changes using Alzheimer's disease biofluid, PET, postmortem pathology biomarkers, and APOE genotype. *International Journal of Molecular Sciences, 25*. https://www.semanticscholar.org/paper/9ac336aeac39d808e9e05df27dba101f2dd95d84 (accessed on 29 May 2025).

49. Keenan, S. W., & DeBruyn, J. M. (2019). Changes to vertebrate tissue stable isotope (δ15N) composition during decomposition. *Scientific Reports, 9*. https://doi.org/10.1038/s41598-019-46368-5.

50. Kinney, J. W., Bemiller, S. M., Murtishaw, A. S., Leisgang, A. M., Salazar, A., & Lamb, B. T. (2018). Inflammation as a central mechanism in Alzheimer's disease. *Alzheimer's & Dementia: Translational Research & Clinical Interventions, 4*, 575–590. https://doi.org/10.1016/j.trci.2018.06.014.

51. Kodama, W. A., Xu, Z. Z., Metcalf, J. L., Song, S. J., Harrison, N. L., Knight, R., Carter, D., et al.

(2018). Trace evidence potential in postmortem skin microbiomes: From death scene to morgue. *Journal of Forensic Sciences, 64*, 791–798. https://doi.org/10.1111/1556-4029.13949.

52. Langit, K. S., Prabowo, Y. B., & Shifa, L. L. (2024). Analysis of changes in oral microbiota for interval of post-mortem estimation: Review article. *Odonto: Dental Journal*. https://www.semanticscholar.org/paper/121b9b3cce2e78b0ee9b67ec2e0f8ca6eabe53e9 (accessed on 29 May 2025).
53. Linstädt, J., Thöne-Reineke, C., & Merle, R. (2024). Animal-based welfare indicators for dairy cows and their validity and practicality: A systematic review of the existing literature. *Frontiers in Veterinary Science, 11*. https://doi.org/10.3389/fvets.2024.1429097.
54. Liu, R., Wang, Q., Zhang, K., Wu, H., Wang, G., Cai, W., Yu, K., et al. (2021). Analysis of postmortem intestinal microbiota successional patterns with application in postmortem interval estimation. *Research Square*. https://doi.org/10.21203/rs.3.rs-411962/v1.
55. Liu, X. B., & Schumann, C. M. (2014). Optimization of electron microscopy for human brains with long-term fixation and fixed-frozen sections. https://core.ac.uk/download/323071028.pdf.
56. Mangin, P., & Palmiere, C. (2018). Postmortem biochemical investigations in hypothermia fatalities. https://core.ac.uk/download/159156050.pdf (accessed on 29 May 2025).
57. Marcos-Zambrano, L. J., Karađuzović-Hadžiabdić, K., Lončar-Turukalo, T., Przymus, P., Trajkovik, V., Aasmets, O., Berland, M., et al. (2021). Applications of machine learning in human microbiome studies: A review on feature selection, biomarker identification, disease prediction and treatment. *Frontiers in Microbiology, 12*. https://doi.org/10.3389/fmicb.2021.634511.
58. Mätlik, K., Pressl, C., & Heintz, N. (2025). Cell type-specific studies of human tissue for investigation of the molecular cell biology of late-onset neurodegenerative disease. *Annual Review of Neuroscience*. https://www.semanticscholar.org/paper/43b7477f2ab283a7d0c1637f7de82b3c29d9afeb (accessed on 29 May 2025).
59. Mee, J. F. (2020). Investigation of bovine abortion and stillbirth/perinatal mortality–similar diagnostic challenges, different approaches. *Irish Veterinary Journal, 73*. https://doi.org/10.1186/s13620-020-00172-0.
60. Novak, S. A., & Willoughby, W. (2014). Resurrectionists' excursions: Evidence of postmortem dissection from the Spring Street Presbyterian Church. https://core.ac.uk/download/215547552.pdf (accessed on 29 May 2025).
61. Oh, S., Ahn, B., Lee, B., & Nam, S. (2024). Effect of humidity on postmortem changes in rats. *Journal of Veterinary Science, 25*. https://www.semanticscholar.org/paper/789e4ad2fc1cc96a702325fd820abcd0ba4044a1 (accessed on 29 May 2025).
62. Palić, M., Šoštarić Zuckermann, I. C., Džaja, P., Ljubić, B. B., & Severin, K. (2024). A biochemical and histological assessment of postmortem changes to the eyes of domestic pigs: A preliminary study. *Animals, 14*. https://www.semanticscholar.org/paper/298c5f55f281eac0d26b9c2126a942321201fbf9 (accessed on 29 May 2025).
63. Parsons, H. R. (2009). *The Postmortem Interval: A Systematic Study of Pig Decomposition in West Central Montana* [Doctoral dissertation, Montana State University]. https://core.ac.uk/download/267575606.pdf (accessed on 29 May 2025).
64. Passalacqua, N. V., Pilloud, M. A., & Congram, D. (2021). Forensic anthropology as a discipline.

Biology, 10, 691. https://doi.org/10.3390/biology10080691.

65. Pinchi, E., Frati, A., Cipolloni, L., Aromatario, M., Gatto, V., La Russa, R., Pesce, A., Santurro, A., Fraschetti, F., Frati, P., & Fineschi, V. (2018). Clinical-pathological study on β-APP, IL-1β, GFAP, NFL, Spectrin II, 8OHdG, TUNEL, miR-21, miR-16, miR-92 expressions to verify DAI-diagnosis, grade and prognosis. *Scientific Reports, 8*(1), 2387. https://doi.org/10.1038/s41598-018-20699-1.

66. Pittner, S., Bugelli, V., Weitgasser, K., Zissler, A., Sanit, S., Lutz, L., Monticelli, F., et al. (2020). A field study to evaluate PMI estimation methods for advanced decomposition stages. *International Journal of Legal Medicine, 134*, 1361–1373. https://doi.org/10.1007/s00414-020-02278-0.

67. Procopio, N., & Bonicelli, A. (2024). From flesh to bones: Multi-omics approaches in forensic science. *Proteomics, 24*. https://doi.org/10.1002/pmic.202200335.

68. Quinn, A. M. (2014). *Identifying Desaparecidos: The Development of Forensic Anthropology in Chile* [Doctoral dissertation, University of Glasgow]. https://core.ac.uk/download/215704516.pdf (accessed on 29 May 2025).

69. Reisdorf, A., & Wuttke, M. (2018). Re-evaluating Moodie's opisthotonic-posture hypothesis in fossil vertebrates Part I: Reptiles—the taphonomy of the bipedal dinosaurs *Compsognathus longipes* and *Juravenator starki* from the Solnhofen Archipelago (Jurassic, Germany). https://core.ac.uk/download/159149524.pdf (accessed on 29 May 2025).

70. Romano, M., Moreira, H. T., Alenezi, F., Saraiva, L. A. L., Schmidt, A., Maciel, B. C., Rassi, A., et al. (2017). Rapid fire abstract session–The prognostic value from echocardiography. https://www.semanticscholar.org/paper/17d8f9b5d29eead3411a788c89a3d18e30922d41 (accessed on 29 May 2025).

71. Rörup, B., He, X., Shen, J., Baalbaki, R., Dada, L., Sipilä, M., Kirkby, J., et al. (2024). Temperature, humidity, and ionization effect of iodine oxoacid nucleation. *Environmental Science, 4*, 531–546. https://www.semanticscholar.org/paper/3e064017081b7ee802cf3bd04106f9e64afe4f45 (accessed on 29 May 2025).

72. Rousseau, G., Reynier, P., Jousset, N., Rougé-Maillart, C., & Palmiere, C. (2018). Updated review of postmortem biochemical exploration of hypothermia with a presentation of standard strategy of sampling and analyses. *Clinical Chemistry and Laboratory Medicine, 56*(11), 1819–1827. https://doi.org/10.1515/cclm-2018-0153.

73. Rubin, G. D., Ryerson, C. J., Haramati, L. B., Sverzellati, N., Kanne, J. P., Raoof, S., Schluger, N. W., et al. (2020). The role of chest imaging in patient management during the COVID-19 pandemic: A multinational consensus statement from the Fleischner Society. *Radiology, 296*, 172–180. https://doi.org/10.1148/radiol.2020201365.

74. Sage, M. (2018). *Neurocognitive Findings in Adults Who Played Youth Football* [Master's thesis, Boston University]. https://open.bu.edu/bitstream/2144/33032/5/Sage_bu_0017N_14075.pdf (accessed on 29 May 2025).

75. Salado Puerto, M., Abboud, D., Baraybar, J. P., Carracedo, Á., Fonseca, S., Goodwin, W., Guyomarc'h, P., et al. (2021). The search process: Integrating the investigation and identification of missing and unidentified persons. *Forensic Science International Synergy, 3*, 100154. https://doi.org/10.1016/j.fsisyn.2021.100154.

76. Sandhi, R. K., Pickens, V., Bello, E., Elzay, S., Salgado, S., Hauri, K., Ternest, J. J., et al. (2023). Entomology beyond research and education: 2022 student debates. *Journal of Insect Science*, (23). https://doi.org/10.1093/jisesa/iead036.

77. Sansola, A. (2015). *Postmortem Iris Recognition and Its Application in Human Identification* [Master's thesis, Boston University]. https://open.bu.edu/bitstream/2144/13975/8/Sansola_bu_0017N_11536_web.pdf (accessed on 29 May 2025).

78. Singla, T., Anandayuvaraj, D., Kalu, K. G., Schorlemmer, T. R., & Davis, J. C. (2023). An empirical study on using large language models to analyze software supply chain security failures. *Proceedings of the ACM Conference*. https://doi.org/10.1145/3605770.3625214.

79. Steuer, A., Wartmann, Y., Schellenberg, R., Mantinieks, D., Glowacki, L. L., Gerostamoulos, D., Kraemer, T., et al. (2024). Postmortem metabolomics: Influence of time since death on the level of endogenous compounds in human femoral blood. Necessary to be considered in metabolome study planning? *Metabolomics, 20*. https://www.semanticscholar.org/paper/334a0d542dd8704dd0536d1d0d1d80bf53aee736 (accessed on 29 May 2025).

80. Stiles, M. K., Wilde, A. A. M., Abrams, D. J., Ackerman, M. J., Albert, C. M., Behr, E. R., Chugh, S. S., Cornel, M. C., Gardner, K., Ingles, J., James, C. A., Juang, J. M., Kääb, S., Kaufman, E. S., Krahn, A. D., Lubitz, S. A., MacLeod, H., Morillo, C. A., Nademanee, K., Probst, V., & Wang, D. W. (2021). 2020 APHRS/HRS expert consensus statement on the investigation of decedents with sudden unexplained death and patients with sudden cardiac arrest, and of their families. *Heart Rhythm, 18*(1), e1–e50. https://doi.org/10.1016/j.hrthm.2020.10.010.

81. Sun, X., Song, Z., Tang, Z., Yu, J., Fan, X., Yang, Y., Yuan, S., et al. (2024). Effects of different post-harvest processing methods on changes in the active ingredients of licorice based on LC-MS and plant metabolomics. *Phytochemical Analysis*. https://www.semanticscholar.org/paper/fa6a02c62e41fa861e466611b3952398952d54f5 (accessed on 29 May 2025).

82. Taskent, I., Başer, S., Ece, B., Kılıç, S., Akpulat, U., Cinar, I., & Sarikaş, N. (2025). Postmortem temporal changes in liver and spleen stiffness: Evaluation with shear wave elastography in a rat model. *Diagnostics*. https://www.semanticscholar.org/paper/834cb972ed26217239dad6b37fe8201e98dc96ca (accessed on 29 May 2025).

83. Turysbek, R. B., & Zhanibekov, A. K. (2024). Peculiarities of investigating the basis and significance of evidence in legal proceedings. *Eurasian Scientific Journal of Law*. https://www.semanticscholar.org/paper/c779a054cc51cc0b3f8da7f2285732fddcfd57f9 (accessed on 29 May 2025).

84. Ubelaker, D. H., & Khosrowshahi, H. (2019). Estimation of age in forensic anthropology: Historical perspective and recent methodological advances. *Forensic Sciences Research, 4*, 1–9. https://doi.org/10.1080/20961790.2018.1549711.

85. Wagensveld, I. M. (2020). *Hospital Implementation and Acceptance of Minimally Invasive Autopsy* [Doctoral dissertation, University of Amsterdam]. https://core.ac.uk/download/287757145.pdf (accessed on 29 May 2025).

86. Wallace, J., Receveur, J., Hutchinson, P. H., Kaszubinski, S. F., Wallace, H. E., & Benbow, M. (2021). Microbial community succession on submerged vertebrate carcasses in a tidal river habitat: Implications for aquatic forensic investigations. *Journal of Forensic Sciences, 66*, 2307–2318. https://www.semanticscholar.org/paper/dc0e7721620880b083eeeb4b6d3a4ac535f28cf9 (accessed on 29 May 2025).

87. Wang, Q., Wang, S., Zhu, S., Meng, S., Yu, H., & Yu, J. Z. (2024). Exploring the effect of environmental conditions on decay kinetics of aerosol unsaturated fatty acids: New insights gained from long-term ambient measurements. *Environmental Science & Technology*. https://www.semanticscholar.org/paper/ec672a1d0e3856d2f4d20b13cde3e57aeea73e9b (accessed on 29 May 2025).

88. Westling, L. (2012). *Underwater Decomposition: An Examination of Factors Surrounding Freshwater Decomposition in Eastern Massachusetts* [Master's thesis, Boston University]. https://open.bu.edu/bitstream/2144/12670/4/Westling_Lauren_2012_web.pdf (accessed on 29 May 2025).

89. Young, S. T. (2011). *RNA in Forensic Science: Novel Techniques for Biological Evidence* [Doctoral dissertation, University of Glasgow]. https://core.ac.uk/download/230456785.pdf (accessed on 29 May 2025).

90. Zuckerman, M. K., Marklein, K., Austin, R. M., & Hofman, C. A. (2024). Exercises in ethically engaged work in biological anthropology. *American Journal of Biological Anthropology*. https://www.semanticscholar.org/paper/4beea2b9e1e856b3ff8eab1f2c53a047b174b644 (accessed on 29 May 2025).

MEDICO-LEGAL AUTOPSY

6

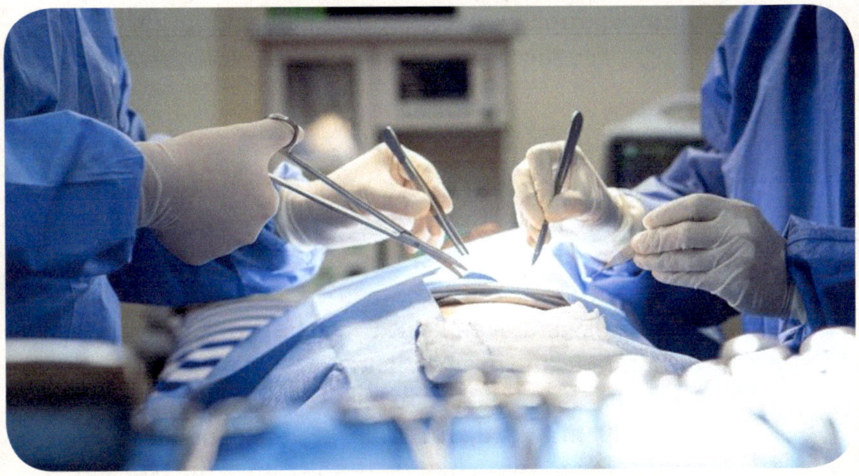

LEARNING OBJECTIVES

After studying this chapter, you will be able to:

1. Know the process of medico-legal autopsy;
2. Explain the legal implications of medico-legal autopsy;
3. Identify challenges and controversies;
4. Appreciate how medico-legal Autopsy is used in public health.

Introduction

There are times when medicine and law meet unexpectedly such as when a death is difficult to explain. A medicolegal autopsy is usually relied upon—it is used to determine what happened, mainly when there are signs of wrongdoing or mistakes in care. This process usually does two things: it unravels the medical details and also makes sure all legal requirements are met. Lately, as new tech like artificial intelligence finds its way into these procedures, extra challenges have started popping up—issues like privacy worries and ethical debates over using data (Singh et al., 2025). Even older methods, such as diatom testing in drowning scenarios, still stir up debates about how reliable or conclusive they are (Singh et al., 2025). All these aspects make it obvious that having clear standards and teamwork is very important in dealing with medicolegal autopsies.

Definition of Medico-legal Autopsy

Forensic experts are very important now, especially when there are both health and legal issues involved. A mix of medicine and law in autopsies reveals the cause of death and also helps solve legal questions about the case. They do not just use one routine; they look at what is visible and also what is hidden, checking for anything that could suggest a crime or legal problem. The COVID-19 crisis basically forced forensic science to switch gears on the fly, changing how autopsies were done and pushing stricter safety rules for everyone involved (Nunno et al., 2022). Plus, new tools like post-mortem computed tomography (PMCT) have popped up, adding fresh insights by spotting injuries that can slip past a regular exam (Arcangeli et al., 2020). To summarize, this mixed approach shows how vital these medico-legal autopsies are in defending both our community's health and its legal standards (Figure 6.1).

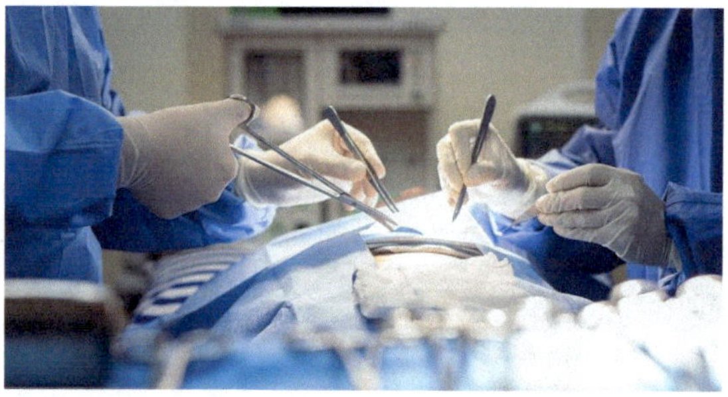

Figure 6.1. Medico-legal autopsy.

Source: https://cdn.expresshealthcare.in/wp-content/uploads/2019/12/03141319/surgery-750x396.jpg.

Importance in the Legal System

Lately, medicine and law are working more closely together, mainly in investigating deaths. Medico-legal autopsies are not simply tests, but an important source of evidence for handling legal cases when the cause of death is unclear. Most of the time, finding out the cause and manner of death can confirm or contradict what is said in the courtroom which can result in big changes. Some recent research even nudges us to dig deeper into how medico-legal evidence works, like looking at how medical cues are read inside legal debates (Renzi et al., 2007). A study from Nepal, for instance, shows that while people often speak positively about these autopsies, there's still a lot of uncertainty about what they actually try to accomplish (Chudal et al., 2018). When medicine and law work together, they perfect the law and gradually help people trust autopsies as an important legal resource.

Historical Background

Medicine and law have been intertwined since ancient times. In the early days, forensic work leaned on very basic methods; yet a look at late imperial China shows that coroners, legal officials, and even literati-officials once handled examinations in surprisingly refined ways (Asen et al., 2012). Over time, as these practices slowly matured, forensic genetics ushered in transformative changes—shifting from simple blood group antigen tests to newer, more intricate molecular techniques—which, in most cases, improved the accuracy, and dependability of medico-legal autopsy findings over the past century (Kozma et al., 2018). Many scientific discoveries and law changes became linked as time passed and this helped investigations and changed society's view of justice and accountability in the law. Medico-legal autopsy has shown, in its own history, how important it has been for medical and legal knowledge to come together.

Overview of the Process

The autopsy helps to reveal the reason and way someone died by looking closely at the body. After all the legal procedures are done, the pathologist starts by examining the body's outside, noting down any marks, injuries or signs that something may be wrong. In many cases, checking delicate areas, like the mouth which, frankly, can be a real pain when rigor mortis sets in Roy et al. (2021), requires not only the right tools but a fair bit of ingenuity. After that, the examiner goes inside to see if everything matches up with the first suspicions which can be just as important as it is hard to predict. Odd anatomical quirks—say, a sternal foramen—might sometimes be mistaken for signs of trauma (Singh et al., 2022), so there's a natural need for caution. To summarize, the mix of detailed dissection, up-close visual checks, and even radiographic analysis (when it seems necessary) collectively builds a case that underpins the entire forensic investigation.

Key Stakeholders Involved

Many people with different roles come together in a medico-legal autopsy and their contributions are usually essential. For example, forensic pathologists inspect the bodies and determine the cause of death which usually guides all the other actions.

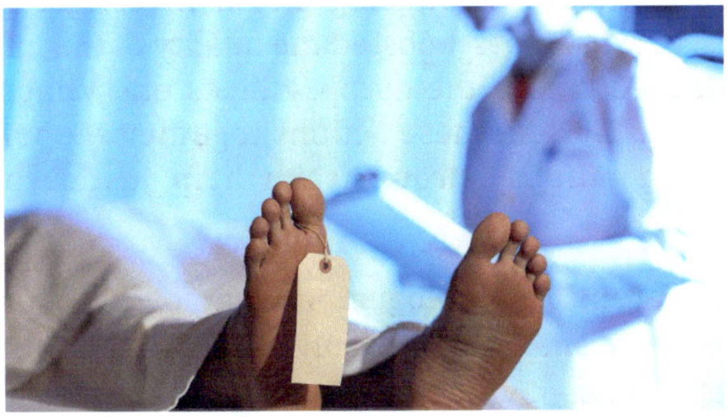

Figure 6.2. Forensic pathologists lead the charge by examining bodies and figuring out the cause of death; their work, quite often, sets the tone for everything that follows.

Source: https://cdn.hswstatic.com/gif/body-autopsy.jpg.

Then police or investigators collect evidence and make sure the chain of custody is not broken which is very important for legal reasons. There are also prosecutors and defense attorneys, who interpret the results of the autopsy in terms of the crime. Family members are involved in the story, even if their part sometimes seems less important than the main characters. In recent chats about advancing forensic methods, people have noted that innovative imaging technologies are starting to boost how accurately investigations are carried out (Villa et al., 2024). And, in many cases, when ethical and human rights questions crop up—especially around prisoner deaths—public health experts are brought into the conversation, typically aiming to stop similar tragedies from happening again (Tomczak et al., 2023) (Figure 6.2).

Ethical Considerations

Medico-legal autopsies are more complicated than they seem; besides knowing the technical part, you must be familiar with the ethical aspects in both practice and teaching. A lot of medical students start out with the belief that the human body is sacred which often makes them feel uncomfortable about doing autopsies. In most cases, research shows that—even if these students understand the basic goal of forensic postmortem exams—they still trip up when it comes to the legal and procedural side of things, which points to a clear gap in what they're being taught (Maqsood et al., 2024). Plus, the medico-legal realm can be a real minefield, because mistakes in diagnosis sometimes lead to serious fallout—not only hurting patient outcomes but also throwing healthcare professionals into legal trouble too (Albano et al., 2024). It is clear then that updating our teaching methods for these issues is necessary to ensure future practitioners are ready for the complexities of forensic pathology and that the field upholds respect and integrity.

Differences from Clinical Autopsy

Investigating strange deaths usually reveals that the work done for legal reasons is very different from normal clinical checks. In cases like sudden cardiac stoppages, the exam must dig deeper than usual—often, the lack of earlier health records only makes it trickier, especially when strange genetic hints such as variants in the PRKAG2 gene Ariza et al. (2024) come into play. It's interesting how things like a duplex kidney—an anomaly that might slip by in a standard checkup—suddenly matter a lot in legal investigations by pointing out pre-existing conditions that could tip the scales in court (Bhargava et al., 2024). Generally, all of these details stress that medico-legal autopsies are designed to address both medical and legal questions about a death.

6.1. The Process of Medico-Legal Autopsy

Learning Outcome

1. Perform initial investigation and scene assessment;
2. Collection of evidence;
3. Examination of the body;
4. Discuss documentation and photography;
5. Explain toxicology testing;
6. Focus on histopathological analysis;
7. Describe report writing and findings;
8. Understand communication with law enforcement.

In forensic science, nothing is ever quite straightforward. An autopsy can often find clues about what happened to the person before they died which can be important for legal cases. Even so, things can be very complicated; decomposition is a big problem for forensic pathologists, especially when parts of the body decay at various rates, making it harder to understand what happened. At times, mixing other fields—like forensic entomology and histopathology—is generally necessary to sort through this confusion (Ambica et al., 2024). And then there's anatomy itself: small quirks such as a sternal foramen may sometimes be misread as gunshot wounds, so knowing these oddities is pretty important (Singh et al., 2022). Being very careful and paying attention to every detail is most important, since that's what helps an autopsy fully explain the death.

6.1.1. Initial Investigation and Scene Assessment

Starting with a good examination of the scene is very important, especially during a medico-legal autopsy. Initially, forensic experts examine a crime or suspicious death site which helps them do a better analysis and interpretation later on. Forensic doctors, pathologists and at times coroners cooperate to collect evidence that could alter the outcome of the case. Generally speaking, the European Council of Legal Medicine suggests a step-by-step inspection process; they offer detailed pointers on how to gather evidence, keep records, and even recommend that different experts, like anthropologists and toxicologists, pitch in (Anzillotti et al., 2022). In places facing bigger systemic troubles, like South Africa, introducing Death Investigators has, in most cases, boosted the quality of the info gathered before the autopsy kicks off (Villiers et al., 2020). All these actions together support a solid autopsy process and help justice be achieved.

Forensic pathologists are important from the first scene check, not only during the autopsy. Many times, by noticing the environment and available clues, we can understand better what happened to the person. In one striking case, an expert found that a death, nonviolent in nature, was linked to cavernous tuberculosis—a connection revealed after a detailed look at the scene (Crisan, 2019). In many cases, though, when deaths turn violent—as you might see with mechanical asphyxia—the role of these experts becomes even more crucial in piecing together the messy details (Rathnaweera, 2016). In general, their thoughts help the judicial system understand the situation better, especially as trauma and illness often overlap. Ultimately, mixing autopsy results with the firsthand observations of a forensic pathologist shapes our overall grasp of these key medico-legal cases (Figure 6.3).

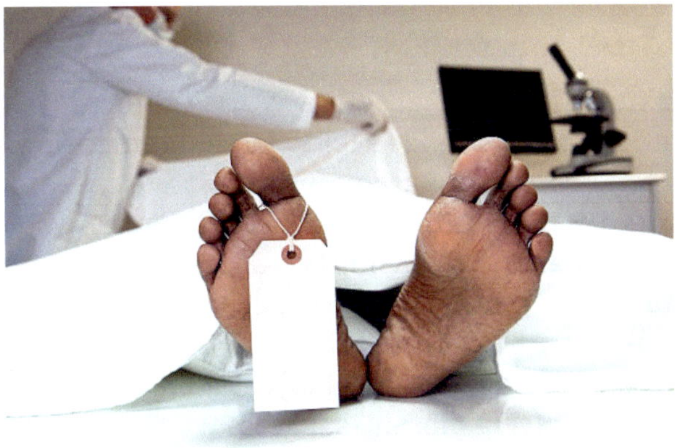

Figure 6.3. A careful look at the surroundings and available clues can give us a clearer idea of what led to a person's death.

Source: https://media.istockphoto.com/id/173056887/photo/mortician-coroner-covering-dead-body-in-morgue-feet-toe-tag.jpg?s=612x612&w=0&k=20&c=nZmVLRBim79NEbyNkrh8Hbu2tQUZMtjNKdOvAqsWs30=.

6.1.2. Collection of Evidence

Since a medico-legal autopsy helps to find out the cause of death, it must be done with great care. The way blood, tissue or hair is found can have a big impact on the rest of the forensic investigation. Many people say that if the environment is not perfectly clean and organized, even the most advanced DNA tests can give unclear results which highlights the importance of sample collection. And yes, contamination isn't just a minor worry—especially with decayed remains, it can seriously throw off the dependability of the findings (Argo et al., 2019). Ultimately, solid evidence collection not only backs up potential malpractice claims but also boosts quality checks during procedures in forensic pathology, trimming down the chances of deaths that might have been avoided (Argo et al., 2019) (Figure 6.4).

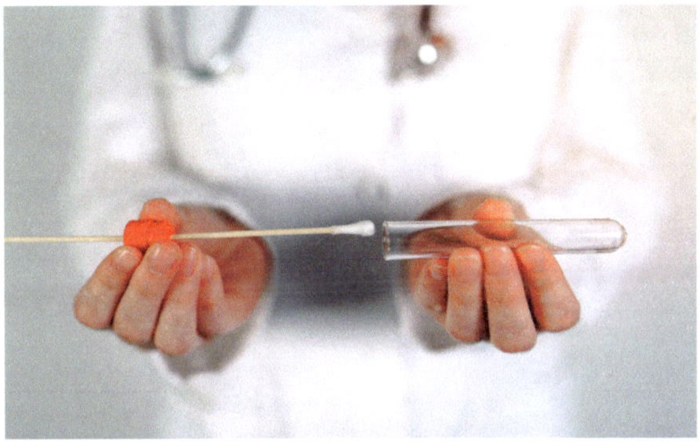

Figure 6.4. The way biological samples like blood, tissue, or hair come out can majorly sway what follows in a forensic investigation.

Source: https://dbgp98ysvt3y0.cloudfront.net/blog/SvdV7Nnt6F3Xta87tlIiQHOy3EIPDPX1yQ6AJJv1.jpg.

6.1.3. Examination of the Body

Finding out the cause of death usually involves a careful examination of the body during a medico-legal autopsy which is especially necessary in questionable cases. Being careful when collecting and examining biological samples is important, since their state can strongly affect the forensic results; usually, having good quality samples is very important. The way samples are taken changes greatly when comparing a living person with a deceased person, so using the correct methods is very important. The body's condition or exposure to the environment can limit your options which adds difficulty to the process. Getting reliable evidence—think blood, soft tissues, and other remains—mostly depends on sticking to strict, well-practiced protocols to dodge contamination and keep results trustworthy (Kozma et al., 2018). Overall, this broad yet detail-oriented approach generally shows us just how critical examining the body is in the bigger picture of medico-legal investigations (Valck et al., 2011) (Figure 6.5).

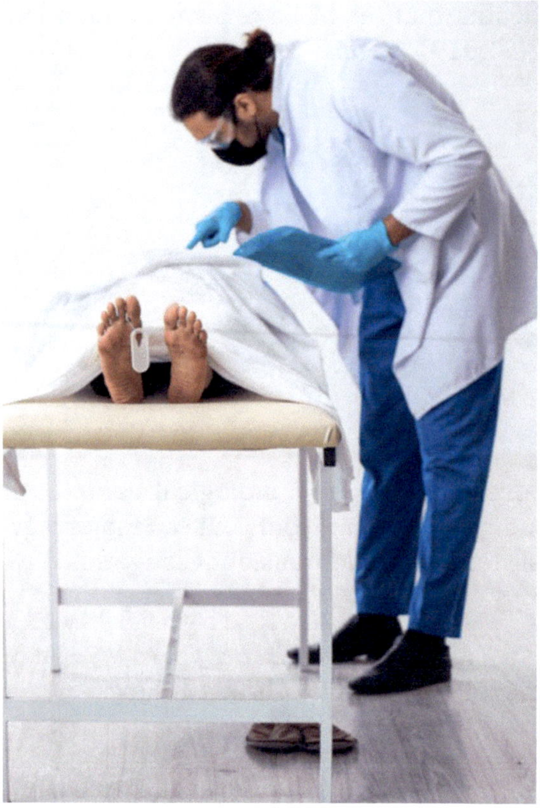

Figure 6.5. Examination of the body.

Source: https://www.shutterstock.com/image-photo/police-coroner-examining-dead-body-600nw-1736119679.jpg.

6.1.4. Documentation and Photography

The records from a medico-legal autopsy matter because they both describe findings and support them in court. Photos taken often do not show the fine details of human anatomy which can make important evidence hard to understand. Some people are now using 3D models instead of traditional images which often brings together technology and everyday life. When LiDAR is used in an autopsy, it produces detailed and repeatable 3D scans that make the entire process better, although it can feel like a big change from the usual way. The new way of examining autopsies allows experts to see more details which helps them make better forensic conclusions. In many cases, mixing these modern approaches could shake up how medico-legal documentation is handled, plugging gaps left behind by traditional methods (Ciallella et al., 2022; Larraguibel et al., 2023).

6.1.5. Toxicology Testing

Toxicology tests are now very important in understanding the events of a medico-legal autopsy. New research on near-body screening tests is suggesting that there are other ways to do toxicology. In many cases, these newer methods line up quite well with the tried-and-true liquid chromatography coupled with mass spectrometry (LC-MS) (Hansmeyer et al., 2016), which generally suggests we might boost diagnostic accuracy in forensic work. At the same time, the field's eye on sudden cardiac death has led to innovative ideas that start uncovering hidden contributing factors (Basso et al., 2017). To summarize, pushing forward toxicology testing not only makes investigations run smoother but also tackles legal and public health issues, steadily raising the bar for forensic pathology (Figure 6.6).

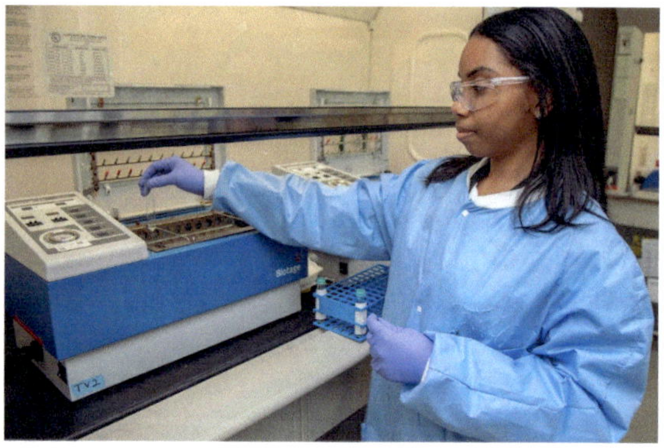

Figure 6.6. Toxicology tests now play a big role in figuring out what happened in medico-legal autopsies.

Source: https://media.defense.gov/2023/Dec/08/2003354945/1280/1280/0/191031-F-BH656-1008C.JPG.

6.1.6. Histopathological Analysis

If it is thought that a crime might have taken place, looking at tissue samples is a very important part of the investigation. They look at these samples to spot any signs of trauma or disease and also to put together a basic timeline of the events that led to the person's death. Many times, forensic tests can make clear injuries that were not originally visible which can help or contradict the assumed reasons for someone's death. For example, when a body is buried, the analysis could show signs of blunt force trauma or asphyxiation which are then related to the rest of the case. Generally speaking, mixing modern techniques with old-school histology tends to boost the accuracy of these findings, which can sway judicial outcomes and clarify the messy dynamics of a case, as highlighted in detailed forensic reports (Berloco et al., 2024; Faur et al., 2021).

6.1.7. Report Writing and Findings

Medico-legal autopsy is more than just checking boxes; it uses various ways to find out the true cause of a death. One study showed that postmortem computed tomography (PMCT)—a modern scan technique—matched up about 92% with traditional dissection autopsies when they looked at custodial torture cases in Karachi jails (Khan et al., 2010). Then there's another look at iatrogenic deaths in Finland: roughly 75% of those cases went through a full medico-legal autopsy, which helped clear up how the death actually happened (Kuvaja et al., 2022). Using high-tech imaging and detailed studies of tissue usually helps separate the confusing elements of a case. This kind of framework helps identify what causes deaths and also supports a bigger discussion about patient safety and medical responsibility. To summarize, even if it's not flawless, this mix of old and new methods brings a refreshingly human touch to forensic investigations (Figure 6.7).

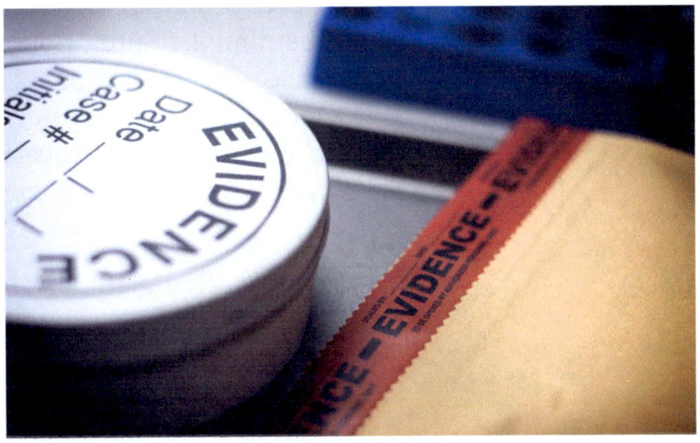

Figure 6.7. Medico-legal autopsy work isn't just about ticking off boxes—it mixes different investigative methods to shed light on the real story behind a death.

Source: https://murderpolicepodcast.com/wp-content/uploads/2022/01/files-and-evidence-bag-in-a-crime-lab-conceptual-2021-10-13-19-33-16-utc-scaled.jpg.

6.1.8. Communication with Law Enforcement

In many difficult cases, forensic experts and police join forces. The COVID-19 pandemic is a good example - the usual ways of doing things no longer work when everything is disrupted. Forensic specialists communicate with law enforcement a lot which helps investigations continue smoothly and safely. Take body handling for instance; when it comes to dealing with the deceased, folks need to be crystal clear about risks like those from post-mortem exams, which can sometimes generate aerosols (Shrestha et al., 2021). The safety of the forensic team is important, but police officers who may be exposed to danger are involved as well. Generally speaking, figuring out how the pandemic messes with forensic work, such as the scramble for personal protective gear, calls for careful coordination (Esposito et al., 2022). In short, when these groups are honest with each other, even if the exchange is not always perfect, it greatly helps ensure safety and trust in medico-legal investigations.

Test Your Knowledge

1. What is a medico-legal autopsy?
2. Who is legally authorized to perform a medico-legal autopsy?

6.2. Legal Implications of Medico-Legal Autopsy

Learning Outcome

1. Explain the role in criminal investigations;
2. Discuss use in civil litigation;
3. Focus on the chain of custody;
4. Describe the admissibility of autopsy findings in court;
5. Analyze expert testimony;
6. Know the impact on legal outcomes;
7. Learn privacy concerns and family rights;
8. Explain ethical dilemmas in legal contexts;
9. Learn case studies illustrating legal implications.

Death investigations rarely follow a neat, predictable path. Problems with the law can happen when an autopsy is not performed correctly. A case where a 70-year-old man's death was first thought to be accidental could be used as an example. That early mistake meant no proper forensic exam took place—and in most cases, that oversight delayed uncovering clear signs of foul play (Campobasso et al., 2015). It proves that if any step is overlooked in an autopsy, it can disrupt the process, prevent justice and make the law unclear. Using biological evidence also brings certain difficulties. The reliability of statistics depends a lot on the proper collection and management of samples. If the collection spot isn't kept in tip-top shape, even top-notch forensic DNA tests might falter, potentially skewing criminal case outcomes (Kozma et al., 2018). All in all, if medico-legal autopsies are not done with great care, the whole process of seeking justice and following the law may fail.

6.2.1. Role in Criminal Investigations

In criminal investigations, autopsies are very important because they help explain the circumstances of a person's death. Examinations are used by law enforcement to find important clues which may reveal wrongdoing or carelessness. Take, for example, the challenge of dealing with healthcare-associated infections (HAIs) during an autopsy; such infections can blur our understanding of the decedent's health before death and, generally speaking, force investigators to use in-depth methods like histopathological tests paired with microbiological swabs. On the legal side, things aren't always straightforward; family consent issues and statutory rules often add extra layers of complication, yet in many cases, investigators may press ahead with an autopsy when it's deemed essential for justice (Isnaeni, 2024). Ultimately, a medico-legal autopsy not only shines a light on the circumstances surrounding a death but also bolsters the integrity of the overall investigation—helping to ensure that conclusions drawn are both reliable and, well, actionable (Figure 6.8).

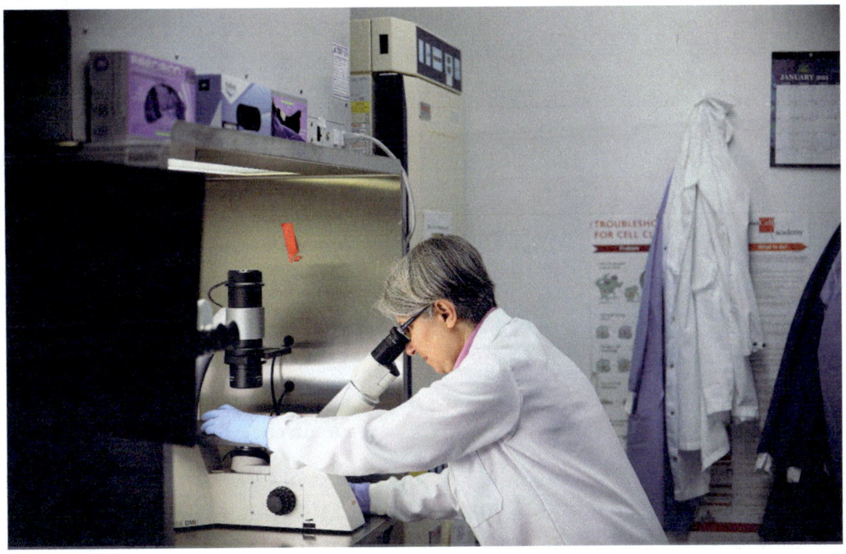

Figure 6.8. Autopsies play a key role in criminal investigations—they're the breakthrough tool that helps unravel what happened when someone dies.

Source: https://www.statnews.com/wp-content/uploads/2023/01/ManaParast_055.jpg.

6.2.2. Use in Civil Litigation

Autopsy reports are usually important pieces of evidence that can change the outcome of a trial. They examine the day-to-day aspects of care such as the treatments used and how they were given and this can show cases of negligence or errors that others may not notice. One study, for example, looked into hospital claim records and found that when you sort through medical events in less expected ways, hidden malpractice issues start becoming clearer, which then helps shape practical improvement plans and guides smarter resource use (Fazio et al., 2023). Paying attention to patterns in poisoning cases—whether they seem like accidents or lean toward intentional self-harm—also builds the groundwork for arguments about who's responsible, stressing why it's so important to collect as much data as possible in these medico-legal scenarios (Dhara, 2023).

6.2.3. Chain of Custody

Evidence preservation is non-negotiable, especially in medico-legal autopsies. The main idea that keeps all evidence safe and pure during an investigation is called the chain of custody. Because of technology, we now have to pay close attention to every single action from the crime scene to the courtroom. Usually, the people working on these tasks are required to follow well-known procedures since small mistakes can seriously reduce the value of the evidence. Nowadays, as digital data gains more weight, setting up internationally accepted guidelines is pretty essential to maintain forensic standards in both the physical and electronic realms (Can et al., 2014; D'Anna et al., 2023) (Figure 6.9).

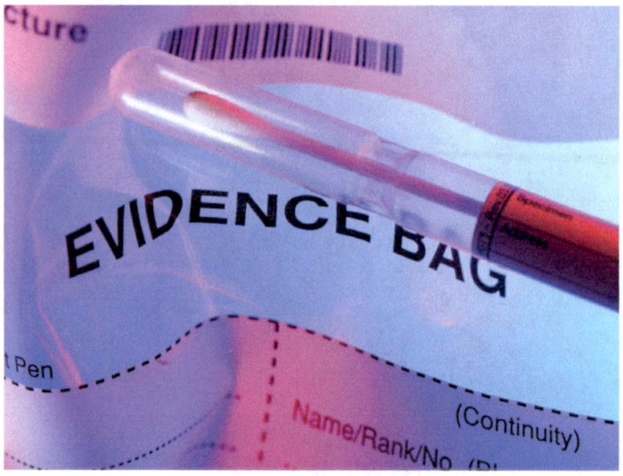

Figure 6.9. Chain of custody.

Source: https://www.thoughtco.com/thmb/8k6FFjuXsmNi-lui3oBS2ODlGKI=/1500x0/filters:no_upscale():max_bytes(150000):strip_icc()/bag-5c8909b5c9e77c0001f2ad4f.jpg.

6.2.4. Admissibility of Autopsy Findings in Court

There are many times when forensic science and law get mixed and this is especially true when autopsy results are presented in court. Autopsy results are often central to a criminal investigation when death seems suspicious or unnatural. Courts use these reports to determine how someone died, look for signs of trauma and sometimes suggest if a crime took place, but their usefulness depends on being done step by step. Sometimes, if evidence is mishandled or even misinterpreted—say, in cases that require examination—it can end up being ruled inadmissible, which then throws a serious wrench into the pursuit of justice (Khurshid et al., 2021). On another front, innovative ideas like using 3D printing to showcase autopsy details are being explored as a way to help jurors get a better grip on the evidence while still keeping in line with legal norms (Carew et al., 2022). Overall, whether autopsy findings stick in court remains a major issue in medico-legal matters, continuously shaped by evolving forensic practices and ongoing judicial oversight (Figure 6.10).

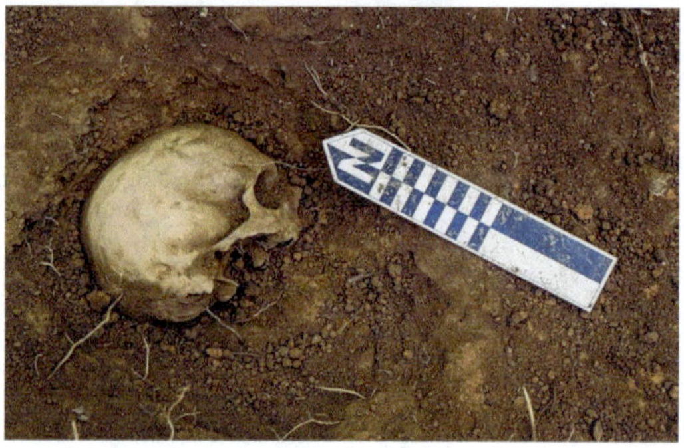

Figure 6.10. Forensic science and law often mix in ways that aren't so cut-and-dry—especially when autopsy findings get pulled into court.

Source: https://undark.org/wp-content/uploads/2019/10/Skull2-e1573062396605.jpg.

6.2.5. Expert Testimony

Expert testimony is very important in investigating difficult death cases. Consider a situation where a 70-year-old man was first ruled an accidental death simply because a quick check missed some clear stab wounds (Campobasso et al., 2015). It is obvious that the experience and knowledge of forensic examiners play a big role—if they lack proper training in autopsy, key details could be missed. Voices from victims, doctors, and other parties often jumble together, painting a messy picture that, in many cases, is further complicated by denial and even state-inflicted violence (Can et al., 2014). Most of the time, the input of experts is vital in making sure investigations are thorough, honest and based on real medical facts. By being so involved, officials ensure better legal results and help increase public trust in our justice system.

6.2.6. Impact on Legal Outcomes

Sometimes when surgery ends in death, the autopsy results play a big role in legal matters. For example, if a review of coronary bypass procedures reveals that sudden problems with grafts caused patients' hearts to fail—this seems to have contributed greatly to the high number of deaths. Autopsy reports even hinted that nearly half of those who died were plagued by graft problems that went unnoticed during treatment; investigators uncovered these clues using both traditional methods and newer approaches like postmortem cast angiography (Karhunen et al., 2010). Examining a body after death can show mistakes in medical care that may affect the outcome of malpractice cases. In most cases, using advanced imaging in these investigations can further sharpen diagnostic accuracy—a crucial step when figuring out liability in clinical errors (Zinno et al., 2018). To summarize, medico-legal autopsies not only help explain medical failures, they also end up reshaping the legal landscape around malpractice and patient safety (Figure 6.11).

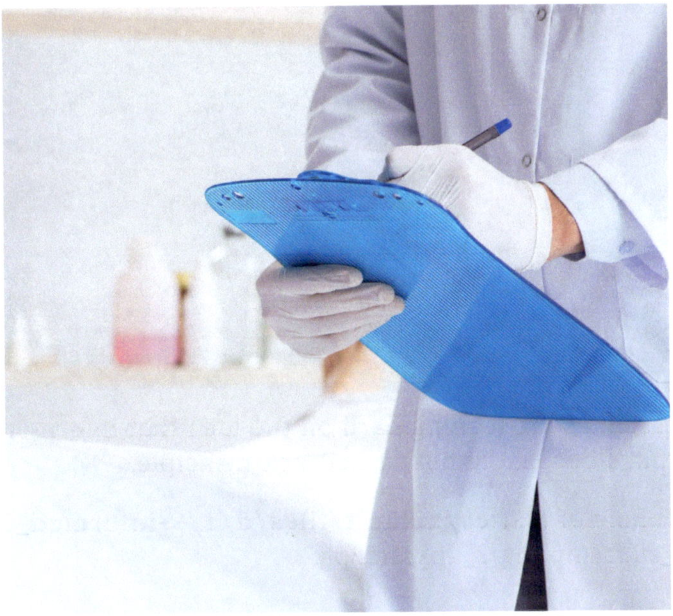

Figure 6.11. Autopsy reports.

Source: https://jp4.mctx.org/wp-content/uploads/2021/01/autopsy-reports.jpg.

6.2.7. Privacy Concerns and Family Rights

The concerns of privacy and family rights in medico-legal autopsies are not always in agreement. When someone in a family passes away, they usually face both grief and the confusing rules and paperwork around post-mortem privacy. New tech, like AI-driven Patient Preference Predictors, pops up unexpectedly; while such tools can help sort out tough decisions, they also tend to put patient autonomy and data security on shaky ground (Refolo et al., 2025). In multidisciplinary team meetings, things can get even murkier as debates over informed consent sometimes leave families unclear about who's allowed to see which bits of medical data or join in on decision-making (Mahani et al., 2024). All in all, it is very important to manage these factors to maintain trust between families and healthcare providers during a hard time.

6.2.8. Ethical Dilemmas in Legal Contexts

It is obvious that handling human remains for a medico-legal autopsy involves many difficult ethical and legal questions. In the past, taking bodies for scientific purposes often meant body snatching which clearly went against consent and respect for the dead; in general, these early methods made a lot of people doubt if respect was ever considered. Today, most professionals are leaning hard on the idea that informed consent should be the rule of thumb, a point that's become almost a bedrock principle (Jones et al., 2011). And now, with new tech like 3D printing stepping into forensic labs, fresh debates pop up about issues such as anonymity, personal autonomy, and the simple concept of not causing harm (Carew et al., 2023). All of this suggests that we should have more flexible rules that focus on ethics and also support strong forensic practices. Ultimately, navigating this ethical maze is crucial for anyone in the medico-legal field—it's key to ensuring that respect for the deceased sticks around even as scientific practices move forward (Figure 6.12).

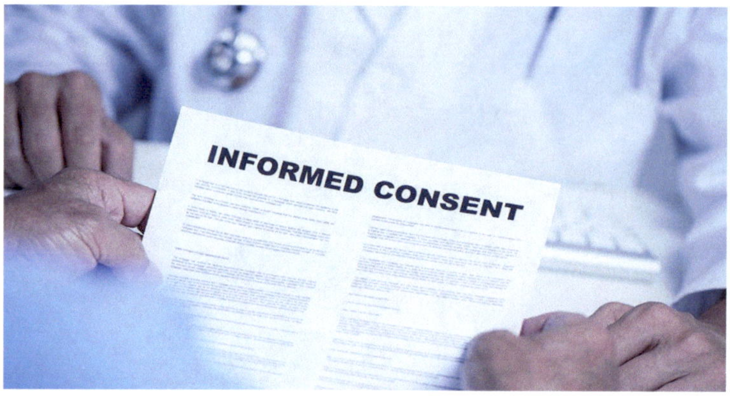

Figure 6.12. Most professionals are leaning hard on the idea that informed consent should be the rule of thumb, a point that's become almost a bedrock principle.

Source: https://www.aamc.org/sites/default/files/d/1/9-informed_consent_redboxxmain.jpg__992x558_q85_crop_subsampling-2_upscale.jpg.

6.2.9. Case Studies Illustrating Legal Implications

Medico-legal autopsies tend to bring up many medical and legal issues. An example is a murder case in South Korea—the victim had no visible symptoms despite having a lot of nicotine in their system which raised questions about how the poisoning could have happened. This kind of case generally shows just how important solid scientific testing is for legal matters; forensic clues end up being key in supporting convictions (Yoo et al., 2024). Healthcare-associated infections also add to the problem—it is necessary to find out how and where the infection started to decide on liability. All in all, these cases suggest that sometimes the details of forensic work can have a subtle impact on the outcomes of court cases.

Test Your Knowledge

1. Under what circumstances is a medico-legal autopsy legally mandated?
2. Can the family's consent be ignored for a medico-legal autopsy? Explain.

6.3. Challenges and Controversies

Learning Outcome

1. Understand variability in autopsy practices;
2. Explain the misinterpretation of the findings;
3. Knowing public perception and media influence;
4. Focus on resource limitations in forensic facilities;
5. Discuss cultural and religious considerations;
6. Know the role of technology in autopsy;
7. Identify training and education of forensic professionals;
8. Addressing biases in autopsy conclusions;
9. Understand future directions for improvement.

There are many difficulties in performing medico-legal autopsies and it seems that problems and disputes keep arising. A big issue is how forensic work gets mixed up with public health concerns—take, for example, those unexpectedly high SIDS rates in places like Cape Town that point to the urgent need for routine autopsy methods (Dempers et al., 2016). Then there's the whole matter of epilepsy treatments; you see, antiepileptic drugs sometimes behave quite aggressively, which, in many cases, ends up muddying the waters when it comes to making a clear diagnosis during autopsies (Brodie et al., 2016). It can be difficult at times, since all these complexities can make it tricky to find justice and lead to debates on if our current methods are adequate and if medical examiners are behaving ethically. In short, dealing with these issues is very important for making sure medico-legal autopsies are reliable and useful in many situations.

6.3.1. Variability in Autopsy Practices

It is often challenging to determine how a person died and this can show how different autopsy approaches are in different places. Local habits, different legal standards and the abilities of those doing the exams make each situation different. In most cases, debates about brain death—an issue that's been talked about a lot lately—seem to suffer from a lack of consistent standards and might even spark ethical concerns when it comes to organ donations (Kellehear et al., 2009). Historical accounts, too, remind us that the line between an autopsy and a dissection tends to blur, which can throw off the way skeletal findings are understood (Vanni et al., 2024). All these obstacles make it harder for pathologists and can weaken faith in the medico-legal system and legal duties. When you look at it all, there's an ever-growing push for clear and steady guidelines—ones that keep autopsy results honest and help the whole system deliver justice (Figure 6.13).

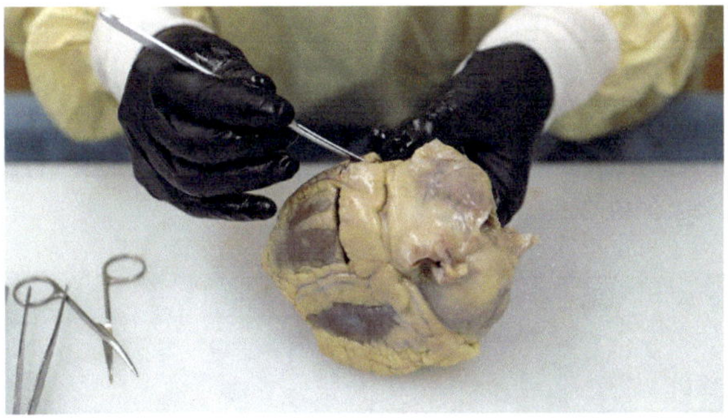

Figure 6.13. Figuring out how someone died is never simple—it often reveals just how different autopsy practices can be from one region to another.

Source: https://undark.org/wp-content/uploads/2020/10/covid_autopsy-scaled.jpg.

6.3.2. Misinterpretation of Findings

Mistakes in reading autopsy results can lead to major changes in both forensic analysis and the law. Generally speaking, when experts rely only on neuropathological exams, they sometimes mix up traumatic axonal injury (TAI) with vascular axonal injury (VAI), which might lead to an incorrect diagnosis of axonal injury (AI). Recent injuries often come with clues like a subdural hemorrhage, so a little extra care is needed—otherwise, there's a risk of wrongly pinning down the cause or how the injury happened (Narayan et al., 2025). Take, for instance, a postoperative patient who developed a pseudoaneurysm; it was first observed by imaging but only later verified during an autopsy, a slip-up that shows why it's so important to line up autopsy results with clinical data to avoid misleading legal conclusions (Pelletti et al., 2025). It is usually very important to get these details correct to ensure both the forensic process and justice remain intact.

6.3.3. Public Perception and Media Influence

Cultural views and medical practices often blend which can influence how people see medico-legal autopsies. Because Islam plays a big role in daily life in Pakistan, the concept of doing a post-mortem exam leads to many debates about ethics, as the legal rules often clash with religious beliefs.

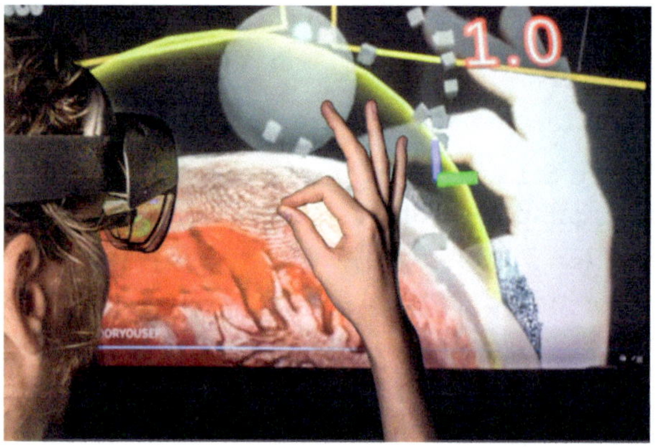

Figure 6.14. Cultural beliefs and everyday medical practices mix together in ways that can change how people view medico-legal autopsies.

Source: https://liu.se/dfsmedia/dd35e243dfb-7406993c1815aaf88a675/71531-50063/viir-tuell-obduktion-2023-06-12-tb-dsg6414.

This clash tends to spark suspicion and even fear about the procedure, even though these examinations play a key role in figuring out why someone passed away and in boosting medical progress (Cassum et al., 2014).

At the same moment, media stories may exaggerate events which only increases confusion and stigma. It's crucial for medico-legal experts to get a handle on these complicated, and sometimes messy, dynamics as they navigate issues of public trust, healthcare practices, and ethical dilemmas—especially when dealing with sepsis tied to hospital infections, where autopsy findings might just inform better risk management and guide clinical updates (Cassum et al., 2014) (Figure 6.14).

6.3.4. Resource Limitations in Forensic Facilities

Forensic labs that do not have enough resources can cause many problems with medico-legal autopsies. Besides missing or underperforming equipment, there are not enough experienced people to handle things which makes toxicology tests take longer and slows down case processing. You can see this firsthand in the Forensic Chemistry Laboratory (FCL), where backlogs not only slow down justice but also create messy legal outcomes and community frustration (Hansmeyer et al., 2016).

Rapid changes in forensic radiography seem to hint, in most cases, that bringing in new technology mixed with some fresh standard practices might ease these burdens (Viner et al., 2020). Mostly speaking, if labs improve their training and review their daily routines, their diagnostic abilities could improve. In short, dealing with these issues is very important for ensuring the whole autopsy process works well and remains sound.

6.3.5. Cultural and Religious Considerations

When you add various cultural and religious beliefs to medico-legal autopsies, unexpected ethical issues may occur. In several communities, the idea of not separating the body is very important which makes some traditional surgeries seem inappropriate. For many faiths, respecting the body is very important, so an autopsy might be viewed as a violation. The different ideas about death and what follows make it harder for families to accept the need for an autopsy. Take South Africa: the Inquests Act 58 of 1959 gives a lot of freedom to those in charge of autopsies, yet it still sparks debates about balancing these cultural sensitivities with what the law demands (Singh et al., 2021). Plus, medical education, all too often, skirts around these cultural layers, subtly shifting how students view and engage with forensic medicine (McNamee et al., 2007).

6.3.6. The Role of Technology in Autopsy

Technology has pushed autopsy practices in unexpected directions. Experts can now use virtual autopsy and CT scans to inspect bodies closely without always cutting them which helps keep the body's natural features intact. AI has also joined the mix, generally helping in analysis, spotting odd changes, and even highlighting patterns; algorithms sometimes step in to estimate post-mortem intervals and aid forensic identification, which can trim down human error and bias (Piraianu et al., 2023). The COVID-19 crisis, in most cases, forced forensic teams to adjust their methods, relying on these tech tools to keep things safe and efficient, a shift that shows just how vital modern technology has become in autopsy work (Esposito et al., 2022) (Figure 6.15).

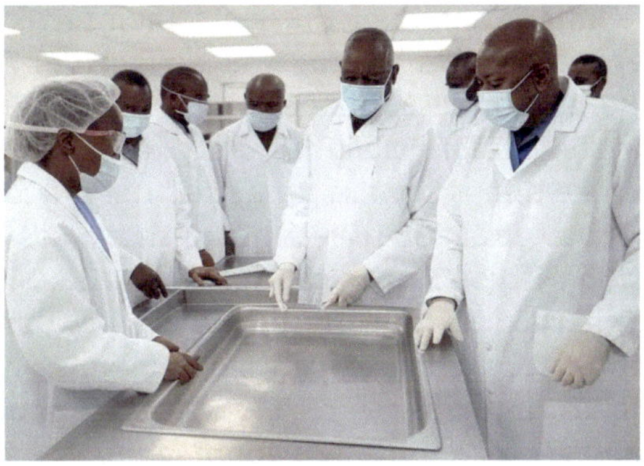

Figure 6.15. Forensic science keeps changing these days, and solid training for those working in the field is becoming a must.

Source: https://thekenyatimes.com/wp-content/uploads/2025/02/image-4.jpg.webp.

6.3.7. Training and Education of Forensic Professionals

These days, forensic science is always evolving which means those working in it must have strong training. With the COVID-19 crisis emerging, people had to adjust quickly which made having both old and new skills necessary. Experts doing medico-legal autopsies now have to mix a deep knowledge of traditional techniques with the latest practices, like proper infection prevention (it's kind of a balancing act). Practices differ a lot from one country or legal system to another, and you can see that in how forensic reports vary with their legal fallout (Meilia et al., 2018); generally speaking, there's a growing push for more standardized training that leans on evidence, smart thinking, and clear communication. To summarize, a well-rounded education is key to keeping consistency and quality in forensic work (Esposito et al., 2022).

6.3.8. Addressing Biases in Autopsy Conclusions

Autopsy findings can be very difficult; people's biases can easily affect the outcome of legal cases. How the evidence is interpreted is usually more important than the facts themselves in determining if a death was an accident or deliberate. In cases like severe poisoning, for example, factors such as drug dependence often tilt things toward an accidental outcome (Bjornaas et al., 2010)—a detail that's easy to overlook if you're not careful. With kids, it is often harder to know if injuries are accidental or not, because biases can make us miss real, inflicted injuries. Forensic experts should usually use a step-by-step approach to examine evidence, so their own opinions do not influence the results. In short, handling these biases is crucial for ensuring medicolegal autopsies are accurate and fair.

6.3.9. Future Directions for Improvement

Medico-legal autopsies are changing these days and it's obvious that new approaches could make them more effective. Experts are now mixing methods from other areas which is helping us better understand health, sickness and the many small things that lead to death. This kind of mix, which you can see hints at the ideas in Ruberg et al. (2023), brings in social, economic, and cultural angles that sit at the heart of medical work. Usually, considering ethical matters based on cultural and religious customs, mainly within Islamic societies, makes the rules for post-mortem exams appear much more detailed. Research noted in Azizet al. (2023) suggests that when we tackle these moral aspects, we not only pay proper respect to the deceased and their families, but we also help build trust between communities and medical professionals. In short, applying these approaches may make medico-legal autopsies more relevant and helpful to people in our society.

Test Your Knowledge

1. What are the usual difficulties that come up during a medico-legal autopsy?
2. What effect does poor preservation of bodies have on the dependability of autopsy results?

6.4. The Role of Medico-Legal Autopsy in Public Health

Learning Outcome

1. Learn contribution to epidemiology;
2. Identification of public health trends;
3. Explain the role in preventing future deaths;
4. Know collaboration with health organizations;
5. Discuss the impact on policy-making;
6. Focus on education and awareness initiatives;
7. Learn case studies of public health interventions;
8. Explain the importance of data collection and analysis;
9. Identify future challenges in public health integration.

Forensic science and public health come together in medico-legal autopsies, giving a clear view of mortality and disease patterns. Usually, when there is a global crisis like COVID-19, autopsies are used in ways that were not expected before to help with new health problems and collect essential epidemiological data. For example, forensic teams have taken on the task of looking into how long SARSCoV2 RNA sticks around in bodies after death, an effort that generally ends up feeding valuable clues back into public health planning (Nunno et al., 2022). At times, newer analytic frameworks like Bayesian networks are thrown into the mix to demystify post-mortem drug levels, which can tweak mortality stats in ways that might affect future health policies (Bolton et al., 2015). While helping families, these autopsies also give us important findings that help us improve public health.

6.4.1. Contribution to Epidemiology

Thorough autopsies subtly help us understand changes in diseases and public health issues. In a bustling city like Kanpur—where the population grows almost overnight and urban challenges come in droves—the frequent cases of fatal poisoning seem to offer raw hints about the economic and social troubles behind them (Bajpai et al., 2017). Usually, researchers look into these events, connecting bits of information to notice patterns that could stop similar disasters in the future. In the same way, unexpected cases like cardiac cysticercosis, which too often slip by unnoticed amidst sudden deaths, remind us that a careful forensic look can sometimes uncover treatable issues even in the most crowded neighborhoods (Hamukale et al., 2022). These examinations, sharing the health stories of individuals, also encourage public health actions to prevent unnecessary deaths and they slightly improve how community healthcare is carried out.

6.4.2. Identification of Public Health Trends

Autopsies in medicine help us see the development of health trends by showing how many and how severe certain diseases are. Thorough post-mortem checks allow researchers to learn about problems like atherosclerosis which is now being seen more often in young people. For example, one recent study found that 60.9% of young individuals examined after death had aortic lesions; It even hinted at ties between atherosclerosis and everyday habits like smoking and drug use (Asok et al., 2024). It's also curious that many people can't quite tell the difference between clinical autopsies and medico-legal ones; even though fewer than half know the details, lots of folks still see the potential benefits of these exams in helping to ward off future health crises (Naz et al., 2023). In short, medico-legal autopsies don't just spell out what caused an immediate death—they also illuminating broader trends that can shape community health strategies (Figure 6.16).

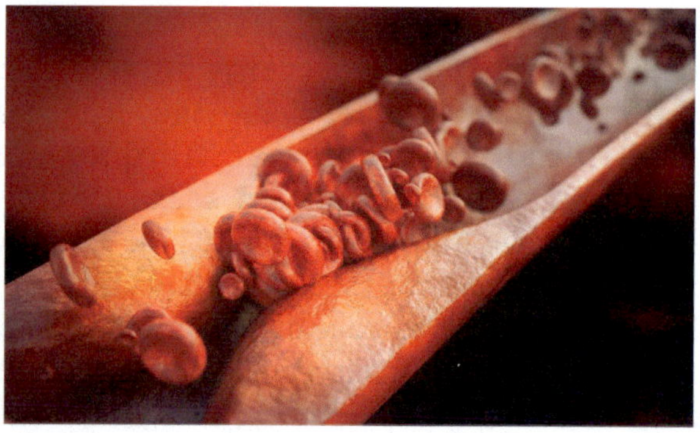

Figure 6.16. Detailed post-mortem checks help researchers grab vital clues about issues like atherosclerosis, a condition that generally speaking, has been popping up more often among younger people.

Source: https://d14d5nk8lue86f.cloudfront.net/s3fs-public/2018-11/artery%20image.jpg.

6.4.3. Role in Preventing Future Deaths

Medico-legal autopsies help prevent more deaths by finding out the details of untimely deaths. They work hard to understand the details—mainly when cases involve issues like sepsis which, in most cases, remains a major cause of death worldwide. Investigators in this area frequently spot hospital-acquired infections which explain some tragedies and help form new health policies. Their work, contributing to assessments of clinical risks, ends up guiding patient safety protocols and fostering improved healthcare practices (Dell'erba et al., 2019). Besides this, addressing malpractice concerns helps promote accountability across healthcare systems—a key factor in gradually rebuilding public trust (Dell'erba et al., 2019). All in all, autopsies can lead to more than just the first investigation, sometimes inspiring changes that may prevent similar disasters in the future.

6.4.4. Collaboration with Health Organizations

Medico-legal autopsies are not simple and need a different approach for each case—it helps to rely on health organizations. Working with these organizations improves the care for victims and their families and also helps gather information about injuries or deaths. In many cases, partnering with non-governmental organizations that focus on animal care can ease public health issues like dog bites, offering balanced solutions for both those hurt and the animals involved (Vural et al., 2024). Similarly, organizations dedicated to suicide prevention can shed light on the deeper causes behind such tragedies and, drawing on a wealth of clinical and demographic data, help craft effective intervention strategies (Sofi et al., 2024). To summarize, these kinds of collaborations let us look at victims' needs in a more rounded way and open doors to preventive measures that cover both physical and psychological aspects, ultimately bridging different facets of public health (Figure 6.17).

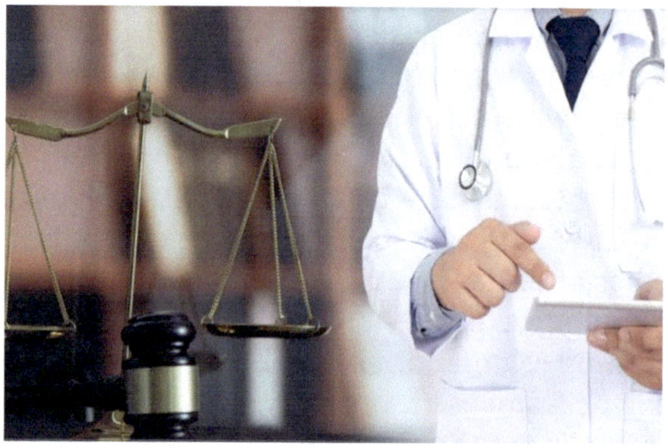

Figure 6.17. Medico-legal autopsies are complicated and call for more than a one-size-fits-all plan—it pays to work with health organizations.

Source: https://www.financialexpress.com/wp-content/uploads/2021/06/pharma-1.jpg.

6.4.5. Impact on Policy-making

When a crisis happens, forensic science and public health often join forces which can lead to changes in the law. For example, the COVID-19 pandemic caused labs to make quick changes which made it clear that rules are needed to address health issues and legal requirements together. In many cases, experts had to deploy new protocols under intense pressure, balancing immediate public health needs with the complexities of forensic work; this balance eventually steered lawmakers toward revamping autopsy practices (Nunno et al., 2022). At the same time, making sure these vital tests are done with respect for different cultural and religious beliefs about death has led to continuous debates about policies which seem to change as fast as the problems they deal with. Recent legal tweaks show a growing trend toward involving families more directly in autopsy decisions, although these changes can sometimes run headlong into established medico-legal customs, further muddling the policy scene (Carpenter et al., 2014). All in all, these linked challenges underline the importance of a thoughtful and detailed approach when making policies for medico-legal autopsies.

6.4.6. Education and Awareness Initiatives

The rapid progress in forensic science has pushed for changes in teaching and now more hands-on and practical approaches are being used for medico-legal autopsy. There's been a growing buzz—yes, —that groups such as the European Council of Legal Medicine (ECLM) have been keen on smoothing out forensic training across countries; in most cases, this has meant taking a fresh look at how undergraduates get introduced to forensic medicine. They even rolled out detailed surveys to capture opinions from a wide range of stakeholders, hoping to design a curriculum that better fits local needs and meshes with established forensic setups (James et al., 2024). Then, when you throw the COVID-19 crisis into the mix, its challenges made it plain that educational resources were crucial in handling unexpected hurdles—training had to shift just enough to keep public health in check without ditching rigorous academic standards (Esposito et al., 2022). To summarize, these varied initiatives end up being pretty key in shaping a forensic community that's as informed as it is prepared to deal with the tangled issues of today's medico-legal investigations (Figure 6.18).

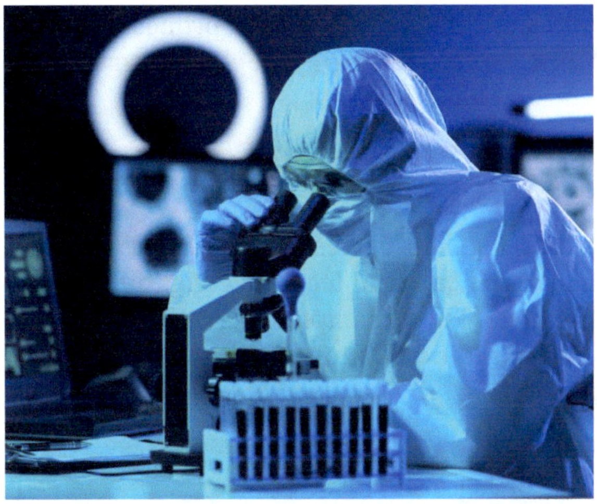

Figure 6.18. Forensic science is moving at a breakneck speed these days, and that shift has spurred efforts to mix hands-on learning with more practical approaches to medico-legal autopsy.

Source: https://www.aafs.org/sites/default/files/styles/fifty_fifty/public/media/images/AdobeStock_334068669.jpeg?itok=bE5E3TCC.

6.4.7. Case Studies of Public Health Interventions

Occasionally such autopsies demonstrate the positive results of public health actions by showing how many lives were saved. Looking into the details from post-mortem reports, researchers have started to figure out that tools like PMCT and PMCTA, those imaging techniques used during autopsies, can boost how accurately we diagnose tricky cases of suspected malpractice (Zinno et al., 2018). And when you dig into suicide investigations, you uncover this messy mix of violence, mental health issues, and even money problems—this jumble drives home that our public health strategies need to be broad and all-embracing (Brew et al., 2022). Experts regularly create case studies by mixing statistics with personal experiences which helps them understand how different actions can reduce both disease and death. In short, it is very clear from these findings that joining efforts in medico-legal probes and public health projects is highly beneficial.

6.4.8. Importance of Data Collection and Analysis

Medico-legal autopsies rely heavily on accurate data which can lead legal investigations to new directions. Taking samples correctly is important because their condition can decide the outcome of a case.

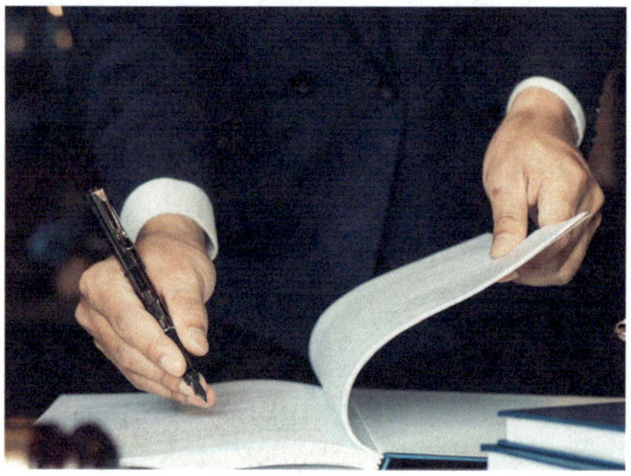

Figure 6.19. Medico-legal autopsies lean on precisely gathered data—a fact that steers legal investigations in unexpected ways.

Source: https://legaldesire.com/wp-content/uploads/2020/05/AdobeStock_295873176-scaled-e1622524869279.jpeg.

For instance, consider forensic DNA analysis that tells us that if samples aren't handled just right, they can become contaminated or even degrade, which in turn lessens their value in a criminal case (Kozma et al., 2018). Also, to determine drug levels after someone has died, all the collected data must be carefully analyzed. The approach presented in Bolton et al. (2015) shows that Bayesian networks might shed more light on drug-related deaths—particularly when record keeping is meticulous and the sample origins are clear. In most cases, carefully gathering and checking every bit of data not only builds a stronger legal case but also makes the medical findings from autopsies more reliable, reminding us again how vital good data is to fair judicial decisions (Figure 6.19).

6.4.9. Future Challenges in Public Health Integration

Medico legal autopsy and public health are closely connected which leads to tough challenges we must address. With elder abuse rising in Japan and similar places, there is a stronger push for forensic checks which should be included in overall health plans. Autopsy details—especially those pointing to neglect within families—keep reminding us again and again that leaning on solid data is key (Kato et al., 2013). When you look back, the slow shift in forensic practices shows, in most cases, that our systems need an update to handle modern health worries while still sticking to ethical standards (Asen et al., 2012). There are many obstacles for healthcare systems using forensic knowledge: working with other fields, handling limited resources and ensuring public health professionals get adequate training. In short, dealing with these problems is very important if we aim to create public policies that help prevent unnecessary deaths.

Test Your Knowledge

1. In what ways does a medico-legal autopsy affect public health surveillance?
2. Why should autopsy results be communicated to public health officials?

Summary

If we look at medico-legal autopsies carefully, we can see that they help clear up what happened in cases that end up in court. New methods, like those Bayesian network frameworks (which, generally speaking, have been a game-changer), now make it possible to get a more solid read on drug levels found after death, adding extra depth to our understanding of fatalities involving various substances (Bolton et al., 2015). Forensic science, when teamed with legal steps, helps fix death reporting and also influences public health data, although the connections are not always clearly defined. Studies from Nepal hint at this mix too: many people show a positive vibe about autopsies, though there's still a fair bit of fuzziness about what they actually entail (Chudal et al., 2018). Filling in these knowledge gaps among regular people, even if sometimes the explanation is not perfect, could encourage more people to accept autopsies as an important part of justice.

Multiple stab wounds and other traumatic injuries, can help us understand the events leading to a death. Many times, these wounds suggest that violence was involved which means investigators need to find out if the person caused them or someone else did. Autopsies are not only standard—they show how deep the injury was and the route it took which can help explain the events that caused the death. At the same time, new ways of radiocarbon dating are being used to find out how long the skeletal remains have existed which is often an important legal point. Bringing together these approaches—closely examining wounds and using radiocarbon dating—generally strengthens legal proceedings while also boosting the teamwork between forensic anthropologists and archaeologists when they're trying to crack cases with unidentified remains (Asif , 2025; Bertrand et al., 2024).

KEY TERMS FROM THIS CHAPTER

- Artificial intelligence
- Communication
- Diatom testing
- Pathologist
- Sternal foramen
- Blood group antigen tests
- COVID-19 crisis
- Evolution
- Public trust
- Teamwork
- Caution
- Criminal behavior
- Medicine
- Radiographic analysis

Short Answer Questions

1. What are the main objectives of a medico-legal autopsy?
2. What documents are required before conducting a medico-legal autopsy?
3. What is the significance of external examination during autopsy?
4. Why are the organs inside the body sometimes needed for an autopsy?
5. How is the autopsy report used in solving crimes?
6. How is it determined how long it has been since the person died during an autopsy?
7. What results from an autopsy can suggest the reason for the person's death?
8. What problems do regions face because of a lack of standardization in medico-legal autopsies?

Critical Thinking Questions

1. **A medico-legal autopsy is performed primarily to:**
   a. Study anatomical abnormalities
   b. Determine cause and manner of death
   c. Preserve organs for donation
   d. Treat undiagnosed medical conditions
2. **None of the following is considered a feature of a medico-legal autopsy.**
   a. Requires police requisition
   b. Performed by a forensic expert
   c. Conducted only when family gives consent
   d. Aimed at aiding legal investigations
3. **In a medico-legal autopsy which of the following is normally saved for examination by a toxicologist?**
   a. Brain, heart, liver
   b. Skin, muscles, bone
   c. Viscera, blood, urine
   d. Hair, nails, tears
4. **The final report produced in a medico-legal autopsy is called:**
   a. Certificate of death
   b. Autopsy summary
   c. Medico-legal death record
   d. Postmortem report
5. **Which one of these is required for carrying out a medico-legal autopsy?**
   a. Birth certificate
   b. Police inquest report

c. Death certificate
d. Prescription slip

Answers to Critical Thinking Questions

1. (b); 2. (c); 3. (c); 4. (d); 5. (b)

References

1. Albano, D., Argo, A., Bilello, G., Cumbo, E., Lupatelli, M., Messina, P., Sciarra, F. M., et al. (2024). Oral squamous cell carcinoma: Features and medico-legal implications of diagnostic omission. *Case Reports in Dentistry, 2024*. https://www.semanticscholar.org/paper/5323431fa8ecb0e827e2a2e32b8f3086d78da94c (accessed on 29 May 2025).
2. Ambica, K., & Khan, T. (2024). Challenges presented by decomposition in medico-legal autopsies–A case series. *IP International Journal of Forensic Medicine and Toxicological Sciences*. https://www.semanticscholar.org/paper/646d4bc25737b9f80377eea6f7537c9afb58977f (accessed on 29 May 2025).
3. Anzillotti, L., Cattaneo, C., Cecchi, R., et al. (2022). European Council of Legal Medicine (ECLM) on-site inspection forms for forensic pathology, anthropology, odontology, genetics, entomology and toxicology for forensic and medico-legal scene and corpse investigation: The Parma form. https://core.ac.uk/download/534988556.pdf (accessed on 29 May 2025).
4. Arcangeli, M., De Matteis, A., Del Fante, Z., Di Fazio, N., Fazio, V., La Russa, R., & Quattrocchi, A. (2020). The importance of post-mortem computed tomography (PMCT) as a complementary diagnostic technique to traditional autopsy in a case of asphyxia related-death. https://core.ac.uk/download/326235075.pdf (accessed on 29 May 2025).
5. Argo, A., Buscemi, R., Karch, S. B., Lanzarone, A., Roccuzzo, R., & Zerbo, S. (2019). Perioperative and anesthetic deaths: Toxicological and medico legal aspects. https://core.ac.uk/download/224993621.pdf (accessed on 29 May 2025).
6. Ariza, J. A., Duran-Tellez, Y. X., & Bermúdez-Santana, C. (2024). Case report: Molecular complement to the medico-legal autopsy in a case of unexplained death. *ARC Journal of Forensic Science*. https://www.semanticscholar.org/paper/b2f3fff8706b83980ab5ec1501eba94e010c4737 (accessed on 29 May 2025).
7. Asen, D. (2012). *Dead Bodies and Forensic Science: Cultures of Expertise in China, 1800–1949*. https://core.ac.uk/download/161440673.pdf (accessed on 29 May 2025).
8. Asok, A. V., George, N., & Maheshwari, U. (2024). A comprehensive investigation of atherosclerosis in the 10–25 age group through medico-legal autopsies. *Sri Lanka Journal of Forensic Medicine, Science & Law*. https://www.semanticscholar.org/paper/cc6edfc26d891c30ea337291c1f6ace53669b828 (accessed on 29 May 2025).
9. Aziz, D. A., Haider, W. A., Baig, H., Naz, S., & Haider, W. (2023). Post-mortem in Islamic jurisprudence: Examining perspectives, principles, and practices. *Russian Law Journal*. https://doi.org/10.52783/rlj.v11i4.3538.
10. Bajpai, A., Dev, R., Awasthi, P. M., et al. (2017). Trend of fatal poisoning in Kanpur: A two-year autopsy-based study. https://core.ac.uk/download/539910795.pdf (accessed on 29 May 2025).

11. Basso, C., Aguilera, B., Banner, J., Cohle, S., d'Amati, G., de Gouveia, R. H., di Gioia, C., Fabre, A., Gallagher, P. J., Leone, O., Lucena, J., Mitrofanova, L., Molina, P., Parsons, S., Rizzo, S., Sheppard, M. N., Mier, M. P. S., Kim Suvarna, S., Thiene, G., van der Wal, A., & Association for European Cardiovascular Pathology. (2017). Guidelines for autopsy investigation of sudden cardiac death: 2017 update from the Association for European Cardiovascular Pathology. *Virchows Archiv: An International Journal of Pathology, 471*(6), 691–705. https://doi.org/10.1007/s00428-017-2221-0.

12. Berloco, T., Bolino, G., Bolino, G., Del Prete, et al. (2024). Fire and blood: The dynamic reconstruction of a double murder with different attempts to conceal the corpses. https://core.ac.uk/download/638807907.pdf (accessed on 29 May 2025).

13. Bertrand, B., Clauzel, T., Richardin, P., Bécart, A., Morbidelli, P., Hédouin, V., & Marques, C. (2024). Application and implications of radiocarbon dating in forensic case work: When medico-legal significance meets archaeological relevance. *Forensic Sciences Research, 9*. https://www.semanticscholar.org/paper/f71993cf5ce191e912a2544c0785fd34c10cccce (accessed on 29 May 2025).

14. Bhargava, D., Nair, A. S., Meshram, V., Rao, M., & Kanchan, T. (2024). Duplex kidney: An incidental autopsy finding of clinical and medico-legal significance. *The Medico-Legal Journal*. https://www.semanticscholar.org/paper/4a0b6aed870e7a8b44389ae012f58d5bb1a43845 (accessed on 29 May 2025).

15. Bjornaas, M. A., Teige, B., Hovda, K. E., et al. (2010). Fatal poisonings in Oslo: A one-year observational study. *BMC Emergency Medicine, 10*, 13. https://doi.org/10.1186/1471-227X-10-13.

16. Bolton, J., Carlin, M., Langford, A., et al. (2015). Post-mortem toxicology: A pilot study to evaluate using a Bayesian network to assess the likelihood of fatality. https://core.ac.uk/download/41072180.pdf (accessed on 29 May 2025).

17. Brew, B. K., Fitzpatrick, S. J., Handley, T., et al. (2022). Men, suicide, and family and interpersonal violence: A mixed methods exploratory study. https://core.ac.uk/download/534041317.pdf (accessed on 29 May 2025).

18. Brodie, M. J., Besag, F., Ettinger, A. B., Mula, M., Gobbi, G., Comai, S., Aldenkamp, A. P., et al. (2016). Epilepsy, antiepileptic drugs, and aggression: An evidence-based review. *Pharmacological Reviews, 68*, 563–602. https://doi.org/10.1124/pr.115.012021.

19. Campobasso, C. P., Dell'Erba, A., Grattagliano, I., Laviola, D., & Strada, L. (2015). Undetected patricide: Inaccuracy of cause of death determination without an autopsy. https://core.ac.uk/download/132564083.pdf (accessed on 29 May 2025).

20. Can, B. (2014). State-making, evidence-making, and claim-making: The cases of torture and enforced disappearances in post-1980 Turkey. https://core.ac.uk/download/76388827.pdf (accessed on 29 May 2025).

21. Carew, R. M., French, J., & Morgan, R. M. (2023). Drilling down into ethics: A thematic review of ethical considerations for the creation and use of 3D printed human remains in crime reconstruction. https://core.ac.uk/download/564422041.pdf (accessed on 29 May 2025).

22. Carpenter, B., Quadrelli, C., & Tait, G. (2014). The body in grief: Death investigations, objections to autopsy, and the religious and cultural "other". https://core.ac.uk/download/19966054.pdf (accessed on 29 May 2025).

23. Cassum, L. A. (2014). Refusal to autopsy: A societal practice in Pakistan context. https://core.ac.uk/download/47263681.pdf (accessed on 29 May 2025).

24. Chiara Villa, S. T., Larsen, K., Hansen, M. C., Rohde, M. K., Haahr, L. W. T., Boel, P. M., et al. (2024). Forensic imaging in Denmark, 20-year experience: Status and future directions. *Forensic Imaging, 36*, Article 200583. https://doi.org/10.1016/j.fri.2024.200583.

25. Chudal, A., Kandel, D., Paudel, I. S., et al. (2018). Knowledge and perception of public towards medico-legal autopsy in Nepal. https://core.ac.uk/download/235170473.pdf (accessed on 29 May 2025).

26. Ciallella, C., Fineschi, V., Maiese, A., et al. (2022). The introduction of a new diagnostic tool in forensic pathology: LiDAR sensor for 3D autopsy documentation. https://core.ac.uk/download/599305397.pdf (accessed on 29 May 2025).

27. Crisan, C. (2019). The significance of death-scene investigation in determining cause and circumstances of medico-legal death. *Journal of Legal Studies, 24*, 53–62. https://www.semanticscholar.org/paper/f43c27f45fdbc6555e4af6eea70d9704da5bc922 (accessed on 29 May 2025).

28. D'Anna, T., Puntarello, M., Cannella, G., Scalzo, G., Buscemi, R., Zerbo, S., & Argo, A. (2023). The chain of custody in the era of modern forensics: From the classic procedures for gathering evidence to the new challenges related to digital data. *Healthcare, 11*(5), 634. https://doi.org/10.3390/healthcare11050634.

29. De Renzi, S. (2007). Medical expertise, bodies, and the law in early modern courts. https://core.ac.uk/download/1405.pdf (accessed on 29 May 2025).

30. De Valck, E., Beauthier, J. P., & Lefevre, P. (2011). Autopsy and identification techniques. https://core.ac.uk/download/322392483.pdf (accessed on 29 May 2025).

31. De Villiers, K. (2020). Assessing the functionality and value of introducing death investigators into forensic pathology service in South Africa. https://core.ac.uk/download/528261014.pdf (accessed on 29 May 2025).

32. Dell, F., Ferorelli, D., Gasbarro, A., Solarino, B., et al. (2019). Sepsis and nosocomial infections: The role of medico-legal experts in Italy. https://core.ac.uk/download/351122729.pdf (accessed on 29 May 2025).

33. Dempers, J. J., Coldrey, J., Burger, E., Thompson, V., Wadee, S. A., Odendaal, H. J., Sens, M. A., et al. (2016). The institution of a standardized investigation protocol for sudden infant death in the Eastern Metropole, Cape Town, South Africa. *Journal of Forensic Sciences, 61*, 1508–1514. https://doi.org/10.1111/1556-4029.13204.

34. Di Fazio, N., Scopetti, M., Delogu, G., La Russa, R., Foti, F., Grassi, V. M., Vetrugno, G., et al. (2023). Analysis of medico-legal complaint data: A retrospective study of three large Italian university hospitals. *Healthcare, 11*. https://www.semanticscholar.org/paper/7fdb5c93be78e21846fa2267e24af9155dadc185 (accessed on 29 May 2025).

35. Di Nunno, N., Esposito, M., Salerno, M., et al. (2022). The impact of the COVID-19 pandemic on the practice of forensic medicine: An overview. https://core.ac.uk/download/521187203.pdf (accessed on 29 May 2025).

36. Errickson, D., Carew, R. M., Collings, A. J., Biggs, M., Haig, P., O'Hora, H., Marsh, N. P., et al. (2022). A survey of case studies on using forensic three-dimensional printing in England

and Wales. *International Journal of Legal Medicine, 136*, 1605–1619. https://doi.org/10.1007/s00414-022-02872-4.

37. Esposito, M., Salerno, M., Scoto, E., Di Nunno, N., & Sessa, F. (2022). The impact of the COVID-19 pandemic on the practice of forensic medicine: An overview. *Healthcare, 10*, 319. https://doi.org/10.3390/healthcare10020319.

38. Faur, M., Mohor, C., Moisin, A., et al. (2021). A rare complication in a COVID-19 positive patient with sigmoid colon cancer—Hemoperitoneum due to gallbladder necrosis following micro-thrombosis. https://core.ac.uk/download/482003362.pdf (accessed on 29 May 2025).

39. Hamukale, A., Himwaze, C., Kapata, N., et al. (2022). Cardiac cysticercosis and neuro cysticercosis in sudden and unexpected community deaths in Lusaka, Zambia–A descriptive medico-legal post-mortem examination study. Retrieved from: https://core.ac.uk/download/519716192.pdf (accessed on 29 May 2025).

40. Hansmeyer, C. G. (2016). Near-body drugs of abuse testing in a post mortem medico-legal population in South Africa: A pilot study. Retrieved from: https://core.ac.uk/download/188770368.pdf (accessed on 29 May 2025).

41. Hussain, A. (2025). Forensic insights into multiple stab wounds: Autopsy findings from a case of sixty stab wounds. *Journal of Forensic Science and Research*. https://www.semanticscholar.org/paper/92b63c20cf1a4d68d8f9bf5822902e83e22ba79e (accessed on 29 May 2025).

42. Isnaeni, B. (2024). The role of forensic autopsy in pursuit of material truth in optical evidence for negative legal proof in the cyanide coffee murder case. *Sinergi International Journal of Law*. https://www.semanticscholar.org/paper/d6a3f9306daed28db19bd91e93917c9ca54818be (accessed on 29 May 2025).

43. Jadav, D. M. R. (2023). Study of deaths due to poisoning among the autopsies conducted at Civil Hospital Ahmedabad. *International Journal of Science and Research (IJSR)*. https://www.semanticscholar.org/paper/4f414d22a135be6290ed159f0f0f9920a52f8b46 (accessed on 29 May 2025).

44. Jones, D. G. (2011). The centrality of the dead human body for teaching and research–Social, cultural and ethical issues. Retrieved from: https://core.ac.uk/download/478413707.pdf (accessed on 29 May 2025).

45. Karhunen, J. P., Karhunen, P. J., Raivio, P. M., Sihvo, E. I., Vainikka, T. L., & Salminen, U. S. (2011). Medico-legal autopsy in postoperative hemodynamic collapse following coronary artery bypass surgery. *Forensic Science, Medicine, and Pathology, 7*(1), 9–13. https://doi.org/10.1007/s12024-010-9189-2.

46. Kato, G., Matsuzawa, A., Tamiya, N., et al. (2013). Family caregiving problems of suspected elderly neglect: A review of forensic autopsy cases in Japan. Retrieved from: https://core.ac.uk/download/234673542.pdf (accessed on 29 May 2025).

47. Kellehear, A., Zeman, A., Walker, A. E., Capron, A. M., Owen, A. M., Joffe, A. R., et al. (2009). Brain death, states of impaired consciousness, and physician-assisted death for end-of-life organ donation and transplantation. https://core.ac.uk/download/pdf/8348722.pdf.

48. Khan, Q. S., Mirza, F. H., & Sohail, S. (2010). Postmortem computed tomography for diagnosis of cause of death in male prisoners. Retrieved from: https://core.ac.uk/download/334961540.pdf (accessed on 29 May 2025).

49. Khurshid, A., Shah, M. U. F. A., Khurshid, M., Sohail, A., & Ali, G. (2021). Diatom-positive cadaver: Drowning or homicide? *Cureus*. https://doi.org/10.7759/cureus.18312.

50. Kozma, Z., Pádár, Z., & Zenke, P. (2018). Forensic DNA technological advancements as an emerging perspective on medico-legal autopsy: A mini review. Retrieved from: https://core.ac.uk/download/322434894.pdf (accessed on 29 May 2025).

51. Kuvaja, P., Keinänen, N., & Pakanen, L. (2022). The incidence of iatrogenic deaths in the Finnish cause-of-death statistics; A retrospective study. *Journal of Forensic and Legal Medicine, 86*, 102302. https://doi.org/10.1016/j.jflm.2021.102302.

52. Larraguibel, D. (2023). Behind the image–Cerebral reflections. Retrieved from: https://core.ac.uk/download/599332375.pdf (accessed on 29 May 2025).

53. Mahani, A., & Zadu, R. (2024). Malpractice litigation in multidisciplinary cancer care: Navigating medico-legal challenges and shared decision making in India. *Indian Journal of Forensic and Community Medicine*. https://www.semanticscholar.org/paper/331ce1a3e681669d7301717ca41bc8731291b7ec (accessed on 29 May 2025).

54. Maqsood, M., Butt, M. K., Adhami, S. U. Z., Hafeez, M. H., Javaid, T., & Sardar, H. (2024). Assessment of understanding and perception of undergraduate medical students regarding medico-legal autopsy. *Esculapio*. https://www.semanticscholar.org/paper/2eeb9ac2f0e0d2303a7800c98bf705d13f040095 (accessed on 29 May 2025).

55. McNamee, L. S. (2007). Students' perceptions of medico-legal autopsy demonstrations as a learning experience at a South African medical school. Retrieved from: https://core.ac.uk/download/196543878.pdf (accessed on 29 May 2025).

56. Meilia, P. D. I., Freeman, M., Herkutanto, & Zeegers, M. P. (2018). A review of the diversity in taxonomy, definitions, scope, and roles in forensic medicine: Implications for evidence-based practice. *Forensic Science, Medicine and Pathology, 14*(4), 460–468. https://doi.org/10.1007/s12024-018-0031-6.

57. Narayan, G., & Oura, P. (2025). Comparison of background characteristics and neuropathology findings between medico-legal autopsy cases with traumatic axonal injury, vascular axonal injury, or absence of axonal injury in β-amyloid precursor protein stain. *International Journal of Legal Medicine*. https://www.semanticscholar.org/paper/5f3a7286046548f08fc55fca9efa17da4f525aaa (accessed on 29 May 2025).

58. Naz, R., Fatima, M., Rehman, S. I., Rasool, R., Imran, S., & Waseem, F. (2023). Unveiling opinions: Exploring the public's view on clinical autopsies. *Pakistan Journal of Medical and Health Sciences*. https://www.semanticscholar.org/paper/bdce62318734a3d59ed3c3668762cb9539d37abf (accessed on 29 May 2025).

59. Payne-James, J., Payne-James, G. J., Cecchi, R., Cusack, D. A., Keller, É., Ludes, B., Madea, B., et al. (2024). Current status of undergraduate teaching in forensic & legal medicine in Europe. *International Journal of Legal Medicine, 138*, 1965–1976. https://doi.org/10.1007/s00414-024-03224-0.

60. Pelletti, G., Sech, M., Montanari, N., Quaia, E., Garcea, D., & Pelotti, S. (2025). Correlation between *in vivo* imaging and post-mortem autopsy findings for the medico-legal evaluation of a right hepatic artery pseudoaneurysm as a fatal complication of laparoscopic cholecystectomy. *Forensic Science, Medicine, and Pathology*. https://www.semanticscholar.org/paper/c356a7fe8aca8e5b02ba53a59b3ca00a42d82fb5 (accessed on 29 May 2025).

61. Piraianu, A. I., Fulga, A., Mușat, C. L., Ciobotaru, O. R., Poalelungi, D. G., Stamate, E., Ciobotaru, O. C., et al. (2023). Enhancing the evidence with algorithms: How artificial intelligence is transforming forensic medicine. *Diagnostics, 13*, 2992. https://doi.org/10.3390/diagnostics13182992.

62. Rathnaweera, R. (2016). Deaths following trivial trauma. *Journal Name*, *3*(1), 25. https://www.semanticscholar.org/paper/3bb17fd1f07323875624b819923b2b9b0c26cac7 (accessed on 29 May 2025).

63. Refolo, P., Sacchini, D., Raimondi, C., Masilla, S. S., Corsano, B., Mercuri, G., Oliva, A., et al. (2025). Should artificial intelligence-based patient preference predictors be used for incapacitated patients? A scoping review of reasons to facilitate medico-legal considerations. *Healthcare, 13*. https://www.semanticscholar.org/paper/85789b79dbe6ed9eeb85d1ccc6e766028dee77ef (accessed on 29 May 2025).

64. Roy, J., Shahu, U., Shirpure, P., Soni, S., Parekh, U., & Johnson, A. (2021). A literature review on dental autopsy – An invaluable investigative technique in forensics. *Autopsy & Case Reports, 11*. https://www.semanticscholar.org/paper/9af1a40c91ad3af3aff98c86c6e74571be5f1b1d (accessed on 29 May 2025).

65. Ruberg, W., Bergers, L., Dirven, P., & Serrano Martínez, S. (2023). *Forensic Cultures in Modern Europe*. Manchester University Press. https://doi.org/10.7765/9781526172358.

66. Shrestha, R., Krishan, K., & Kanchan, T. (2021). Workplace safety concerns in medico-legal death investigations related to COVID-19. *The Journal of Infection in Developing Countries, 15*(2), 247–253. https://doi.org/10.3855/jidc.14584.

67. Singh, R. K., Duchania, S., & Rani, M. (2022). Sternal foramen–Incidence and medico-legal importance. *IP International Journal of Forensic Medicine and Toxicological Sciences*. https://www.semanticscholar.org/paper/110ccfc7dae79c1a1ef4c9fe43966ab2505edd66 (accessed on 29 May 2025).

68. Singh, R. R., Tripathi, S. K., Bharti, A., & Yadav, P. K. (2025). Analyzing the efficacy of artificial intelligence in facilitating medico-legal investigations and enhancing forensic processes for emergency trauma patients: A systematic review. *Journal of Forensic Science and Medicine*. https://www.semanticscholar.org/paper/43b6e94c4f01224ec121d449ebc50f605a5e1d66 (accessed on 29 May 2025).

69. Singh, Y. (2021). The role of the minimally invasive forensic autopsy in South Africa: A legal perspective. https://core.ac.uk/download/517438868.pdf (accessed on 29 May 2025).

70. Sofi, F. M., Wahengbam, U., Singh, K. P., & Raj, T. P. (2024). Retrospective study of suicidal deaths in a tertiary care hospital at Imphal, Manipur, India. *Journal of Medical Society*. https://www.semanticscholar.org/paper/518a8ce7aeb993c705720457d0ecdca178f6f8da (accessed on 29 May 2025).

71. Tomczak, P., & Mulgrew, R. (2023). Making prisoner deaths visible: Towards a new epistemological approach. *Incarceration, 4*. https://doi.org/10.1177/26326663231160344.

72. Tyr, A., Lunetta, P., Zilg, B., Winskog, C., & Heldring, N. (2025). The medico-legal interpretation of diatom findings for the diagnosis of fatal drowning: A systematic review. *International Journal of Legal Medicine, 139*, 729–746. https://www.semanticscholar.org/paper/7fb161ea24c29cb344186008f2a2a7bb42440e92 (accessed on 29 May 2025).

73. Vanni, A., Tesi, C., Licata, M., & Fusco, R. (2024). Autopsy or anatomical dissection? Comparative

analysis of an osteoarcheological sample from an 18th-19th century hypogeal cemetery (Northern Italy). https://core.ac.uk/download/621392912.pdf (accessed on 29 May 2025).

74. Viner, M. (2020). An examination of the development of standards, protocols and standard operating procedures in forensic radiography. https://core.ac.uk/download/574557104.pdf (accessed on 29 May 2025).

75. Vural, T., Erbaş, M., & Baysal, I. (2024). Medical and legal evaluation of injuries due to dog bites: A Türkiye study. *Turkish Journal of Trauma & Emergency Surgery, 30*(1), 43–49. https://www.semanticscholar.org/paper/f71bb892e013de1fcffc8bf3c4d043ca9353b128 (accessed on 29 May 2025).

76. Yoo, S. H., Lee, W. T., & Lee, J. (2024). Evaluating the forensic inferences of oral nicotine ingestion: Autopsy case review, animal experimentation, and legal implications. *Korean Journal of Legal Medicine*. https://www.semanticscholar.org/paper/bef3c6d5f655f507e7ff17ce67f0bbea83c64386 (accessed on 29 May 2025).

77. Zinno, M. A. (2018). Virtual autopsy: Possible applications in cases of presumed medical malpractice. https://core.ac.uk/download/328815004.pdf (accessed on 29 May 2025).

7

CAUSE, MANNER, AND MODE OF DEATH

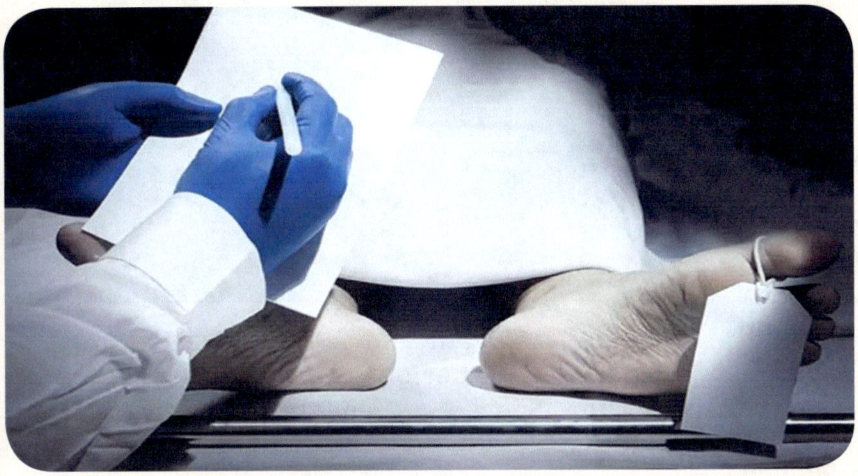

LEARNING OBJECTIVES

After studying this chapter, you will be able to:

1. Identify the cause of death;
2. Understand the manner of death;
3. Know the mode of death;
4. Show how cause, manner and mode of death are related.

Introduction

Mortality is not easy to explain because many different things play a part in it. When trying to work out the cause of a death, we frequently discuss terms like cause, manner and mode. Most of the time, what causes death is the existing injury or disease and the manner describes how the death happened such as naturally, in an accident, by homicide, suicide or sometimes without any clear explanation. Although the mode is often included with cause, it usually involves a wider range of events that can result in death. Take, for example, the situation in some broiler houses. High ammonia levels can mess up livestock health and, over time, result in notably high mortality rates among the birds; this, generally speaking, points to the need for better environmental control practices in agriculture (Xu et al., 2020). Similarly, chronic inflammation—like that seen in diabetic foot ulcers—can sometimes spiral into severe complications and even death, which shows just how deeply connected various health issues can be (Amala et al., 2019). There are moments when the plot is confusing, but it all points out that death is not simple to understand. All of these terms and cases have their own value, showing how small changes in explanations can matter a lot when we try to understand the whole subject.

Definition of Key Terms: Cause, Manner, and Mode of Death

It is important in forensic pathology and legal investigations to tell apart cause, manner and mode of death. Generally, the cause of death is the medical condition or injury that leads to someone's death, for example, a heart attack or a gunshot wound and the manner of death is about the circumstances surrounding the death which might be natural, accidental, suicidal, homicidal or sometimes not determined. How someone dies can also cover social or cultural aspects which may change the way different communities approach and investigate a death. For example, iatrogenic deaths—those linked to medical interventions—raise real concerns about patient safety and ethical practices, as several studies (Kuvaja et al., 2022) have pointed out a strong link to high-risk procedures and medications. Generally speaking, thoughtfully mixing these definitions is key for sound legal decisions and public health assessments (Sansola et al., 2015).

Importance of Understanding Death in Forensic Science

Death and forensic science are linked in a strange way that leads to new discoveries and new ideas about dying. Experts look into all the details related to a death, trying to find out what happened, how it happened and why it happened which is very important for both legal issues and debates about morality. New tools like iris recognition have popped up, opening unexpected routes for identifying someone after they've passed, which shows that personal markings still play a role (Sansola et al., 2015). Step back a bit, and you'll see that death is tied up with wider social and political ideas; these shared assumptions end up molding the stories we tell about accountability, a trend we notice in discussions about reports such as the Hutton Report (Coole et al., 2005). Generally speaking, understanding death goes far beyond simply slotting it into categories – it gradually reveals the layered nuances of human experience and the societal frameworks that shape how we interpret both life and loss (Figure 7.1).

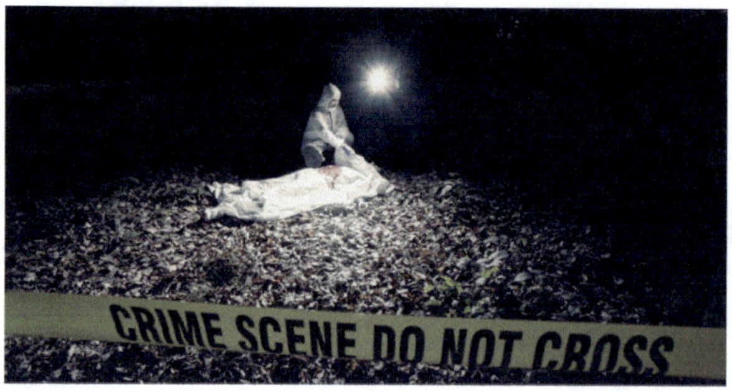

Figure 7.1. Death and forensic science are wedded in a curious dance that sparks breakthroughs and reshapes how we view life's final chapter.

Source: https://www.in-the-loop.net.au/wp-content/uploads/2014/10/featured-forensic.jpg.

Historical Context of Death Investigation

Death investigation didn't just appear overnight. The way we think about death has been influenced by how our culture views dying, law and ethics over time. In the early days, people often thought of death as the result of mysterious powers or divine punishment which meant few attempts were made to investigate it. Then, in general, as Enlightenment ideas appeared, people started believing facts and common sense more than ancient mystical ideas. Because of this focus on evidence, forensic science became the field we know today which combines technical abilities with strong ethical values. It's also interesting to see how this change appears in other debates. In discussions around International Relations (Odysseos et al., 2002), one often finds that modern investigation methods reflect an ever-shifting moral backdrop, hinting that understanding death has always been wrapped up in larger social implications. The way history is woven together points out that our current practices are influenced by many cultural and philosophical ideas which keep coming up in our studies of death.

Overview of the Legal Implications of Determining Death

The decision of when someone is dead has consequences for insurance, law and ethics in healthcare. Generally, a clear legal definition of death is very important; it can influence how court cases are handled and what doctors and other medical staff are required to do. Sometimes, it all hinges on nailing down the exact moment life ends, as seen in the Rus versus Comcare cases (Cardaci et al., 2017) where even hearsay evidence played a decisive role. There are many cases where people argue about end-of-life options, as in Diane Pretty's assisted suicide case which highlights the conflict between personal freedom and strict laws and causes many ethical and practical issues. Death is decided in a variety of ways which can surprise individuals, health professionals and the justice system.

The Role of Medical Examiners and Coroners

We never really understand death and medical examiners and coroners help us learn more about it. Most of the time, these professionals are responsible for finding out what led to the death — choosing the cause, manner and mode, especially when the case is strange or suspicious. Investigations by epidemiologists can change the outcome of court cases and encourage changes in public health policies.

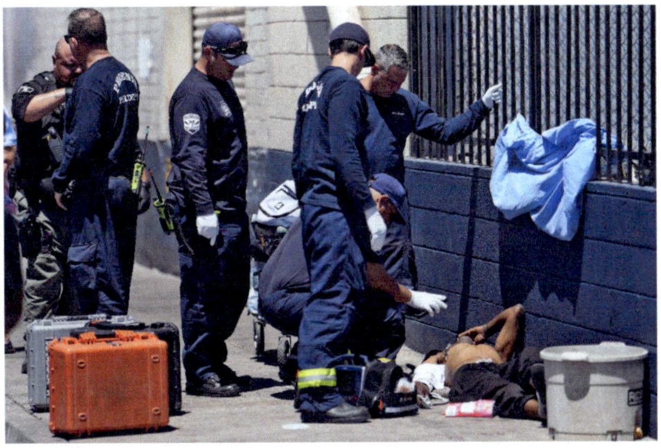

Figure 7.2. Death remains a mystery we never fully grasp, and medical examiners along with coroners play a key role in figuring it out.

Source: https://static.politico.com/54/e0/7dc3b7eb4154a791e7fd4dbfb4dd/extreme-heat-surface-burns-08043.jpg.

For example, the recent uptick in opioid-related fatalities generally reminds us why a careful review is necessary; when med examiners get involved, hidden trends in drug misuse emerge that can help guide preventive measures (Manchikanti, 2017). Also, when looking into suicides, there's a need to dive into the maze of psychological factors, which shows why training in mental health complexities is so important for these professionals (Christine et al., 2017). In close partnership with law enforcement and health departments, their work collectively builds a broader picture of mortality trends and helps shape public health initiatives that make a difference (Figure 7.2).

7.1. Cause of Death

Learning Outcome

1. Give definition of cause of death;
2. Identify types of causes;
3. Know common natural causes of death;
4. Explain common unnatural causes of death;
5. Emphasize the importance of autopsy in finding out how someone died;
6. Learn the impact of underlying health conditions;
7. Describe the influence of environmental factors;
8. Discuss case studies illustrating various causes of death;
9. Identify challenges in determining the cause of death.

In public health and medical research, understanding why death rates occur is very important. It has been observed lately that how people move such as walking or riding a bike, may influence their risk of heart disease and cancer and this can also affect their overall chances of dying. Take one extensive investigation with over 263,000 folks: it found that cycling to work was linked with a noticeably lower chance of dying from both CVD and cancer-related problems, which pretty much highlights how lifestyle choices matter (Celis-Morales et al., 2017). On the flip side, research using canines suggests that early and proper treatment in the preclinical stages of heart problems can extend life and delay harsh symptoms—an indication that a preventive approach isn't just for humans but for animals as well (Boswood et al., 2012). In short, these findings reveal that health risks such as death, are shaped by daily habits and prompt treatment.

7.1.1. Definition of Cause of Death

Death and life go hand in hand which means understanding death is not only about medicine—it's about what it means to exist. In addition to talking about the body's final breakdown, this explanation touches on questions that are almost philosophical. Some contemporary thinkers think that we must deal with the contradictions in death, since it is always present and affects our lives and culture. The details of a death in hospitals and crime labs can show if the death was caused by natural factors or by violence such as a homicide. You could see that the way we discuss these causes often reflects our society's values which influences discussions about laws, ethics and health. And now, as more of our conversations move online, the way we define and look at death seems to pick up fresh twists that, in most cases, are definitely worth a deeper look (Gábor et al., 2017; Ntelia et al., 2015).

7.1.2. Types of Causes: Natural Versus Unnatural

There are only two main ways in which death can happen and this makes it tricky. At times, the body simply gets tired—diseases such as heart problems or infections cause it to wear out over time which leads to a natural and unavoidable collapse. In some cases, accidents, suicides or homicides reveal that things outside the person's control can lead them to commit a crime. The difference is important for people in the law and medicine who rely on these clues to understand the outcome. Recent research, for example, hints that everyday environmental issues—microplastics being just one example—might be nudging our health in unexpected (and sometimes unnatural) directions (Yuan et al., 2022); and increasingly, our views on death are shifting as cultural trends spill over into new digital spaces like the Metaverse (Park et al., 2022) (Figure 7.3).

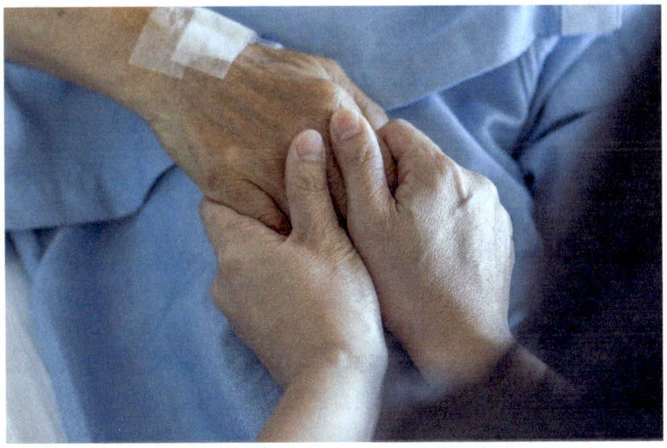

Figure 7.3. Natural death.

Source: https://nouvelles.umontreal.ca/fileadmin/_processed_/csm_20220531_soins_palliatifs_e77395f048.jpg.

7.1.3. Common Natural Causes of Death

Life and death are always mixed in nature and this idea appears in our daily lives. Heart trouble, lung problems and various cancers are common examples and they happen because of what we inherit and the lifestyle we choose. Sometimes, our environment makes things more complicated by making these issues worse and mixing up personal health with the world we live in. Medicine is always trying to get ahead by introducing new studies and technology and this is usually necessary. While trying to solve the problem, we can forget to ask the deeper question: what is death? Spinoza once hinted that maybe we're not ever going to fully grasp its true nature—which makes us wonder if our chase for neat answers might miss the point (Toth et al., 2017). This thought, oddly enough, brings out the many layers of mortality and underscores that understanding death's natural causes is key to seeing the whole picture (Bourdieu et al., 2014).

7.1.4. Common Unnatural Causes of Death

It is important to understand why people die unnaturally to design better health policies. Accidents top the charts in many cases; one analysis shows they make up about 38.4% of these cases, and oddly enough, road mishaps alone clock in at around 67.6% (Mayedo et al., 2017). Violence, too, leaves its mark—another study found that injuries from firearms account for roughly 46.4% of fatal incidents, a detail that tends to hit young men particularly hard (Saghir et al., 2020). Suicide and hanging being a common method, only makes the situation more complicated and tragic. All these issues, if you think about it, make it clear that public health officials should increase safety and educate people. In most cases, addressing these issues means taking a comprehensive approach rather than relying on one-size-fits-all solutions, which just don't seem to capture the full, messy picture (Figure 7.4).

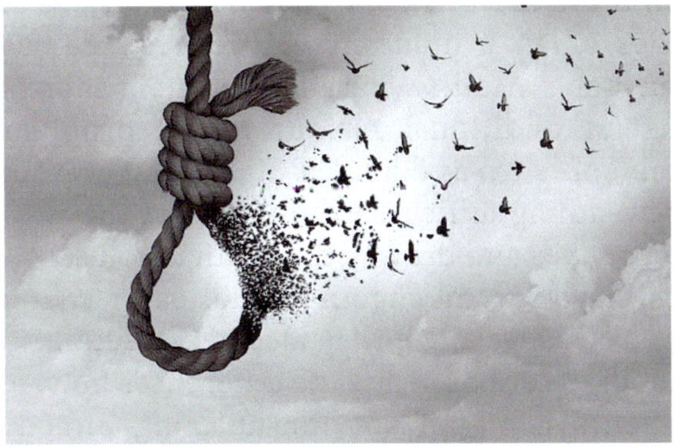

Figure 7.4. Understanding what drives unnatural deaths is key to shaping better public health policies.

Source: https://www.moh.gov.rw/index.php?eID=dumpFile&t=p&p=305965&token=6ed7d33459550f117a0f88029a908ce81a40fbfc.

7.1.5. Role of Autopsy in Determining Cause of Death

Autopsies help link medicine and law by noticing details that could be missed in regular checks. The procedure is meant to find out the cause of death and also to discover hidden illnesses that are often missed. Sometimes, what doctors initially assume clashes with what the autopsy reveals, nudging healthcare practices in surprising new ways (Silas et al., 2009). It helps solve difficult problems in diagnosis and also provides information that affects health statistics and planning.

What is found in an autopsy can be important for investigations and may lead to changes in public health. And then there's emerging tech like iris recognition which, in most cases, seems to open up fresh routes for postmortem identification, potentially sharpening forensic work overall (Sansola et al., 2015).

7.1.6. Impact of Underlying Health Conditions

Many different things can affect health outcomes and these are often why people die. There are times when a hidden condition can damage a person's health which makes them more at risk for additional serious health problems. Problems such as diabetes, high blood pressure or breathing difficulties both impact the way a person dies and the way the death unfolds. Folks who have several ongoing issues can face a lot of risks, especially if they also get infections. In a lot of situations, fixing the differences between patients is important for building effective care plans. Occasionally, healthcare turns to alternative dispute resolution methods to boost communication among all involved, which can help ease non-litigable disputes in health policy reforms (Ljung et al., 2005; Rabinovich-Einy et al., 201) (Figure 7.5).

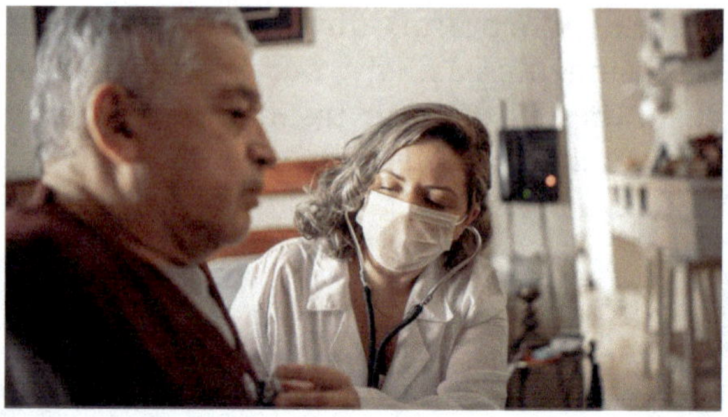

Figure 7.5. Chronic ailments like diabetes, high blood pressure, or breathing troubles don't just change how someone passes away – they also shape the way these events actually happen.

Source: https://www.grxstatic.com/4f3rgqwzdznj/12nmMh8I9OYmI83Q1FP0yv/ffad61dd2ef9ba291a19b8d1ddd942a4/patient_stethoscope_1218253271.jpg?format=pjpg&auto=webp&width=704.

7.1.7. Influence of Environmental Factors

There is a strong link between the environment and health which means we should examine many different causes when trying to find out what leads to death. Some research has found that even very common daily toxins can increase your risk of getting cancer. Some estimates suggest that roughly 7%–19% of cancer cases are linked to these environmental toxins (Hamid et al., 2015). Chemicals usually work together in ways that are hard to notice and their small impacts on our health make us question the total effect on our well-being. Social issues such as your income level or the continuing impact of racism make it even harder to get the best results from treatment. These pressures can mix in unpredictable ways, sometimes messing up how well medicine works and even leading to unexpected adverse reactions (Wallace et al., 2003). Usually, being clear about these factors is important for creating successful strategies that support health and improve outcomes in many communities.

7.1.8. Case Studies Illustrating Various Causes of Death

Death is not solved by one answer—it is explained by a variety of stories that include changes in society, the environment and personal decisions. Instead of neatly lining up causes, each case seems to spill over into another, like when a sudden accident shows that a momentary lapse (or getting too caught up in your phone) can lead to catastrophe, nudging us to wonder who bears the blame (Bernstein et al., 2019). Sometimes, people have to fight for years with serious illnesses and problems like money and social barriers can make it very hard for them to get the care they require. At times, the stories you tell overlap and the result is a view that's as surprising as real life. Most of the time, these accounts are not simple and instead weave together many different moments and meanings. In most cases, such mixed narratives end up reshaping our look at death—and, by extension, how we appreciate the twists and turns of life (Ntelia et al., 2015).

7.1.9. Challenges in Determining Cause of Death

It's not easy to figure out the cause of death, since many different experts contribute and sometimes the results are unclear. Most of the time, forensic pathologists and medical examiners are given only a limited amount of a person's medical history which can be very important for understanding the case. Then there are outside influences, like environmental hardships and social pressures, which tend to complicate things even more, especially for folks in marginalized communities where systemic bias often makes health disparities worse (as seen in the study on lupus prevalence among African-American women (Wallace et al., 2003). Legal and ethical issues, too, throw their weight around; in situations with suspected foul play, judicial decisions sometimes tip the scales and nudge forensic methods off balance, raising concerns about objectivity (Aarons et al., 2008). To summarize, determining a cause of death remains a layered, tricky puzzle that resists a neat, one-size-fits-all explanation (Figure 7.6).

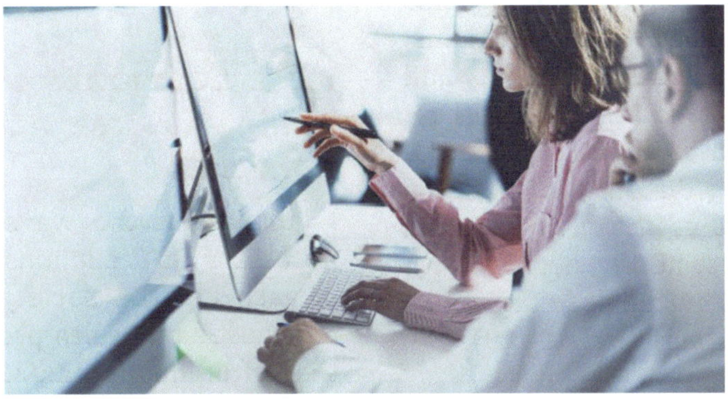

Figure 7.6. Challenges in determining cause of death.

Source: https://www.rgare.com/images/default-source/kc-article-images/suicide-claims-thumb.jpg?sfvrsn=d3e50fd6_2.

Test Your Knowledge

1. List any three natural causes of death.
2. Name two examples of mechanical causes of death.

7.2. Manner of Death

Learning Outcome

1. Give the definition of the manner of death;
2. Know categories of the manner of death;
3. It is important to know the difference between cause and manner of death;
4. Explain legal implications of the manner of death;
5. Be aware of how forensic evidence helps determine the way the death occurred;
6. Identify psychological factors influencing the manner of death;
7. Discuss cultural perspectives on death and dying;
8. Learn case studies highlighting different manners of death;
9. Identify challenges in classifying the manner of death.

One of the main tasks in forensics is to find out how the death occurred which reveals what happened beforehand. Usually, calling a death natural, accidental, self-inflicted, homicidal or undetermined helps experts begin their investigation. Forensic anthropology, for instance, jumps in to check out skeletal remains; it not only helps pinpoint a person's identity and unique features but also lends clues about how things unfolded (Mishra et al., 2021). Marine scientists are now using diatom analysis as a method. This technique digs into environmental traces that might connect human activity with drowning, showing just how tangled our actions can be with nature (Barbieri et al., 2018).

7.2.1. Definition of Manner of Death

Death has many aspects that need us to examine it more closely. Usually, determining the manner of death such as by natural causes, accident, suicide, homicide or something uncertain, is very important in forensics. The labels direct how the law handles cases, how doctors treat patients and how we interpret death. Usually, the ending of someone's life gets us to think about matters that are bigger and more meaningful such as what it means to die. Now, because of the digital world, ideas about life and death are being reconsidered all the time. Getting a grip on these classifications helps in piecing together the ongoing conversation about death (Boros Gábor et al., 2017; Ntelia et al., 2015) (Figure 7.7).

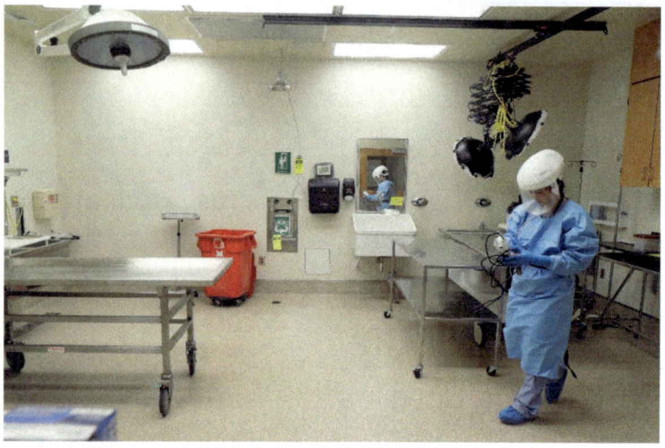

Figure 7.7. Manner of death.

Source: https://npr.brightspotcdn.com/legacy/sites/kplu/files/202011/AP_20197022058021.jpg.

7.2.2. Categories of Manner of Death: Natural, Accidental, Suicidal, Homicidal

Figuring out the ways we classify death is necessary, as it explains the causes and effects of each type on society. Many natural deaths are caused by health problems or illnesses and they often happen more often in older people. Accident-related deaths, like those from car crashes or unexpected falls, make up a big share of cases and point to the need for better safety measures for vulnerable groups (Vadysinghe et al., 2018). Suicidal deaths usually stem from many complex mental struggles and substance misuse (in some instances, gabapentin misuse has been a notable factor (Tharp et al., 2019), which adds another layer of difficulty. Homicidal deaths which are not as frequent, often bring attention to social violence and suggest that solutions should be put in place at the community level. All in all, dividing deaths into different groups helps report accurately and also guides the development of public health programs that support and prevent similar deaths.

7.2.3. Distinction between Cause and Manner of Death

It's sometimes hard to know when someone is dead which can lead to small but important differences in how forensic experts proceed. Being aware of these subtle points is important for both legal and medical professionals, in many situations. Instead of seeing "cause of death" as a dry label, consider it to be the main health issue or injury that resulted in death, for example a bullet wound or a serious disease; "manner of death," on the other hand, gives a broader view, showing if death happened naturally, accidentally, through suicide or even by homicide. It's interesting how anthropologists while studying trauma, can sometimes tease apart if an injury comes from an explosion versus a gunshot (Dussault et al., 2016). This kind of insight isn't only key in forensic labs—it can also, quite significantly, influence courtroom decisions (Grossman et al., 2014). All in all, considering both sides helps us see death in more detail and learn how serious injuries can influence society.

7.2.4. Legal Implications of Manner of Death

It is very important in the legal system to know how a person died. Once a death is labeled as homicide, suicide, accident or natural, it frequently starts a process that affects the justice system. A homicide call can result in criminal charges, but an accidental death can lead to suits related to negligence. Sometimes, since the cause is unclear, it becomes difficult in cases of medical malpractice. In many cases, trying out alternative ways to settle these disputes might help, assuming the conversation space is open enough (Rabinovich-Einy et al., 2011). Ultimately, the way a death is classified shows how law, public policy, and ethical concerns get all mixed up when we're dealing with mortality (Wood et al., 2017) (Figure 7.8).

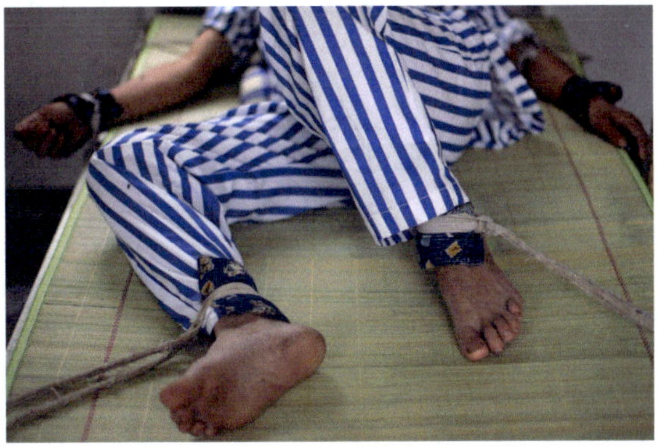

Figure 7.8. Legal implications of manner of death.

Source: https://blog.ipleaders.in/wp-content/uploads/2019/01/schizophrenia.jpg.

7.2.5. Role of Forensic Evidence in Determining Manner of Death

Forensic clues are very important in determining the cause of death—they help reveal if the cause was natural, an accident, murder or suicide. They do not just list the injuries, toxicology results and environmental signs; they put all these details together in ways that can seem a bit unexpected. Usually, putting the events back together helps investigators see more details—each clue moves them closer to the whole story. Generally speaking, the careful use of forensic methods helps establish a timeline that then offers the context needed for legal cases (Coole et al., 2005). At the same time, the trust we put in forensic evidence depends not only on the lab techniques but also on how those methods are read and interpreted (Lewis et al., 2020). In the end, forensic data is not only information—it helps reconstruct the story of death which can affect court decisions and the way society views mortality.

7.2.6. Psychological Factors Influencing Manner of Death

Mindset and emotion strongly color final life decisions. People don't follow a neat, step-by-step process; they flip back and forth between a firm life-affirming YES and a resolute death-affirming NO—a pattern underscored in Gaiseanu et al. (2018)—as personal history and raw beliefs come into play. Many times, especially when people choose voluntary euthanasia, they say they are tired of living or feel that their life is finished which leads them to seek help with dying. This mix of inner well-being, familiar societal pressure, and a sense of personal autonomy as discussed in Richards et al. (2017) hints at a tangled web where mental states shape how one exits life. Generally speaking, grasping these inner mechanisms is key to understanding how our most private thoughts echo both individual will and broader cultural values (Figure 7.9).

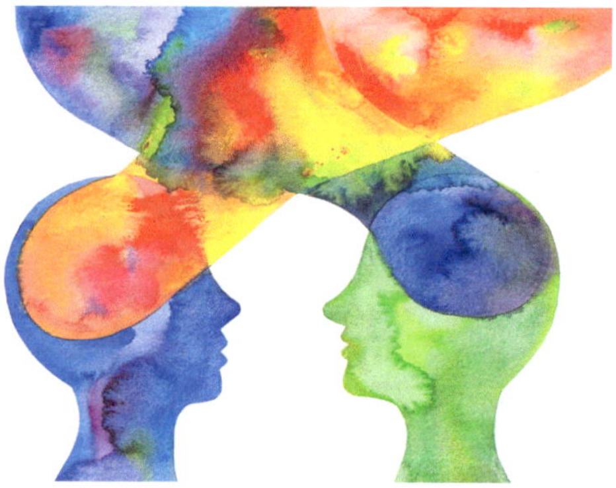

Figure 7.9. Mindset and emotion strongly color final life decisions.

Source: https://www.verywellmind.com/thmb/Khr6WbpyiWSHHfmZu7jgB8yCdGI=/2049x0/filters:no_upscale():max_bytes(150000):strip_icc()/KaterynaKovarzh-1ba05508b85442b499a1ac2a9e324e8b.jpg.

7.2.7. Cultural Perspectives on Death and Dying

Culture has an unpredictable effect on how people view death which affects their last moments and the memories we keep. Various backgrounds bring different thoughts on death, sometimes combining personal emotions with community rituals which impacts how loss is processed and how society responds. Many Western places often use a clinical, almost distant way; people rely on medical solutions and focus on living longer which can make the process feel too much about the science of dying. In most Indigenous communities, death is considered a natural part of life and it is celebrated in rituals that bring together the community to remember the elderly and help everyone grieve gently. Most of the time, the way people think about death plays a role in how we grieve and what we believe about the end of life. In most cases, getting a handle on these views matters a lot—if we aim to offer care that fits into each cultural picture, helping medical staff to meet both the emotional and spiritual needs of those in their final moments along with their families (Željko Reiner et al., 2011).

7.2.8. Case Studies Highlighting Different Manners of Death

Death can be hard to define and often you discover new things about it by studying different cases that show unexpected problems in society. For example, looking back at autopsy records shows that about 46.4% of fatal injuries come from firearms—mostly hitting young men aged 21–40 (Saghir et al., 2020)—which is pretty shocking. At the same time, our shared, culturally shaped ideas about death come through in modern digital stories; these narratives, especially seen in digital games, seem to completely retool how we interact with the concept (Ntelia et al., 2015). Rather than sorting things into categories such as homicide and accident, these studies usually mix together different cultural, social and psychological factors in unexpected manners. In general, noticing the many forms of death helps us see how complex life can be and it reminds us that being cautious and informed could be very useful.

7.2.9. Challenges in Classifying Manner of Death

Determining the cause of death is hard, mainly if health problems are involved and make the process more complicated than usual. It happens a lot with people who have heart issues, especially those using cardiac devices which makes things confusing. Factors related to mental health such as suicidality, usually increase uncertainty and need a team effort from experts in various fields. Doing this kind of thorough evaluation helps ensure legal documents are in order, but it also benefits public health by helping prevent suicide and boosting research on therapy. For instance, the odds of finding a suicide note can differ wildly between methods – cases involving drug intoxication often show higher chances than the more obvious methods like firearms, especially when there isn't a clear forensic autopsy (Caine et al., 2018). Likewise, with our aging population, figuring out whether death was more medical or intentional is becoming increasingly important (Federspiel et al., 2023) (Figure 7.10).

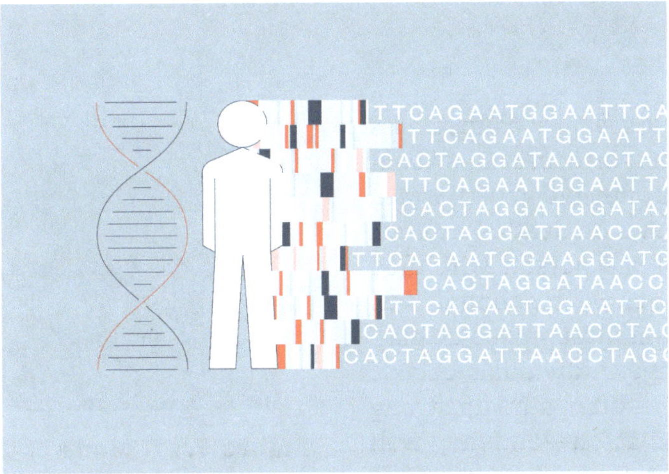

Figure 7.10. Deciding how someone died is tricky, especially when underlying health issues get in the way, making the classification harder than expected.

Source: https://www.adalovelaceinstitute.org/wp-content/uploads/2024/09/Report-Predicting-the-future-of-health.png.

Test Your Knowledge

1. List the five commonly accepted manners of death.
2. How are the manner of death and the cause of death different?

7.3. Mode of Death

Learning Outcome

1. Explain the definition of the mode of death;
2. Be able to tell the difference between a mode and a manner of death.
3. Give examples of modes of death;
4. Be able to use forensic methods to find out the manner of death.
5. Explain why the way a person dies is important for criminal investigations.
6. Appreciate how technology shapes the way we find out about the cause of death.
7. Choose case studies that illustrate many methods of dying.
8. Consider the ethical aspects when deciding how death should occur;
10. Find out the difficulties in correctly determining the cause of death.

Understanding how people see the circumstances of a death is very important in discussions about mortality—as these ideas often blend with wider, sometimes confusing, views on death. Research suggests that the age of the person who died often determines how people respond which shows the mix of grief and acceptance at play. For example, when younger individuals choose voluntary assisted dying, it often stirs up strong feelings—anger, fear, and so on—and may well call for specially tailored support for grieving families (Breen et al., 2021). On top of that, some odd disparities in suicide statistics hint at potential misclassifications that seem tied to race and economic factors, thereby influencing how different groups are seen about their mode of death (Rockett et al., 2010). In other words, how a person dies affects their own feelings and also influences the way society views loss and grief.

7.3.1. Definition of Mode of Death

Death is not only a moment in life but also affects our daily lives and others' views of us. Whether a death is natural, accidental, by suicide or a homicide, it tells us not only about the details of the event but also about the consequences that spread out from it. Basically, these types which we often call "ways of dying," reveal our inner beliefs about death and what is right or wrong. Looking closely at such an event can show that it raises deeper questions about life. Today, our conversation about death is also being nudged (sometimes quite unexpectedly) by the digital age, where online narratives and virtual memorials are reshaping old ideas and forging new ones (Ntelia et al., 2015). To summarize, teasing apart these nuances is key if we want to get a grip on not only the intricate nature of human experience but also the evolving norms that bind us together (Noonan et al., 2013) (Figure 7.11).

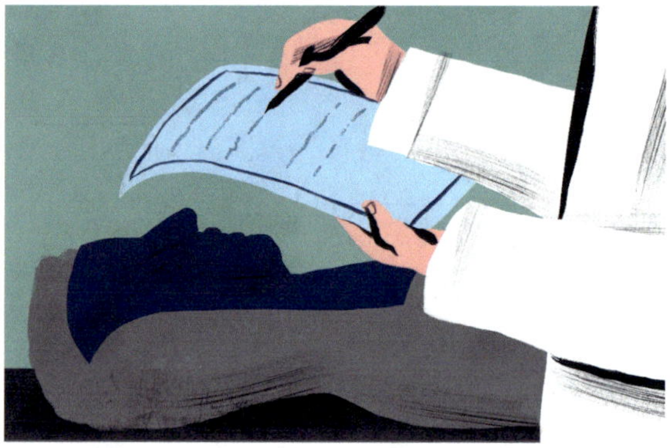

Figure 7.11. Mode of death.

Source: https://static01.nyt.com/images/2022/02/15/science/14sci-brody-death/14sci-brody-death-superJumbo.jpg.

7.3.2. Relationship between Mode and Manner of Death

Determining the cause of death is a main focus in forensics. An important point is called the manner of death which means classifying a death as natural, accidental, self-inflicted, homicidal or undetermined. The next factor is how the body dies such as not receiving enough oxygen or a sudden heart failure. Understanding this series of physical changes can sometimes clear up the reason for the incident. For instance, in a suspected homicide, if investigators can separate the external circumstances from what exactly happened inside the body, that can guide them toward clearer ideas about motive and responsibility (Horgan et al., 2016). And new advances, like iris recognition, are starting to make a difference too—they're boosting efforts in postmortem identification and honing the accuracy of death classification in legal and medical settings (Sansola et al., 2015).

7.3.3. Examples of Modes of Death: Blunt Force, Sharp Force, Asphyxiation

They examine the cause of death to spot hints that may not be noticeable at the start. A fall or collision might result in bruises and fractures and these often suggest blunt trauma without giving all the details.

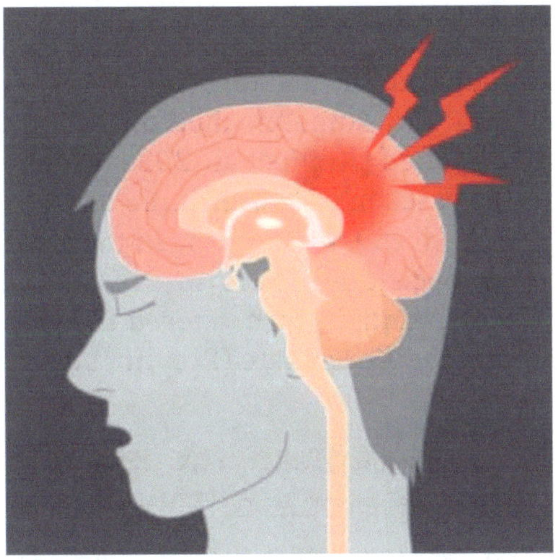

Figure 7.12. A hard knock from a fall or collision leaves behind bruises and broken bones—those marks often hint at blunt trauma without spelling out the whole story.

Source: https://apexbraincenters.com/wp-content/uploads/2015/12/concussion-ep-43-300x300.jpg.

You could then spot cuts or stabs made by a knife or other sharp object which may reveal what was used and sometimes the purpose of the attack. In other instances, a shortage of oxygen, whether from strangulation or drowning, forces investigators to take a close look at the breathing passages; occasionally, they even spot signs like aquaporins that suggest drowning (Alfieri et al., 2024). Generally speaking, the way these specialists work through autopsies and painstaking checks sort of builds a roadmap of what happened, which not only supports legal proceedings but also helps keep the community safe (Abrol, 2024) (Figure 7.12).

7.3.4. Forensic Techniques used to Determine Mode of Death

The way a person died is key to understanding the full story and different forensic methods are used to find out. Using modern tools such as checking the fluids from dead bodies, often offers vital information about what happens after death. In most cases, recent studies suggest that when soft tissue breaks down, it goes through a raft of intricate biochemical reactions that hint at both the elapsed time and the conditions at death (Forbes et al., 2010); these details can be indispensable for a careful investigation. Techniques that assess the risk of danger or criminal intentions usually bring an extra challenge to cases with violent outcomes. Expert opinions, drawn either from handson clinical insights or from more formal, structured assessments, can shift how a suspect's risk is gauged—sometimes influencing legal outcomes in subtle ways (Gamache et al., 2013). All in all, using multiple forensic approaches gives investigators a better, though sometimes confusing, idea of the cause of death which is important for justice and the public's safety.

7.3.5. Importance of Mode of Death in Criminal Investigations

Discovering the way someone died can have a

major impact on an investigation. Detectives can often adjust their approach and use resources differently if they know the death was caused by homicide, suicide, accident or natural causes. This is very important, especially when big social issues are present – such as fatal encounters which can affect public opinion and possibly lead to policy changes. There's also the messy layer of race and class, with talks about the political lives of marginalized communities (Soss et al., 2017) showing how these factors sometimes steer the actions of law enforcement. Overall, digging into the specifics of a death not only helps build solid evidence but also supports accountability in society, tying a clearer picture of the event to the broader story of justice and community care (Bronisław Malinowski, 2018) (Figure 7.13).

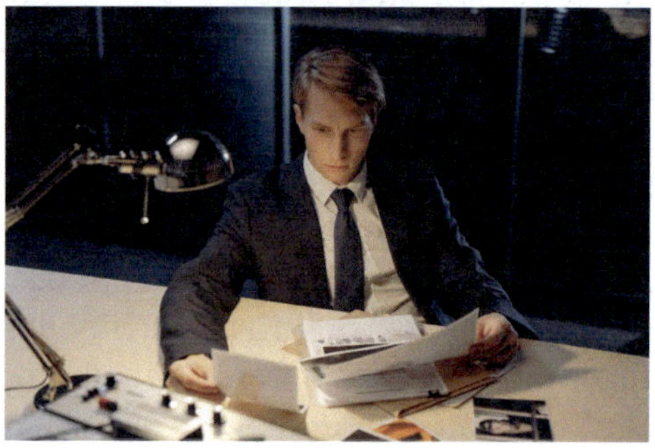

Figure 7.13. In many cases, knowing if a death was from homicide, suicide, accident, or just natural causes gives detectives the chance to change tactics and focus resources where they're needed.

Source: https://financialcrimeacademy.org/wp-content/uploads/2023/10/6142365f-4423-4b05-aed7-67f85b58abe1.png.

7.3.6. Influence of Technology on Understanding Mode of Death

Technology's surge has changed how we think about death. Nowadays, investigators can use digital imaging and 3D reconstruction to record crime scenes more accurately and details that could be overlooked with older methods may be noticed. PMCT is a good example; usually, it provides non-invasive scans of the body that help detect hidden problems inside which could be important for the investigation. Because of these new tools, researchers are questioning past ideas about what counts as a way to die, especially when cases are not simple. Several studies even suggest that, given how varied human experiences can be, our conclusions about death need a more flexible and nuanced approach (Berg et al., 2010; Henrich et al., 2010).

7.3.7. Case Studies Demonstrating Various Modes of Death

It's not always easy to study death and different investigations look at things like train accidents and putting animals to sleep. An investigation of 107 fatal railway incidents showed that men were the main victims, most often between 21 and 40 years old and 66.4% of the accidents resulted in injuries to the brain and liver. This kind of work generally shows that digging into the fine details at the scene (like injury patterns and surrounding circumstances) can help figure out not only why someone died but also exactly how it happened (Khilji et al., 2024). Looking at euthanasia cases in Italy over three decades, it is clear that Law 189/2004 changed the situation. It pushed decision-makers to see animals as truly sentient and, in turn, altered the way life-ending choices were made (Previti et al., 2024).

7.3.8. Ethical Considerations in Determining Mode of Death

Exploring what death involves often leads to questions about morality that are not always easy to solve. Debates about when someone is considered dead such as brain death versus a stopped heart, can become very complicated in places like hospitals. Most of the time, honesty is needed, as patients and families should understand what each definition means. Clinical guidelines often remind us that, in most cases, it's not just about strict medical rules but also about balancing those with cultural backgrounds—a point (Aristovnik et al., 2020) that shows how ideas of dignity can shift from one group to another. On top of that, healthcare providers find themselves wedded to both their professional judgments and the raw emotions of grieving families, trying to merge clear ethical standards with respect for personal beliefs (McClave et al., 2016). To summarize, the ethics involved in defining death remain a tangled, multifaceted subject that calls for careful—and sometimes imperfect—consideration (Figure 7.14).

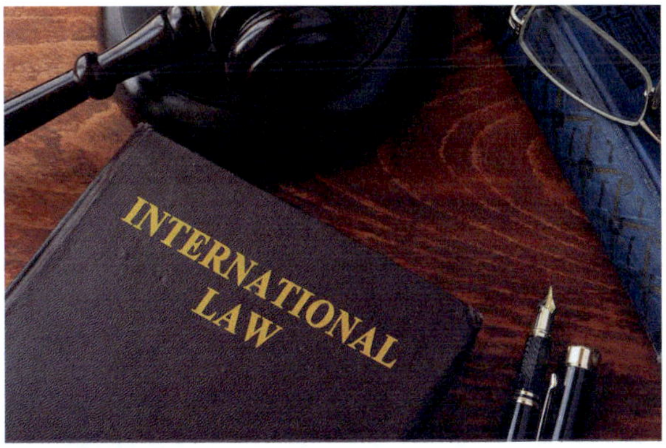

Figure 7.14. Clinical guidelines often remind us that, in most cases, it's not just about strict medical rules but also about balancing those with a cultural background.

Source: https://blog.ipleaders.in/wp-content/uploads/2020/09/International-Law.jpg.

7.3.9. Challenges in Accurately Identifying Mode of Death

Figuring out exactly how someone dies isn't easy. Many things can make things complicated – the circumstances around a death can make it hard to tell if it was homicide, suicide or an accident. In most cases, differing approaches to measuring long-term illnesses can hide clear death trends; for instance, research looking at how diet affects health outcomes (Ard et al., 2016) shows that the way chronic diseases are assessed often blurs usual mortality patterns. Advances in medical technology, along with our growing grasp of brain disorders, further complicate things, particularly when deaths involve several factors like those linked with human immunodeficiency virus (Saunders et al., 2009). All these aspects – the confusing mix of symptoms and the overall situation – prove why careful investigation is necessary. Basically, improving how we identify the manner of death is necessary for fair justice and better health in the community.

Test Your Knowledge

1. Define the term mode of death in forensic medicine.
2. List the common modes of death associated with trauma.

7.4. Interconnections Between Cause, Manner, and Mode of Death

Learning Outcome

1. Explain how cause, manner, and mode are interrelated;
2. Understand the importance of forensic pathology for these ideas.
3. Discuss the impact of misclassification on legal outcomes;
4. Discover the role of proper documentation in death investigations;
5. Understand case studies illustrating interconnections;
6. Examine how what the public thinks affects how death is classified.
7. Know the challenges faced by forensic professionals;
8. Describe future trends in death investigation;
9. Pay attention to how working with different experts improves the accuracy of the findings.

Mortality doesn't come with a neat instruction manual. The way we see things is nudged by understanding the cause, manner and mode of death. The main reason is usually that trigger which may be biological or environmental, that starts the process; the way the end happens often suggests whether it was an accident or something planned.

Then we have the mode which, in a broader sense, deals with the social and ethical aspects that influence our view of death. You see, almost without thinking, that these ideas show up over and over in our stories and discussions. For example, Updike's narratives often show how a fading trust can spiral into a sort of uneasy feeling about existence, highlighting life's inherent fragility (Duffy et al., 2012). Similarly, in more philosophical circles, discussions – like Hessens' critique of Newton – generally suggest that linking motion to cause might open up bigger, more puzzling questions about who we are and how we live with our mortality (Trisokkas et al., 2019).

7.4.1. How Cause, Manner, and Mode are Interrelated

Death can happen in ways that are hard to explain easily. The puzzle-like quality comes from blending cause, manner and mode which all play a role in telling the story. For example, the cause refers to what happened inside the body which is usually a clear problem like an injury or illness, but can also be less noticeable. Then there's the manner, which is all about the context: most often we split it into bouts like natural, accidental, suicidal, or even homicidal (in most cases, these labels help frame what happened). In contrast, mode makes the environment a key part of the process, including things from the environment that may add more to the investigation. For example, evidence isn't just one thing—it can pop up in unexpected places, like witness testimonies from parts of the scene that seem almost overlooked, yet are key to putting the picture together (Schuppli, 2020). All these elements, put together, help forensic experts solve cases. They also spark deeper questions about how we see and understand death—about accountability and the tales we weave around it—which, in a way, reveal how death impacts society (Fei-Wang et al., 2023).

7.4.2. The Role of Forensic Pathology in Understanding These Concepts

There are many parts to death such as what brought it about, how it developed and the way it ended. Forensic pathology becomes very important when things surrounding a sudden death are not clear. With careful study of the evidence left after death, experts can usually distinguish between a natural, accidental, self-inflicted or unnatural death. In general, they look at the evidence with a level of care that sometimes seems natural. Cutting-edge biometric methods, such as iris recognition, are showing promise too, adding a fresh twist to identifying the departed in real-world situations (Sansola et al., 2015). It's not only human cases that get noticed; vet forensic pathology shows how important scene investigations are. In many cases, digging into an animal death may reveal links to abuse—an issue that unexpectedly bleeds into wider societal concerns (Marchetti et al., 2023). In essence, forensic pathology extends far beyond the routine of autopsies, offering a richer, layered understanding of death's complicated nature (Figure 7.15).

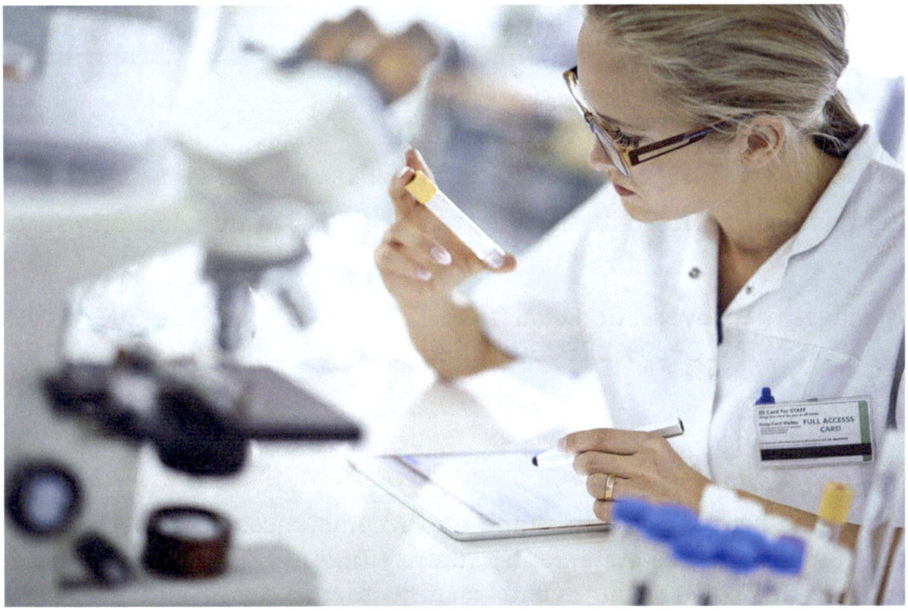

Figure 7.15. The role of forensic pathology in understanding cause, manner, and mode of death.

Source: https://collegeeducated.com/wp-content/uploads/2021/09/How-to-Become-a-Medical-Examiner.jpg.

7.4.3. Impact of Misclassification on Legal Outcomes

Sorting injuries and understanding their true purpose can change the legal results in ways that are not expected. When labels are wrong, everyone can misunderstand the situation - this is an even bigger problem in death investigations. A major problem is that there are often no clear definitions; many studies show this can make the data courts use less clear. If there is no clear way to tell apart accidental, suicidal and homicidal deaths, it becomes hard for the law to decide who is at fault and what punishment should be given. Not analyzing the data by intent can result in many errors that might affect justice. In most cases, experts note that this fuzzy way of talking about injury causes calls for legal and medical teams to come together and hash out a common standard, which should lead to a fairer legal process and better-informed decisions (Bebbington et al., 2023; Chino et al., 2010) (Figure 7.16).

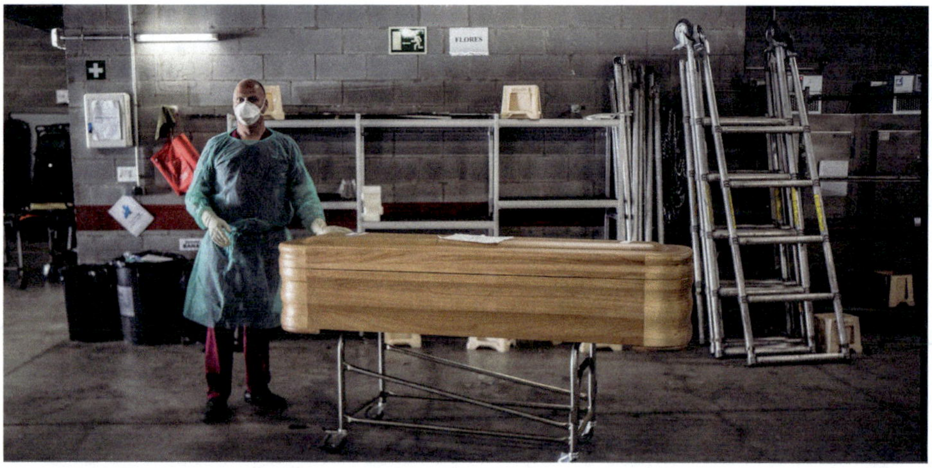

Figure 7.16. Classifying injuries and figuring out their real intent can tip legal outcomes in unexpected ways.

Source: https://images.theconversation.com/files/326115/original/file-20200407-74220-elf1i1.jpg?ixlib=rb-4.1.0&rect=44%2C329%2C5000%2C2500&q=45&auto=format&w=1356&h=668&fit=crop.

7.4.4. Importance of Accurate Documentation in Death Investigations

Gathering and recording proof helps determine the circumstances, reasons and time of the death. Everyday records such as witness statements, autopsy findings and scene analysis, help forensic investigators build a story about the events leading to the death and prepare for later legal action. Often, keeping all the information safe helps avoid minor mistakes that can later lead to misunderstandings; even little mistakes can affect the outcome in the wrong way. When records contain errors, it's thought that these errors can influence court decisions which is another reason for attention to detail. Even when it means changing to fit different areas, making this process standard helps experts from different places cooperate more easily. To summarize, keeping careful records does more than address single cases—it feeds into a larger picture of public health and safety in today's complex socio-legal landscape (Joglar et al., 2023; Manyi-Loh et al., 2018).

7.4.5. Case Studies Illustrating Interconnections

It's not only about the one moment of death—it's also about all the different things that happen around it. Case studies clearly demonstrate how these areas overlap, especially by comparing the actual cause, the manner and the way death occurs. Often, a detailed study of clinical workflows finds that a small error or mistake can quickly spread and cause serious, even deadly, results. Generally speaking, this idea kind of mirrors what Hessen points out when critiquing Newton's old framework; not noticing all the subtle shifts in motion ends up being similar to missing how small, overlooked interactions in a medical setup can suddenly trigger major issues (Trisokkas et al., 2019). Moreover, using automated tools to sift through safety data in hospitals can boost our ability to pinpoint what went wrong—helping to carve out more targeted steps to reduce risks and, ideally, get better results overall (Al-Qora'n et al., 2014). All in all, understanding how all these details are linked is very important for understanding mortality.

7.4.6. The Influence of Public Perception on Death Classification

Classifying death is mainly influenced by regular people's opinions which are shaped by their culture and personal experiences, rather than just by doctors or specialists. How people see things affects which types of deaths and causes are given priority, even though the process may look technical. Usually, views on health impact how we understand deaths from genetic conditions. For example, adults with cystic fibrosis blur the old picture of the disease as a childhood tragedy; their lived experiences push us toward a more layered idea of survival and quality of life (Lowton and Gabe, 2003). In mixed-use areas, too, public take on different transportation methods can, rather interestingly, alter perceptions of risk and even steer policy decisions (Belz et al., 2018). To summarize, the back-and-forth between common beliefs and death classification remains a fascinating, if sometimes messy, subject for further sociological study (Figure 7.17).

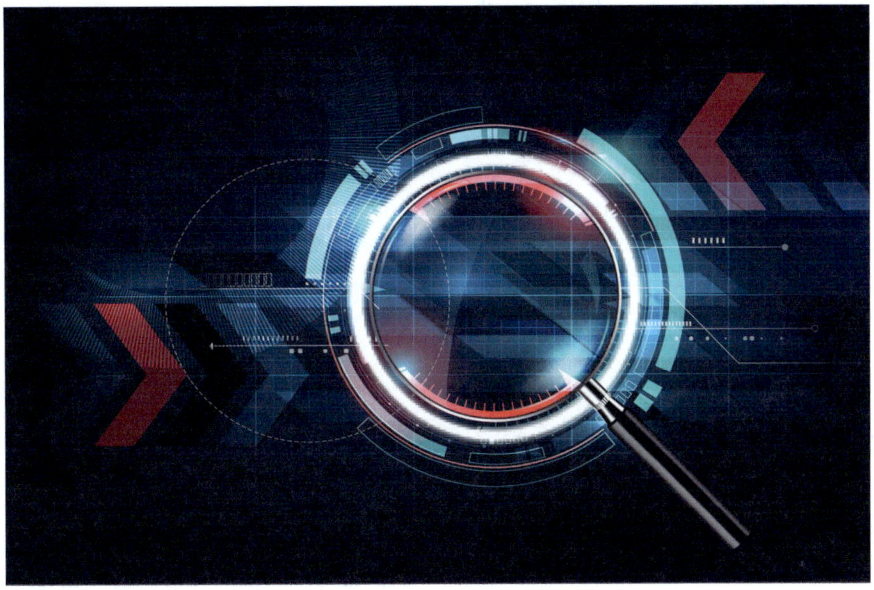

Figure 7.17. People's views end up shaping which causes and manners of death get more attention—even if the process seems technical at first glance.

Source: https://blog.ipleaders.in/wp-content/uploads/2020/09/abstract-arrows_direction_process_magnifying-glass_search_investigate-100777420-large.jpg.

7.4.7. Challenges Faced by Forensic Professionals

It can be very difficult to figure out how a victim died. There are many unpredictable factors at crime scenes now such as changing weather and more technology which make it tough to solve cases. In these situations, forensic practitioners have a hard time determining the cause, manner and mode of death. They're compelled to constantly refresh their skills, a process that, in most cases, is hampered by long-standing resource shortages and insufficient support structures (Fleming et al., 2021). Public views, too, complicate matters; media portrayals often skew the true nature of their work and sometimes pressure labs into rushing their analysis, risking accuracy along the way (Wang et al., 2022). In short, these problems highlight the importance of providing more training, better resources and better information about modern forensic science to the public.

7.4.8. Future Trends in Death Investigation

Technology is transforming everything and that change is touching the way we view deaths. These days, newer and faster methods are being used to work out the cause of death and what happened. For example, AI and machine learning are working with data that is not organized, finding patterns that people might not notice. Occasionally, by mixing advanced imaging with usual toxicology exams, scientists can discover changes in the body and get hints about the environment. The whole scene got extra complicated when events like the SARS-CoV-2 outbreak hit, kick-starting ideas about systems that can quickly track illness and death in real-time (Hu et al., 2020). There's also chatter about research into things like flavonoids, which seems to nudge us toward mixing different fields together in hopes of uncovering more hidden links (Panche et al., 2016).

7.4.9. The Role of Interdisciplinary Collaboration in Improving Accuracy

To find out how, why and in what way a death occurs, investigators look at many different clues. Forensic experts, lawyers and doctors all add their ideas and in general this mix results in a picture that is not always easy to follow or understand. You might find that adding in neurobiological ideas—what some call neurolaw, as noted in Caruso (2024)—can shift the focus on issues like legal insanity and even help predict future behavior. Looking closely at the physical evidence using advanced forensic methods is very important; it helps to understand the events leading up to the death which is why teamwork between forensic pathologists and others is important. As Abrol (2024) points out, this kind of mixing not only ramps up the accuracy of the findings but also holds together the solid integrity of postmortem exams, ultimately lending a hand in the quest for justice. To summarize, when these experts chat and share their points of view—sometimes in a slightly off rhythm—it boosts our ability to understand the messy, complex nature of death and its ripple effects on society (Figure 7.18).

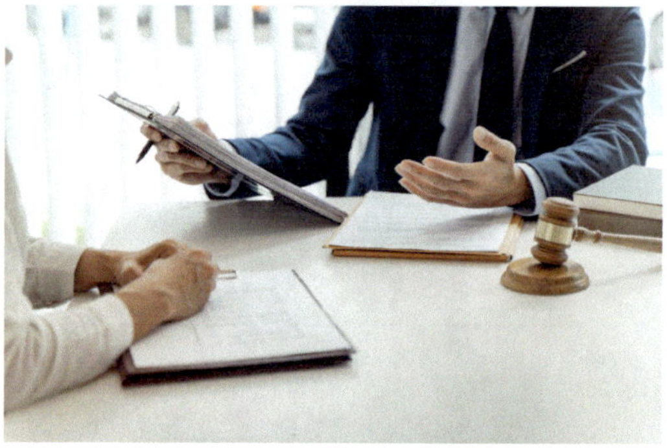

Figure 7.18. Forensic experts, lawyers, and doctors throw their insights into the mix, and generally speaking this mix of perspectives builds a picture that isn't always neat or linear.

Source: https://www.fcpsychexperts.com/wp-content/uploads/2024/09/2-Forensic-psychologist-sitting-at-a-table-talking-to-a-person-while-holding-documents-1024x683.png.

Test Your Knowledge

1. How are the mode of death, the cause of death and the manner of death different from each other?
2. Is it still possible to find out the cause of death if the body is decomposed? Explain.

Summary

Death is never as simple as it seems. When we examine it, understanding cause, manner and mode helps us understand how things end. Think about older patients with heart failure—studies generally show that as overall frailty increases, deaths not tied to heart issues also rise, implying that aging adds extra challenges to understanding mortality (Ohashi et al., 2024). Sometimes, there are even those bizarre cases — like someone ending their own life by, say, using cable ties for self-strangulation — that remind us death can come about in unexpected, if not downright perplexing, ways (Cecannecchia et al., 2024). Usually, these observations suggest that it is important to analyze all the details carefully in both forensic investigations and medical checks, to see what led to the death.

Death is not only about our bodies stopping—it's also about the many ways our lives affect our views on dying. Today, people tend to look at the mind and deeper thoughts as well as just biology when discussing health. Take, for instance, the BBC series In the Flesh; here, the mix of market-driven medical routines with everyday life kind of forces us to rethink what life and death mean, poking holes in those old, Gothic ideas (Murnane et al., 2016). A FOUCAULTian spin on this, in most cases, makes clear that political and moral judgments about death aren't just academic—they actually steer how we talk about and react to it (Kendall et al., 2008). As soon as we look at all these issues together, we realize that why, how and in what way death occurs is influenced by culture and economics, so the only way to understand them is to look at them from many perspectives.

KEY TERMS FROM THIS CHAPTER

Accidents
Cardiovascular issues
Healthcare
Lifestyle choices
Racism
Cancer
Collapse
Heart problems
Momentary lapse
Suicides
Canines
Disease
Infections
Mortality
Transportation habits

Short Answer Questions

1. How does toxicological analysis help to find out why someone died?
2. In forensic science, what is meant by "undetermined cause of death"?
3. How do the findings from the autopsy agree or disagree with the cause of death given by the medical examiner?
4. In sudden death cases which organs are checked to find out the cause?
5. Which person or group is responsible for deciding how a death occurred in a medico-legal case?
6. In what ways can forensic evidence affect the way a death is classified?
7. How does asphyxia relate to the mode of death?

Critical Thinking Questions

1. **The cause of death refers to:**
   a. The underlying physiological process that leads to death
   b. The specific injury or disease that caused the death
   c. The classification of death (e.g., homicide, suicide)
   d. The manner in which death occurred (e.g., asphyxia, drowning)
2. **Which of the following is a way to describe the manner of death?**
   a. Gunshot wound to the chest
   b. Cardiac arrest
   c. Homicide
   d. Hemorrhage
3. **Mode of death is best described as:**
   a. The physiological process leading to death
   b. The underlying disease or injury that led to death
   c. The specific cause of the fatal injury
   d. The manner in which death occurred (e.g., drowning, blunt force trauma)
4. **Which of these is not a usual way people die?**
   a. Natural
   b. Homicide
   c. Suicide
   d. Infection
5. **In a suspected homicide, the reason for death is frequently:**
   a. Trauma
   b. Gunshot wound

c. Poisoning
d. All of the above

Answers to Critical Thinking Questions

1. (b); 2. (c); 3. (a); 4. (d); 5. (d)

References

1. Aarons, D. (2008). The abolitionist's dilemma: Establishing the standards for the evolving standards of decency. https://core.ac.uk/download/72052624.pdf (accessed on 29 May 2025).
2. Ab Hamid, H., Abd Hamid, R., Ahmed, N., Al-Mulla, et al. (2015). Assessing the carcinogenic potential of low-dose exposures to chemical mixtures in the environment: The challenge ahead. https://core.ac.uk/download/29410057.pdf (accessed on 29 May 2025).
3. Abrol, V. (2024). *Forensic science: Revealing the clues*. IntechOpen. https://doi.org/10.5772/intechopen.1003870.
4. Alfieri, L., Montana, A., Frisoni, P., D'Errico, S., & Neri, M. (2024). Application of aquaporins as markers in forensic pathology: A systematic review of the literature. *International Journal of Molecular Sciences, 25*, 2664. https://doi.org/10.3390/ijms25052664.
5. Al-Qora'n, L., Gordon, N., Papadopoulos, et al. (2014). An approach to safety analysis of clinical workflows. https://core.ac.uk/download/151160849.pdf (accessed on 29 May 2025).
6. Ard, J., Atkinson, S., Bier, D., et al. (2016). Options for basing Dietary Reference Intakes (DRIs) on chronic disease endpoints: Report from a joint US-/Canadian-sponsored working group. https://core.ac.uk/download/323080977.pdf.
7. Aristovnik, A., Keržič, D., Ravšelj, D., Tomaževič, N., & Umek, L. (2020). Impacts of the COVID-19 pandemic on life of higher education students: A global perspective. *Sustainability, 12*, 8438. https://doi.org/10.3390/su12208438.
8. Authors Task Force Members, Rydén, L., Grant, P. J., Anker, S. D., Berne, C., Cosentino, F., Danchin, N., et al. (2013). ESC guidelines on diabetes, pre-diabetes, and cardiovascular diseases developed in collaboration with the EASD. *European Heart Journal, 34*(39), 3035–3087. https://doi.org/10.1093/eurheartj/eht108.
9. Barbieri, S., Cozzi, B., Frisoni, P., et al. (2018). The diatoms test in veterinary medicine: A pilot study on cetaceans and sea turtles. https://core.ac.uk/download/159636681.pdf (accessed on 29 May 2025).
10. Bebbington, E., Bibi, F., Kakola, M., et al. (2023). Terminology and methods used to differentiate injury intent of hospital burn patients in South Asia: Results from a systematic scoping review. https://core.ac.uk/download/590715413.pdf (accessed on 29 May 2025).
11. Belz, N., & Chang, K. (2018). Mixed-use safety on rural facilities in the Pacific Northwest: Consideration of vehicular, non-traditional, and non-motorized users. https://core.ac.uk/download/286999908.pdf (accessed on 29 May 2025).
12. Berg, A. T., Berkovic, S. F., Brodie, M. J., Buchhalter, J., Cross, J. H., van Emde Boas, W., Engel, J., et al. (2010). Revised terminology and concepts for organization of seizures and epilepsies:

Report of the ILAE Commission on Classification and Terminology, 2005–2009. *Epilepsia, 51*(6), 676–685. https://doi.org/10.1111/j.1528-1167.2010.02522.x.

13. Bernstein, S. (2019). Moral luck and deviant causation. *Midwest Studies in Philosophy, 43*(1), 151–161. https://doi.org/10.1111/misp.12110.
14. Boros, G., Szalai, J., & Toth, O. I. (2017). *The Concept of Affectivity in Early Modern Philosophy* (ISBN 978-963-284-820-4). https://core.ac.uk/download/131216162.pdf
15. Boswood, A., Braz-Ruivo, L., Culshaw, G. J., Dukes-McEwan, J., et al. (2012). Efficacy of pimobendan in the prevention of congestive heart failure or sudden death in Doberman Pinschers with preclinical dilated cardiomyopathy (the PROTECT study). https://core.ac.uk/download/16458069.pdf.
16. Bourdieu, P., Carey, N., Caruth, C., Cohen, A., Interpol, Lessig, R., Marshall, R. D., et al. (2014). Who knows who we are? Questioning DNA analysis in disaster victim identification. https://core.ac.uk/download/30704511.pdf (accessed on 29 May 2025).
17. Breen, L. J., Eisma, M. C., Johnson, A. R., O'Connor, M., et al. (2021). Does voluntary assisted dying cause public stigma for the bereaved? A vignette-based experiment. https://core.ac.uk/download/519040284.pdf.
18. Caine, E., Connery, H., Jia, H., Lilly, M., et al. (2018). Method overtness, forensic autopsy, and the evidentiary suicide note: A multilevel national violent death reporting system analysis. https://core.ac.uk/download/195692285.pdf (accessed on 29 May 2025).
19. Cardaci, N. (2017). *Rus v Comcare: The Rules of Evidence in the AAT*. https://core.ac.uk/download/213607843.pdf (accessed on 29 May 2025).
20. Caruso, G. D. (2024). *Neurolaw*. Cambridge University Press. https://doi.org/10.1017/9781009271172.
21. Cecannecchia, C., De Simone, S., Baldari, B., Cipolloni, L., & Cioffi, A. (2024). Strangulation using cable ties and a suicidal manner of death: A case report and literature review addressing an atypical suicidal mode. *Forensic Sciences*. https://www.semanticscholar.org/paper/b6d1041541ad2e2a10bd7ea3424e2c7ae8271d79 (accessed on 29 May 2025).
22. Celis-Morales, C. A., Lyall, D. M., Welsh, P., Anderson, J., Steell, L., Guo, Y., et al. (2017). Association between active commuting and incident cardiovascular disease, cancer, and mortality: Prospective cohort study. *BMJ, 357*, j1456. https://doi.org/10.1136/bmj.j1456.
23. Chino, M., Clark, W., Compher, C., Graham, R., et al. (2010). Indigenous health – Australia, Canada, New Zealand and the United States–Laying claim to a future that embraces health for us all. https://digitalscholarship.unlv.edu/cgi/viewcontent.cgi?article=1206&context=community_health_sciences_fac_articles (accessed on 29 May 2025).
24. Christine, B., Franz, P., Guzmán, E. M., Glenn, C. R., Kleiman, E. M., & Nock, M. K. (2017). Annual research review: Suicide among youth–epidemiology, (potential) etiology, and treatment. *Journal of Child Psychology and Psychiatry, 59*(4), 460–482. https://doi.org/10.1111/jcpp.12831.
25. Coole, D. (2005). Agency, truth and meaning: Judging the Hutton report. https://core.ac.uk/download/7337.pdf (accessed on 29 May 2025).
26. Duffy, B. (2012). Loss of trust as disconnection in John Updike's *Trust Me*. *e-Rea, 9*(2). http://journals.openedition.org/erea/2496 https://doi.org/10.4000/erea.2496 (accessed on 29 May 2025).

27. Dussault, M. C., Smith, M., & Hanson, I. (2016). Evaluation of trauma patterns in blast injuries using multiple correspondence analysis. *Forensic Science International, 267*, 66–72. https://doi.org/10.1016/j.forsciint.2016.08.004.

28. Federspiel, J. M., Potente, S., Abeln, K. B., Hennemann, K., Heinbuch, S., Burkhard, K., Richl, M., Kettner, M., Lux, C., Schmidt, P., Verhoff, M. A., & Ramsthaler, F. (2023). Forensic, legal, and clinical aspects of deaths associated with implanted cardiac devices. *Frontiers in Psychiatry, 14*, 1278078. https://doi.org/10.3389/fpsyt.2023.1278078.

29. Fleming, K. A., Horton, S., Wilson, M. L., Atun, R., DeStigter, K., Flanigan, J., Sayed, S., et al. (2021). The Lancet Commission on diagnostics: Transforming access to diagnostics. *The Lancet, 398*(10309), 1997–2050. https://doi.org/10.1016/s0140-6736(21)00673-5.

30. Forbes, S., Lewis, S., & Swann, L. (2010). Analytical separations of mammalian decomposition products for forensic science: A review. https://core.ac.uk/download/195666455.pdf (accessed on 29 May 2025).

31. Gaiseanu, F. D. (2018). Destiny or free will decision? A life overview from the perspective of an informational modeling of consciousness part II: Attitude and decision criteria, free will and destiny. *Gerontology & Geriatric Studies, 4*(1), GGS.000576. https://doi.org/10.31031/GGS.2018.03.000576.

32. Gamache, K., Platania, J., & Zaitchik, M. (2013). Evaluating future dangerousness and need for treatment: The roles of expert testimony, attributional complexity, and victim type. https://core.ac.uk/download/56706256.pdf (accessed on 29 May 2025).

33. Grossman, S. P. (2014). Using the DNA testing of arrestees to reevaluate Fourth Amendment doctrine. https://core.ac.uk/download/144552234.pdf (accessed on 29 May 2025).

34. Henrich, J., Heine, S. J., & Norenzayan, A. (2010). The weirdest people in the world? *Behavioral and Brain Sciences, 33*(2, 3), 61–83. https://doi.org/10.1017/s0140525x0999152x.

35. Horgan, P. G., Mansouri, D., McMillan, D. C., Park, J. J., et al. (2016). Long-term follow-up of patients undergoing resection of TNM stage I colorectal cancer: An analysis of tumor and host determinants of outcome. https://core.ac.uk/download/42372439.pdf.

36. Hu, B., Guo, H., Zhou, P., & Shi, Z. L. (2020). Characteristics of SARS-CoV-2 and COVID-19. *Nature Reviews Microbiology, 19*(3), 141–154. https://doi.org/10.1038/s41579-020-00459-7.

37. Joglar, J. A., Chung, M. K., Armbruster, A. L., Benjamin, E. J., Chyou, J. Y., Cronin, E. M., Deswal, A., et al. (2023). 2023 ACC/AHA/ACCP/HRS guideline for the diagnosis and management of atrial fibrillation: A report of the American College of Cardiology/American Heart Association Joint Committee on Clinical Practice Guidelines. *Circulation, 149*. https://doi.org/10.1161/cir.0000000000001193.

38. Kendall, G., & Wickham, G. (2008). Critical discourse analysis, description, explanation, causes: Foucault's inspiration versus Weber's perspiration. https://core.ac.uk/download/11237206.pdf (accessed on 29 May 2025).

39. Khilji, S., Verma, P. K., Patel, D., & Chouksey, V. (2024). Analysis of injury patterns in railway track death and their correlation with manner of death in the Bhopal region—An autopsy-based study. *Journal of Indian Academy of Forensic Medicine*. https://www.semanticscholar.org/paper/2ee4f161acc931e3c8ec947fbaa12aa79de58955 (accessed on 29 May 2025).

40. Kuvaja, P., Keinänen, N., & Pakanen, L. (2022). The incidence of iatrogenic deaths in the

Finnish cause-of-death statistics; a retrospective study. *Journal of Forensic and Legal Medicine, 86*, 102302. https://doi.org/10.1016/j.jflm.2021.102302.

41. Lewis, D. (2020). *A Profile of Methamphetamine Use in Coronial Cases in South Australia Over the Last 20 Years* (Honors thesis, Adelaide Medical School). https://core.ac.uk/download/482263609.pdf (accessed on 29 May 2025).
42. Ljung, L., Nazin, A., & Roll, J. (2005). Escaping the shadow of malpractice law. https://core.ac.uk/download/62552953.pdf (accessed on 29 May 2025).
43. Lowton, K., & Gabe, J. (2003). Life on a slippery slope: Perceptions of health in adults with cystic fibrosis. *Sociology of Health & Illness, 25*(3), 289–319. https://doi.org/10.1111/1467-9566.00348.
44. Malinowski, B. (2018). *Crime and Custom in Savage Society*. Routledge. https://doi.org/10.4324/9780203794449.
45. Manchikanti, L. (2017). Responsible, safe, and effective prescription of opioids for chronic non-cancer pain: American Society of Interventional Pain Physicians (ASIPP) guidelines. *Pain Physician, 2*, s3–s92. https://doi.org/10.36076/ppj.2017.s92.
46. Manyi-Loh, C. E., Mamphweli, S., Meyer, E. L., & Okoh, A. I. (2018). Antibiotic use in agriculture and its consequential resistance in environmental sources: Potential public health implications. *Molecules, 23*(4), 795. https://doi.org/10.3390/molecules23040795.
47. Marchetti, C., Mastrogiuseppe, L., Vanin, S., Cecchi, R., & Gherardi, M. (2023). On-site inspection form in veterinary cases: The Parma veterinary form. *Animals, 13*(13), 2064. https://doi.org/10.3390/ani13132064.
48. Mayedo, Y. O., Seyoumk, M., & Solano, E. E. (2017). A one-year retrospective study on the pattern of death found at autopsy at Forensic Pathology Department, Menelik II Hospital in Addis Ababa, Ethiopia. https://core.ac.uk/download/478441690.pdf (accessed on 29 May 2025).
49. McClave, S. A., Taylor, B., Martindale, R. G., Warren, M., Johnson, D. R., Braunschweig, C., McCarthy, M. S., et al. (2016). Guidelines for the provision and assessment of nutrition support therapy in the adult critically ill patient. *Journal of Parenteral and Enteral Nutrition, 40*, 159–211. https://doi.org/10.1177/0148607115621863.
50. Mishra, A., & Upadhyay, P. W. (2021). Forensic anthropology. https://core.ac.uk/download/479933772.pdf (accessed on 29 May 2025).
51. Murnane, B. (2016). In the flesh and the Gothic: Pharmacology of everyday life; or into and out of the Gothic. *Text Matters: A Journal of Literature, Theory and Culture,* (6), 227–244. https://doi.org/10.1515/texmat-2016-0014.
52. Noonan, L. (2013). Can human beings truly be considered free? https://core.ac.uk/download/56325485.pdf (accessed on 29 May 2025).
53. Ntelia, R. E. (2015). Death in digital games: A thanatological approach. https://core.ac.uk/download/46604347.pdf (accessed on 29 May 2025).
54. Odysseos, L. (2002). Dangerous ontologies: The ethos of survival and ethical theorizing in international relations. *Review of International Studies, 28*(2), 403–418. https://doi.org/10.1017/S0260210502004035.

55. Ohashi, K., Matsue, Y., Maeda, D., Fujimoto, Y., Kagiyama, N., Sunayama, T., Dotare, T., et al. (2024). Impact of multidomain frailty on the mode of death in older patients with heart failure: A cohort study. *Circulation: Cardiovascular Quality and Outcomes, 17*, e010416. https://www.semanticscholar.org/paper/097f39ef67b4b9350b270fdcf87e4e1e86eaa7bc (accessed on 29 May 2025).

56. Palladino, P. (2003). The politics of death: On life after the 'end of history'. https://core.ac.uk/download/69941.pdf (accessed on 29 May 2025).

57. Panche, A., Diwan, A. D., & Chandra, S. (2016). Flavonoids: An overview. *Journal of Nutritional Science, 5*, e41. https://doi.org/10.1017/jns.2016.41.

58. Park, S., & Kim, Y. G. (2022). A metaverse: Taxonomy, components, applications, and open challenges. *IEEE Access, 10*, 4209–4251. https://doi.org/10.1109/access.2021.3140175.

59. Previti, A., Biondi, V., Pugliese, M., Alibrandi, A., Zirilli, A., Roccaro, M., Peli, A., & Passantino, A. (2024). Canine euthanasia's trend analysis during thirty years (1990–2020) in Italy: A veterinary hospital as case study. *Veterinary Sciences, 11*(5), 224. https://doi.org/10.3390/vetsci11050224.

60. Rabinovich-Einy, O. (2011). Escaping the shadow of malpractice law. *Law and Contemporary Problems, 74*(3), 241–278. https://scholarship.law.duke.edu/lcp/vol74/iss3/10 (accessed on 29 May 2025).

61. Reddy, A., & Sujatha, S. (2019). Presence of pyrroloquinazoline alkaloid in *Adhatoda vasica* attenuates inflammatory response through the downregulation of pro-inflammatory mediators in LPS stimulated RAW 264.7 macrophages. *Bio Impacts: BI, 11*, 15–22. https://www.semanticscholar.org/paper/e299c9570505f2a54c5bf51c88380c4310541a0b (accessed on 29 May 2025).

62. Reiner, Ž., Catapano, A. L., De Backer, G., Graham, I., Taskinen, M. R., Wiklund, O., Agewall, S., et al. (2011). ESC/EAS guidelines for the management of dyslipidemias: The task force for the management of dyslipidemias of the European Society of Cardiology (ESC) and the European Atherosclerosis Society (EAS). *European Heart Journal, 32*(17), 1769–1818. https://doi.org/10.1093/eurheartj/ehr158.

63. Richards, N. (2017). Old age rational suicide. *Sociology Compass, 11*, e12456. https://doi.org/10.1111/soc4.12456.

64. Rockett, I. R., Wang, S., Stack, S., et al. (2010). Race/ethnicity and potential suicide misclassification: Window on a minority suicide paradox? *BMC Psychiatry, 10*, 35. https://doi.org/10.1186/1471-244X-10-35.

65. Saghir, R. (2020). Retrospective autopsy-based analysis of nature and prevalence of fatal injuries in Lahore. https://media.neliti.com/media/publications/301998-retrospective-autopsy-based-analysis-of-ce6fc605.pdf (accessed on 29 May 2025).

66. Sansola, A. (2015). Postmortem iris recognition and its application in human identification. https://open.bu.edu/bitstream/2144/13975/8/Sansola_bu_0017N_11536_web.pdf (accessed on 29 May 2025).

67. Saunders, J. J. (2009). Analysis of quantification methods used for cell viability, cell morphology, and synaptic formation in modeling HIV associated dementia in primary neuronal cultures. https://core.ac.uk/download/12208909.pdf (accessed on 29 May 2025).

68. Schuppli, S. (2020). *Material Witness*. The MIT Press. https://doi.org/10.7551/mitpress/9953.001.0001.

69. Silas, O. A., Adoga, A. A., Manasseh, A. N., Echejoh, G. O., Mandong, B. M., & Olu-Silas, R. (2009). The role of necropsy in diagnostic dilemmas as seen in a tertiary hospital in north central Nigeria. *Journal of Tropical Medicine, 2009*, 718984. https://doi.org/10.1155/2009/718984.

70. Soss, J., & Weaver, V. M. (2017). Police are our government: Politics, political science, and the policing of race–class subjugated communities. *Annual Review of Political Science, 20*, 565–591. https://doi.org/10.1146/annurev-polisci-060415-093825.

71. Tharp, A. M., Hobron, K., & Haupt Wright, T. (2019). Gabapentin-related deaths: Patterns of abuse and postmortem levels. *Journal of Forensic Sciences, 64*(4), 1105–1111. https://doi.org/10.1111/1556-4029.14021.

72. Toth, O. I. (2017). Is Spinoza's theory of finite mind coherent? –Death, affectivity and epistemology in the Ethics. https://core.ac.uk/download/131216013.pdf (accessed on 29 May 2025).

73. Trisokkas, I. (2019). Boris Hessen and Newton's God. *Society and Politics, 13*(1), 64–86.

74. Vadysinghe, A. N., Senasinghe, D. P. P., Sivasubramanium, M., Jayasooriya, P., Premarathna, B. G., Rathnayake, R. M. I. S. D., & Wickramasinghe, M. M. H. P. (2018). Unnatural deaths of the elderly population of Sri Lanka. *American Journal of Forensic Medicine & Pathology, 39*(2), 148–151. https://doi.org/10.1097/paf.0000000000000383.

75. Wallace, R. (2003). Structured psychosocial stress and therapeutic intervention: Toward a realistic biological medicine. Retrieved from: https://core.ac.uk/download/pdf/85483.pdf.

76. Wallace, R. (2003). *Systemic lupus erythematosus in African-American Women: Immune Cognitive Modules, Autoimmune Disease, and Pathogenic Social Hierarchy*.

77. Wang, F. Y., Hu, J., & Lai, J. (2023). Testing intelligence: Accelerating the verification and validation of intelligent vehicles. *IEEE Transactions on Intelligent Vehicles, 8*, 1003–1016. https://doi.org/10.1109/tiv.2023.3246701.

78. Wang, Y., Su, Z., Zhang, N., Xing, R., Liu, D., Luan, T. H., & Shen, X. (2022). A survey on metaverse: Fundamentals, security, and privacy. *IEEE Communications Surveys & Tutorials, 25*(1), 319–352. https://doi.org/10.1109/comst.2022.3202047.

79. Wood, S. K. (2017). *Baptism*. Retrieved from: https://core.ac.uk/download/213087952.pdf (accessed on 29 May 2025).

80. Xu, Z., Zou, X., Yin, Z., Zhang, S., Song, Y., Zhang, J., & Lu, J. (2020). Prediction model of ammonia concentration in yellow-feather broilers house during winter based on EEMD-GRU. *Poultry Science, 61*, 59–70. https://www.semanticscholar.org/paper/2e1096015bb1983273b0b5acfc9015828cf7c3f0 (accessed on 29 May 2025).

81. Yuan, Z., Nag, R., & Cummins, E. (2022). Human health concerns regarding microplastics in the aquatic environment–From marine to food systems. *The Science of the Total Environment, 823*, 153730. https://doi.org/10.1016/j.scitotenv.2022.153730.

MECHANICAL INJURIES

8

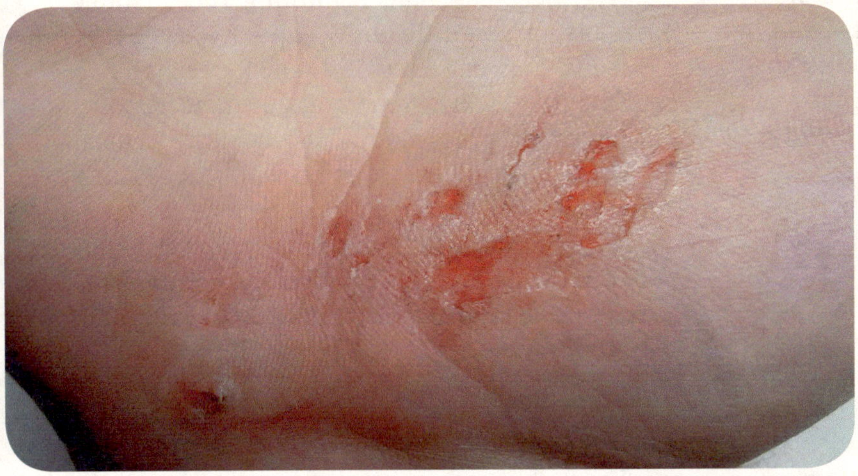

LEARNING OBJECTIVES

After studying this chapter, you will be able to:

1. Identify types of mechanical injuries;
2. Understand the mechanisms of injury;
3. Explain forensic analysis techniques;
4. Learn the legal implications of mechanical injuries.

Introduction

There have been some surprising changes in forensic science, mainly with mechanical injuries. They can happen in many ways and are examined to see what their legal significance might be. Experts carefully examine every aspect of an injury, sometimes using modern equipment and sometimes by doing manual checks, to learn the whole story. It involves digital devices and a lot of training that can point out the injuries and suggest who may be responsible from a legal perspective. Take safety education, for instance; game-based learning now helps people pick up essential skills without any real risk (Jin et al., 2020). And then there's veterinary forensics, which turns the spotlight on how injuries in animals can reveal details about animal-related crimes, expanding the whole idea of what forensic investigations can cover (Viciano et al., 2022).

Definition of Mechanical Injuries

Forensic science focuses on trauma which is often a complicated topic. If something outside the body puts pressure or stretches tissues in an unusual way, it is called a mechanical injury. Sometimes a small-looking scratch can end up as a nasty fracture or a deep cut if the force is strong enough and sudden. Quite often, investigators have to explore these details since each injury appears to reveal its own bit of the story. The situation is not always clear; the environment and social aspects usually add more factors to think about. Take natural disasters, for example—when they hit, they can batter a person's body, complicating how these injury patterns show up and, in most cases, stressing why a thorough look is so crucial in forensic settings (Kishore et al., 2018; Layden et al., 2019) (Figure 8.1).

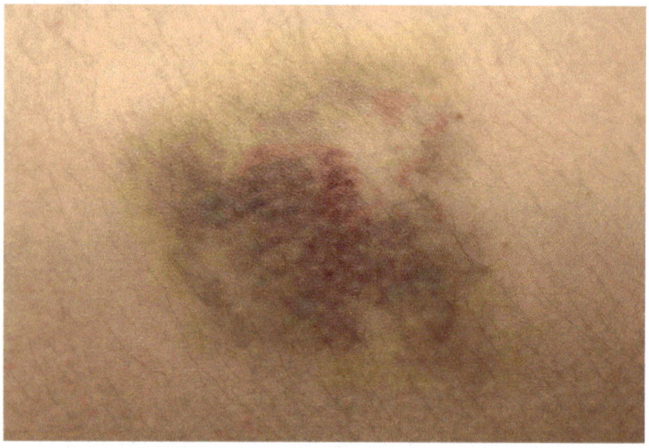

Figure 8.1. When external forces hit body tissues—pressing or stretching them in unexpected ways—the result is what we call mechanical injuries.

Source: https://blogger.googleusercontent.com/img/b/R29vZ2xl/AVvXsEiFhvqM73wKl6d4WItJqHrh-AlfioA7DaerbHd8vJRt96PaQ51xen7jRhWlS6ttdyzTuxAnWJUFS1R4N6gKtQSxT6hbJyaGeoJoSNN986RwZ_RFOxU6uMjW2Nw8Fgjc2_v6gO9uFugSFyBshPkrx1vbeGKKb4S_8c9PYLbXRAXDT9zXjQ7EKbIFstT5/s3600/Bruise.jpg.

Importance of Studying Mechanical Injuries

Injuries to the body can show what happened during an accident. These injuries are rarely random; often, experts see that they reveal details about the events leading up to the trauma. Forensic specialists carefully look at all the bruises and cuts, trying to build a timeline that reveals both the extent of the injury and who might have caused it. Forensic experts often say that examining these injury patterns can guide how an investigation proceeds and can also influence decisions in court. With legal reviews of forensic reports getting stricter nowadays, it's become crucial for these documents to mix plain, accessible language with technical accuracy (Reeder et al., 2024). Looking at mechanical injuries is not only about the injuries themselves—it involves social and legal issues that matter to everyone.

Overview of Types of Mechanical Injuries

Mechanical injuries usually provide special hints that help solve a crime. You see, bruises (or what we call contusions), cuts— more like lacerations—scrapes, broken bones, and even puncture marks each add a layer of meaning. A bruise is usually caused by a blunt object, but a cut is usually caused by something sharp. Most of the time, broken bones point to the presence of a force and sometimes they can even tell us how the force was created such as by looking at patterns in car crashes. Nowadays, experts are even turning to materials that mimic human tissue to get a more detailed examination of the injuries; as some studies show (dos Santos et al., 2025), this approach helps unravel the events leading up to the harm. Head injuries, which quite often come from roadway incidents, also underline a growing call for even more precise forensic profiles to better inform legal decisions (Khan et al., 2024). All these injury types, seen together, can give a clearer, though sometimes complicated, idea of what happened.

Historical Context of Mechanical Injuries

As time has gone on, forensic science has changed the way mechanical injuries are viewed in legal cases. At first, cases depended on what witnesses said; as time went on, experts started to use knowledge of anatomy and basic physics to better understand injuries. Improvements in medical law and advanced methods to examine evidence gradually formed a good foundation for analyzing mechanical damage. A few surveys, for instance, show that roughly 74.2% of forensic experts now use structured assessment tools (Tess Neal et al., 2014). It suggests that people are now using data instead of just their opinions which usually increases the reliability of the results. Meanwhile, machine learning has wedded itself to these techniques, bumping up the whole process, and suggesting that, in the near future, technology might just streamline injury assessments and, perhaps, strengthen judicial outcomes (Das et al., 2015).

Relevance to Criminal Investigations

Mechanical injuries in forensic investigations bring together various clues that make criminal investigations more interesting. Discovering the sequence of events in these injuries can also suggest who was involved, even if things get complicated. Sometimes the way forensic medical experts go about their work ends up giving reports that aren't totally consistent, which can, in many cases, put a dent in how reliable the evidence appears in court (Meilia et al., 2018). Looking closely at the injuries helps distinguish between a deliberate act and an accident which makes the crime scene clearer. On a related note, checking out the behaviors of mentally disordered offenders (MDOs) and weighing their risks provides extra insight into possible future actions, thereby stressing the need for a rounded forensic check-up (Birgit Völlm et al., 2018). To summarize, these jumbled factors remind us—even if it doesn't all come out perfectly neat—that detailed forensic evaluations play a key role in untangling criminal cases (Figure 8.2).

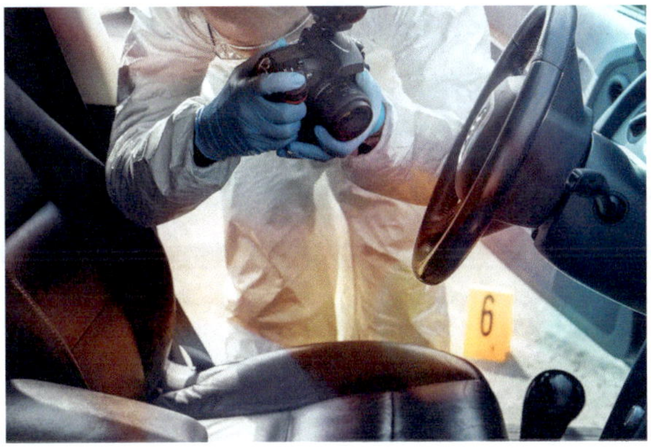

Figure 8.2. Mechanical injuries in forensic work deliver a tangled mix of clues that spice up criminal investigations.

Source: https://s3.us-east-1.amazonaws.com/jensenhughes/1920x1000_Web-Headers/_1920x1350_crop_center-center_80_none/73629/Forensics_Car_InjuryAnalysis_-iStock-669393012_OVL_WEB_1920x1000.webp.

Methodology for Analyzing Mechanical Injuries

To deal with mechanical injuries, a solid way is needed to detect the kind and severity of the injury. In most cases, you first collect data from the real world; occasionally, advanced imaging is used to spot the fine details of the injury. Take bite mark studies, for instance—they've pushed the idea of clever software that helps forensic experts match patterns against huge population databases, which in most cases sharpens the accuracy of pinpointing the injury's source (Ozcanet al., 2014). On another front, research into injuries from low-velocity weapons (say, aluminum arrows) reminds us that details like what someone's wearing and exactly how the weapon is built matter a lot. In some investigations, factors such as the shape of an arrowhead and even how snug the clothing fits can affect how deep something goes and how severe the damage turns out, handing over vital info for forensic analysis (Beattie et al., 2018). When all these techniques are combined, forensic professionals can build a clearer, though not always tidy, description of the events that led to the trauma.

8.1. Types of Mechanical Injuries

Learning Outcome

1. Explain abrasions and their forensic significance;
2. Know lacerations and their characteristics;
3. Discuss contusions and their implications in forensics;
4. Learn fractures and classification in forensic analysis;
5. Focus on penetrating injuries and their forensic relevance;
6. Discuss gunshot wounds and their unique features;
7. Learn to detect thermal injuries and see how they affect the process of investigation.
8. Compare different types of mechanical injuries.

Many cases of mechanical injuries appear in forensic work which makes it tough to understand the details of the trauma and the reason behind the death. You could come across fractures, cuts and bruises and every difference among them can influence an investigation. Take traumatic brain injury; it's a prime example that generally leads to severe outcomes like high mortality and serious disabilities, so experts often dig into its origins and exactly when it occurred (Garazdiuk, 2024). The numbers on violent versus non-violent deaths can change over time, mainly because of changes in transportation and healthcare which usually points to the connection between these injuries and bigger social changes. All in all, being familiar with every type of these injuries guides forensic experts to identify the cause of death and leads to new ways to prevent them in the community.

8.1.1. Abrasions and Their Forensic Significance

Mechanical injuries, mainly abrasions, are important in forensics because they can show what took place during an incident. Abrasions form when the skin rubs against something rough and they could be the result of a fight, a strong impact or touching a weapon which helps professionals understand what occurred. How these injuries appear, their location and how they are grouped can sometimes tell us about the events of the assault and the victim's efforts to defend themselves. Take knife attacks, for example—it's not unusual to see incised cuts along with scratches that tell a story; in most cases, studies show that defensive injuries tend to show up on the hands and forearms (Das et al., 2025). Also, advances in postmortem imaging techniques like PMCT now make it easier to look at abrasions closely, helping investigators figure out the exact causes and circumstances behind the trauma (Wu et al., 2024) (Figure 8.3).

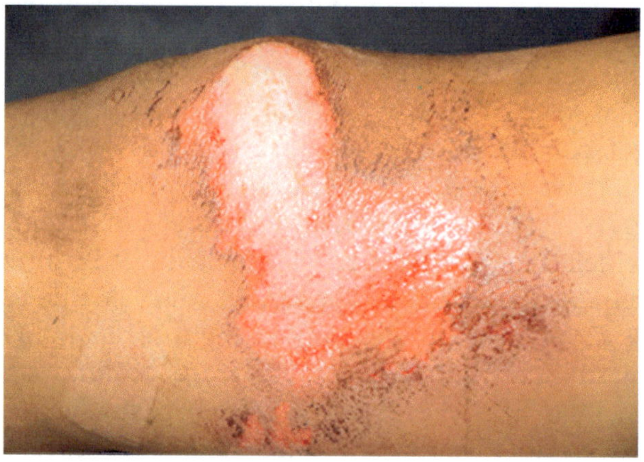

Figure 8.3. Abrasions.

Source: https://www.cfnei.com/forensic_nursing/wp-content/uploads/2016/03/abrasion-C.jpg.

8.1.2. Lacerations and Their Characteristics

A good knowledge of lacerations is very important for forensic work. Such injuries are not clean, but torn which usually means they were caused by a strong impact, not a normal cut. Sometimes, the area and type of laceration can give useful information about what happened during the injury and even hint at the broader situation. Take genital lacerations, for example; their rates can differ a lot between consensual and non-consensual cases, which underlines why detailed documentation during exams is so crucial (Crawford et al., 2024). Looking at the depth of the wound and the type of tissue damage can tell us about the force involved and how long the event lasted which is often important for understanding what happened. To summarize, forensic practitioners need to be on their toes, spotting these subtle features to ensure their assessments hold water in legal investigations (Garazdiuk, 2024) (Figure 8.4).

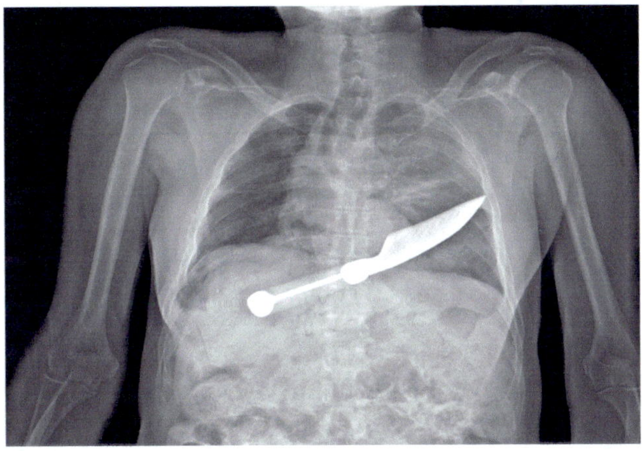

Figure 8.4. Lacerations.

Source: https://www.pathologyoutlines.com/imgau/autopsysharpforceVarious25.jpg.

8.1.3. Contusions and their Implications in Forensics

A bruise or contusion, can often tell us more than just that a mark is on the skin. Most of the time, they show the type, timing and strength of an injury which is very important for understanding what happened before a death. When examined with a microscope, these injuries have similar patterns that appear again and again and together with other methods, they help form the overall picture. One emerging twist is looking at tissues around the gums; this approach, for example, shows how mixing traditional methods with modern science can up the accuracy of trauma analysis (Hadžić et al., 2024). Similarly, ongoing research into biomarkers – including those specific miRNAs linked with traumatic brain injuries – seems to offer extra clues about the cause of death (Boninet al., 2023). To summarize, the way bruises carry these hidden signals points to a real need for more rounded strategies that dig into the messy details of mechanical injuries in forensic science (Figure 8.5).

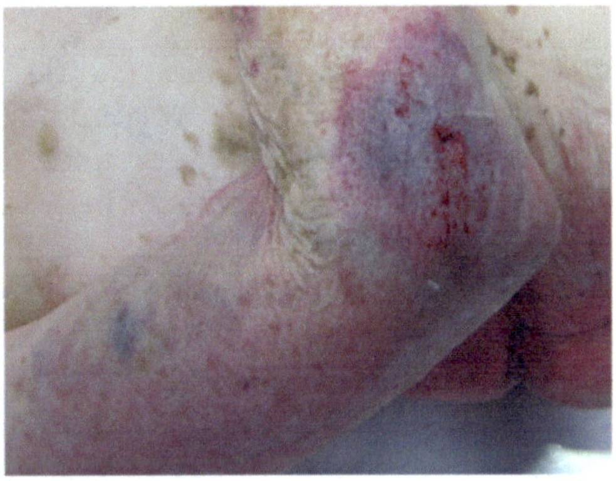

Figure 8.5. Bruises—what many simply call contusions—can reveal a lot more than just a mark on the skin.

Source: https://ars.els-cdn.com/content/image/3-s2.0-B9780128236772000519-f00051-12-9780128236772.jpg.

8.1.4. Fractures and Classification in Forensic Analysis

Forensic investigations depend on understanding how various fractures are sorted—especially because injuries caused by mechanical forces make things more complicated. Fractures may be simple or very complicated and this variety often helps experts find out how and why the person died. Often, forensic professionals mixed many diagnostic tricks, like postmortem computed tomography (PMCT) and even postmortem computed tomography angiography (PMCTA) via angiography, to shed light on what these fractures might truly be signaling in trauma (Wu et al., 2024). Noticing the finer details of these breaks also lets analysts tell if an injury occurred while someone was still alive or only afterward, which is pretty key when piecing together death's circumstances (Varfolomeiev et al., 2024). In brief, this way of grouping fractures is useful for investigations and makes forensic findings more reliable, offering a clearer picture of mechanical injuries in practice.

8.1.5. Penetrating Injuries and their Forensic Relevance

Penetrating injuries provide many subtle hints that can change how forensic work is done. It is often very important to understand these wounds to understand what happened during a violent incident. Whenever you see gunshot marks in the maxillofacial region, you can see that guessing how the tissue will react to various projectiles is difficult and requires advanced modeling techniques. Research generally shows that rounds—a .40-caliber versus a 9x19mm, for example—tend to leave behind unique stress patterns on bones, which can help reconstruct the incident (Costa et al., 2018). At the same time, while our basic insights from human forensic literature lay a decent foundation, the unusual anatomical features of various species mean we often have to tweak our methods to nail an accurate assessment (Piegari et al., 2018). To summarize, bolting together robust analytical frameworks in forensic pathology remains key to boosting the trustworthiness of findings about these injuries and their legal fallout (Figure 8.6).

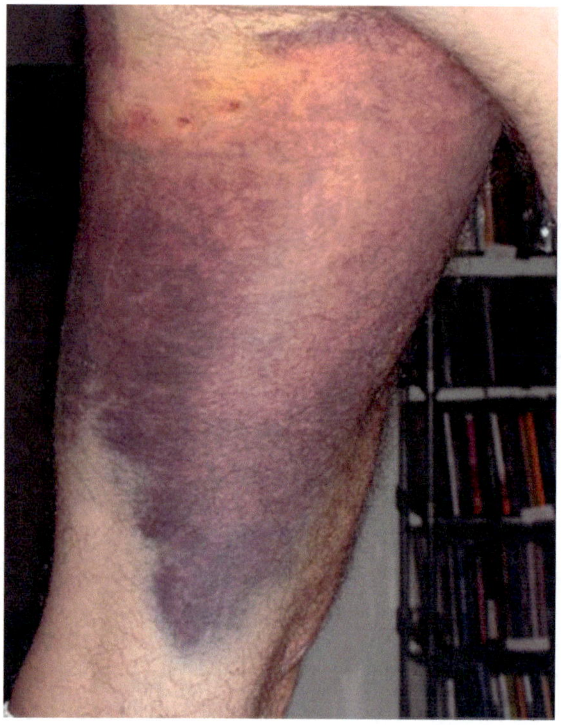

Figure 8.6. Penetrating injuries carry a lot of subtle clues that shape forensic work in unexpected ways.

Source: https://study.com/cimages/multimages/16/13_blunt_trauma_450712408343999272796.jpg.

8.1.6. Gunshot Wounds and their Unique Features

Looking at gunshot wounds can provide important details about a violent incident, especially when studying a crime scene. The type of ammo, the distance and the angle of the shot can all affect the details of the wounds and you'll usually notice a small, clear mark at the entrance, with a bigger, more oddly shaped mark where the bullet came out. Nowadays, residue tests have gotten pretty advanced; experts use tools like scanning electron microscopy to inspect tiny traces that can tie suspects to where the scene unfolded (Ansari et al., 2024). To summarize, nailing these subtle traits not only helps figure out why someone died but also lets investigators rebuild the sequence of events—a vital part of modern forensic science (Drath et al., 2024).

8.1.7. Thermal Injuries and their Impact on Forensic Investigations

It can be very challenging to understand how injuries occurred in forensic investigations. It is not always easy to know if a wound is caused by a hit or by exposure to heat during a fire. Second- or third-degree burns are common in fire incidents which makes it difficult to tell the cause of the damage and death. There are times when burns appear as mechanical injuries which makes it more difficult to figure out the details of the case. Heat can change the way tissues behave which could make a piercing act differently than you would expect. Generally speaking, these little details matter a lot since they affect both the investigation and later legal proceedings; in many cases, a careful, all-around review is needed, especially in instances like (Beattie et al., 2018; Singla et al., 2023.) (Figure 8.7).

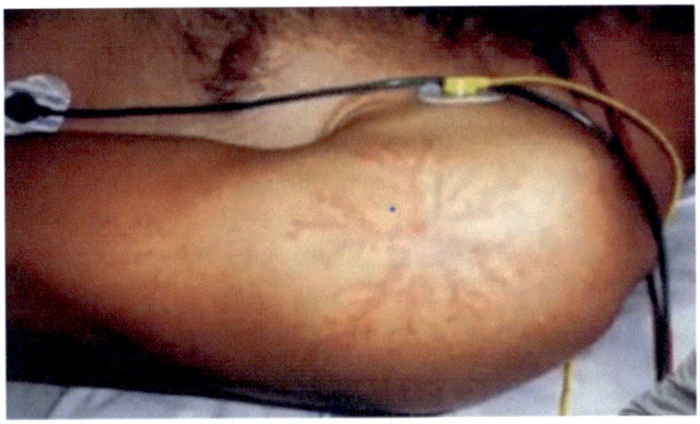

Figure 8.7. Thermal injuries and their impact on forensic investigations.

Source: https://image.prepladder.com/prepladder/2023/05/25052903/Lightning-injuries.png.

8.1.8. Electrical Injuries and their Identification

Electric shock injuries are not always easy to understand; there's more going on than just the first shock. The issue mixes how an injury happens with the surrounding circumstances, and as fire investigations increasingly bump into electrical hazards – in many cases thanks to the growing use of photovoltaic (PV) systems – there's been a fair bit of debate about whether fire examiners can truly pin down incidents tied to electricity. Generally speaking, evidence suggests that when certain parts (like DC isolator switches in PV circuits) give out, they can spark fires that lead to harm; still, quite a few fire scene examiners seem unsure when it comes to nailing down these origins. The uncertainty involved makes it harder to judge injuries and also slows down the effort to create solid safety rules and standards in construction. In most cases, the shifting demands of forensic medicine imply that more thorough training in spotting electrical injuries—alongside other mechanical ones—is needed to support a rounded approach to forensic investigations (Fracasso et al., 2023).

8.1.9. Comparison of Different Types of Mechanical Injuries

Looking at mechanical injuries in forensics is not simple—every wound must be examined closely. Each type of injury, contusions, abrasions and lacerations, may affect a case differently. Take contusions which happen when you get hit hard enough to bruise and abrasions which are caused by scrapes that remove some skin, both are important injuries in sports. But lacerations can be shallow or deep which sometimes makes it hard to figure out the cause of the injury. The environment where the wound happens and the factors nearby can change how the mark looks and heals. With today's forensic techniques sharpening our view, we can piece together events more clearly and even figure out who's to blame (Atzrodt et al., 2017; Layden et al., 2019).

Test Your Knowledge

1. Define mechanical injury in forensic medicine.
2. List all the types of mechanical injuries and give an example of each.

8.2. Mechanisms of Injury

Learning Outcome

1. Learn the kinematics of mechanical injuries;
2. Know the forces involved in producing mechanical injuries;
3. Know how blunt force trauma is used in forensic investigations;
4. Explain sharp force trauma and its forensic implications;
5. Examine how the environment can influence how injuries happen;
6. Perform analysis of injury patterns in forensic cases;
7. Focus on biomechanics of injury and its relevance;
8. Understand the relationship between force and injury severity;
9. Describe case studies illustrating mechanisms of injury.

Understanding the causes of injuries and the approach of forensics is useful for learning why such injuries happen. Forensic experts usually apply several techniques; they depend on PMCT and PMCTA to identify fractures and signs of organ damage. These scans help show where bleeding starts and can even hint at what object might have caused the injury, while also working together with more traditional anatomical checks to give a clearer picture overall (Wu et al., 2024). Some experts have studied head injuries in car crashes and noticed that the seriousness can depend a lot on the type of car that was involved. All of this points out that it is very important to know the details of these injuries. In most cases, getting a solid grasp of how injuries come about not only supports accurate forensic assessments but also ends up influencing legal outcomes and guiding safety measures (Grukhovskiy et al., 2024).

8.2.1. Kinematics of Mechanical Injuries

It is very important in forensics to understand how movement can influence the way injuries happen. How fast, at what angle and how much force are involved in a hit all affect the kind and degree of harm that can occur. Looking at wrist injuries in sports, quick and sudden movements can sometimes cause those hard-to-treat breaks in the small carpal bones. Lately, new 3D scanning methods have upped the game by letting experts take a closer look at the shape and structure of these bones, checking them both before and after a break occurs (Faragó et al., 2020). There's also the rising number of road accidents, which kind of shows why it's important to look at movement in cases like vehicle-pedestrian crashes (Nogayevaet al., 2020). In most cases, combining ideas from different fields gives us fresh insights into injuries and might just open the door to better ways of preventing and investigating them (Figure 8.8).

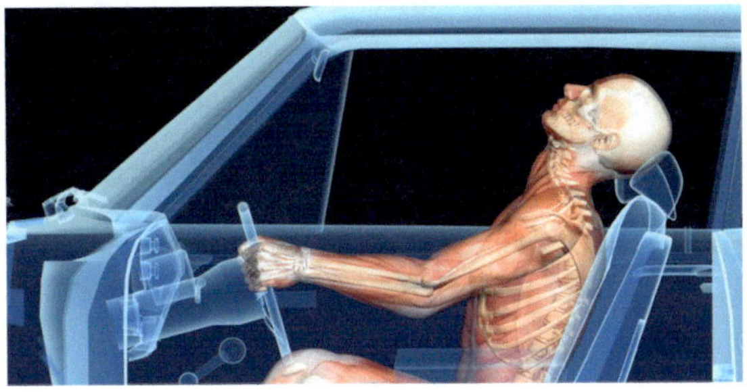

Figure 8.8. Kinematics of mechanical injuries.

Source: https://www.exponent.com/sites/default/files/styles/hero_purple/public/media/images/Biomechanical_Injury_human_anatomy_car_crash%281%29.jpg.webp?itok=63KOeA_l.

8.2.2. Forces Involved in Producing Mechanical Injuries

Forensic investigations depend a lot on a sense of how the different factors in a case interact. It's possible to see that impact, shear and tension don't always behave in a predictable way, but interact in surprising manners. A fast hit to the body usually results in blunt trauma or deep cuts, but shear forces which act from the side, may cause lacerations or even broken bones, especially when a car accident occurs. Biomechanics also helps by revealing the force's character and its small features such as its direction and strength which are key when trying to solve the case. In many forensic cases, these intertwined forces come into sharp focus, reminding us that taking a closer, sometimes messy look is essential, as studies on hybrid threats to law enforcement and military operations have shown (Nyagudi et al., 2013; Singla et al., 2023).

8.2.3. Role of Blunt Force Trauma in Forensics

Fatal injuries are often the result of blunt force trauma which is a major factor in autopsies. A look back at old records shows that roughly 11.9% of deaths involved this kind of trauma (Saghir et al., 2020) – a figure that points to its common presence among various causes of death. Because such injuries can happen in accidents, assaults and other unexpected situations, it is important to check them to learn how and why the person died. It isn't just about deadly wounds either; even cases with non-lethal injuries—say, from offbeat weapons like arrows—reveal that small details such as clothing type and fit can change how bad a wound turns out to be (Beattie et al., 2018). The specifics of a blunt impact, from exactly where the hit lands to just how hard it lands, offer investigators important clues that generally help piece together the story behind a death and ultimately guide efforts toward justice and preventing future violence (Figure 8.9).

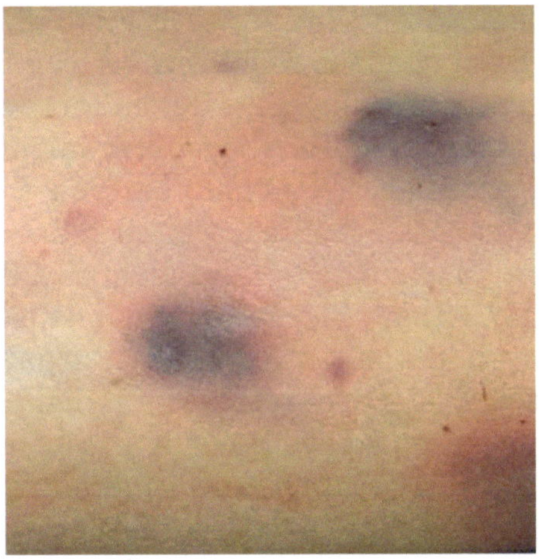

Figure 8.9. Blunt force trauma plays a big role when autopsies dig into fatal injuries.

Source: https://img.medscapestatic.com/pi/meds/ckb/35/9735tn.jpg.

8.2.4. Sharp Force Trauma and its Forensic Implications

If you look at skeletal remains, you could find many signs of how the person died and sharp injuries are usually easy to notice. Forensic work has shown, in most cases, that deliberate assaults leave a very different mark than accidents do; studies have noted that people who are purposely injured often show wounds on the head and neck, almost as if those spots were the easy targets (McNulty et al., 2016). Accidental injuries, by contrast, usually pop up across various parts of the body, especially in the limbs, and are often the result of just a fall or slip (McNulty et al., 2016). The details of the fractures can help too; in some archaeological cases, similar sharp force marks have appeared which tends to prove that the same forensic ideas can be useful for both old and recent cases. All in all, wounds caused by sharp tools play a major role in investigating mechanical trauma cases.

8.2.5. Impact of Environmental Factors on Injury Mechanisms

Forensic experts rely on knowledge of how surroundings and injuries are related. These injuries can be made more serious or different by things happening outside the body. Take, for instance, the habits a mother might have during pregnancy—smoking or even a bit of alcohol use has been linked to birth anomalies like cleft lip and palate (Llerandi et al., 2024)—which hints that everyday environments might set the stage for certain injuries right from the start. Protective gear such as helmets, is not only designed well, but it has to handle the effects of weather and other factors as time goes on. Research generally shows that a bit of regular upkeep can go a long way in keeping a helmet's energy absorption in shape, helping it fend off impacts from both mechanical hits and heat (Walczak, 2024). To summarize, having a broader view of these environmental effects matters for both stopping injuries before they happen and digging deep into forensic investigations (Figure 8.10).

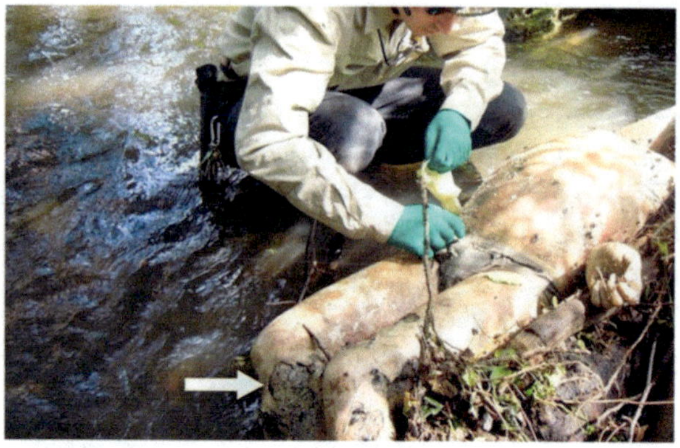

Figure 8.10. Forensic work depends on knowing how our surroundings mix with the ways injuries happen.

Source: Baumjohann K, Benecke M. Mind Your Decompositional Assumptions. *Forensic Sciences*. 2022; 2(4):725-740. https://doi.org/10.3390/forensicsci2040054.

8.2.6. Analysis of Injury Patterns in Forensic Cases

The way injuries happen can tell us a lot about what occurs in traumatic incidents which is especially clear in forensic cases. You can see, for instance, that fatal outcomes often come down to gunshot wounds; one study revealed that roughly 46.4% of such cases involve firearm injuries, usually seen in males aged 21–40 and commonly tied to homicidal acts (Saghir et al., 2020). At the same time, cases of self-inflicted gunshots present their own set of challenges—when there are multiple entrance wounds, investigators need to dive deep into the scene and look closely at the deceased's mental state (Barnes et al., 2015). Overall such details help experts determine if a death was caused by homicide or suicide which is very important for the correct legal categorization. All in all, using this approach to analyze injuries helps us learn more about mechanical injuries, develop ways to prevent them and also affects criminal justice policies.

8.2.7. Biomechanics of Injury and its Relevance

Knowing how injuries happen from a biomechanics perspective is important for forensics because it explains the causes and outcomes of trauma. Generally speaking, research into diffuse axonal injury (DAI) suggests it usually stems from extended acceleration forces; these very forces often lead to marked nerve damage and functional loss. Forensic neuropathological exams play a vital role in spotting such injuries – techniques like immunohistochemistry, for example, often prove crucial in pinpointing specific cellular damage (Davceva et al., 2015). On a related note, looking into mechanical injuries such as traumatic acromioclavicular joint dislocations reveals that different surgical reconstruction methods can offer uneven stability; joint stiffness, it appears, serves as a key hint for predicting recovery outcomes (Nüchtern et al., 2013). All in all, these findings increase our knowledge of injuries and assist in choosing the right treatments and making legal choices in many forensic cases.

8.2.8. Understanding the Relationship between Force and Injury Severity

It matters that force is applied to the body during a traumatic event and it's not only about a single hit. Depending on how strong and what kind of impact it is, it can result in tissue harm or unusual neurological effects. Think about it: studies have repeatedly shown that even small differences in how hard the body is struck can be linked to distinct kinds of injuries—like concussive blows that mess with brain function and may even trigger cognitive impairments (Köcher et al., 2024). In most cases, recent work also points out that rising levels of acoustic pressure seem to boost the chances of tissue damage, an idea proven in animal models (Takayama et al., 2023). All these findings, taken together, remind us that force dynamics are not merely abstract; they offer vital clues that forensic experts lean on when they're trying to understand what exactly happened during an incident, and they help shape the overall approach to analyzing mechanical injuries (Figure 8.11).

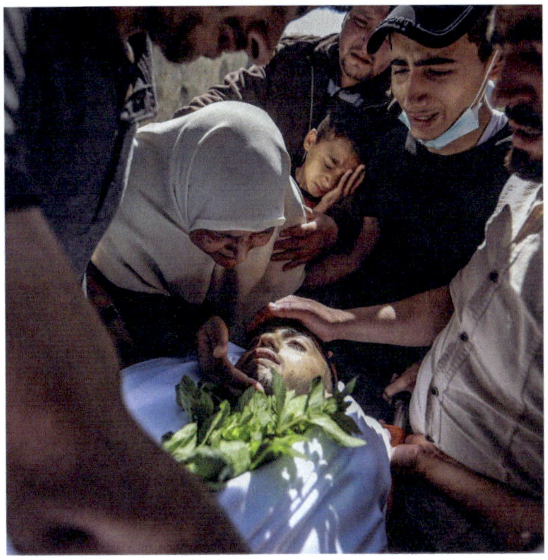

Figure 8.11. Force hitting the body during a traumatic event matters—it isn't just about a simple hit.

Source: https://platform.vox.com/wp-content/uploads/sites/2/chorus/uploads/chorus_asset/file/22527101/gaza_004.jpg?quality=90&strip=all&crop=16.666666666667,0,66.666666666667,100.

8.2.9. Case Studies Illustrating Mechanisms of Injury

Case studies demonstrate that injuries can happen when several different forces interact in ways that are not always clear. A study, for example, generally showed that CT scans are good at detecting skull fractures in the back, but it is harder to see those in the front or in the middle, especially if they are thin and hairline. This kind of finding, in most cases, nudges us toward better imaging and reconstruction techniques (Jacobsen et al., 2009). Viewing bone fractures as an ongoing process instead of clearly defined types gives us a clearer picture of what happens. How intense the force is, the size of the affected area and the speed of the impact all seem to have an effect on the way fractures form. All this, in turn, gives forensic anthropologists a more practical edge when piecing together what happened (Kroman et al., 2007). All in all, these cases make it clear that accurate trauma analysis is very important in forensics.

Test Your Knowledge

1. Distinguish between blunt force trauma and sharp force trauma by their methods of causing injury.
2. What damage does a gunshot wound do at the level of tissue?
3. How do blunt force injuries cause fractures in bones?

8.3. Forensic Analysis Techniques

Learning Outcome

1. Learn documentation of mechanical injuries;
2. Explain photography and its role in forensic analysis;
3. Know the use of imaging technologies;
4. Understand autopsy procedures for mechanical injuries;
5. Pay attention to toxicology and see how it connects to injury analysis;
6. Give expert testimony in court regarding mechanical injuries;
7. Know the part that forensic pathologists play in reviewing injuries;
8. Discuss the collection and preservation of evidence;
9. Identify challenges in forensic analysis of mechanical injuries.

Mechanical injuries in forensic cases are hard to solve and usually require advanced techniques. Investigators now rely on forensic biomechanics which uses basic physics to help make sense of accidents, to help them understand trauma details. In many instances, experts turn to finite element modeling to mimic how forces interact in various real-life scenarios, giving a deeper sense of injury severity and weird patterns that crop up (Chen, 2021). Also, 3D printing is gaining attention; now, we can use it to make models that fit each patient which helps doctors practice more realistic procedures. These detailed recreations, oddly enough, can refine courtroom discussions by presenting evidence in a way that actually makes sense (Aimar et al., 2019). In conclusion, using these techniques appears to fill knowledge gaps and improve the accuracy of investigations, though the results are sometimes unpredictable and still hopeful.

8.3.1. Documentation of Mechanical Injuries

It is not always easy to record injuries caused by machines in forensic cases. Making sure all the details are correct in forensics can change the outcome of a legal case. An example is trauma that happens during pregnancy—it may harm the mother and the baby in ways that are not immediately noticeable. Research generally shows that, in many instances, severe damage from mechanical forces comes about due to car crashes or even certain kinds of assaults (Shatalova et al., 2023). Such note-taking helps explain the reasons behind such injuries and also makes it easier to assess pregnancy results which may result in issues such as intrauterine fetal death or a spontaneous miscarriage. To summarize, methodical documentation amplifies the role of forensic examinations, providing crucial details that stretch far beyond the clinic and into the legal arena (Layden et al., 2019) (Figure 8.12).

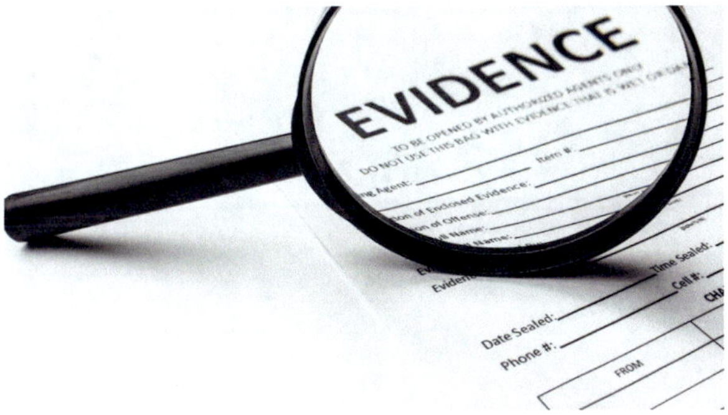

Figure 8.12. Documenting injuries from mechanical trauma in forensic cases isn't as straightforward as it might seem.

Source: https://irp.cdn-website.com/b7db1d7d/dms3rep/multi/Role+of+Forensic+Evidence+Hero.jpg.

8.3.2. Photography and its Role in Forensic Analysis

Tech and forensic science now team up, quietly changing the way investigations take place. With modern photography and imaging, it is possible to see the details of mechanical injuries which helps experts understand what happened and why. Innovations like 3D modeling allow a deep dive into injury patterns and the details of surrounding trauma, adding richer layers to the evolving narrative (Wilhelmson et al., 2015). This way of analyzing allows us to see more clearly what is happening, since it makes the analysis clearer and more objective, even if the details sometimes repeat. Plus, snapping photos isn't only about taking pictures—it plays a key role in preserving evidence so that thorough, remote examinations can occur, all while meeting strict documentation standards (Schweitzer et al., 2018). In short, using these methods together has led to a major and unpredictable progress in forensics, especially with mechanical injuries.

8.3.3. Use of Imaging Technologies (X-rays, Computer Tomography (CT) Scans)

Mechanical injuries can cover up other injuries that are not easy to see at the start; the wounds you can see are usually only part of the problem. Many times, forensic specialists rely on Xrays and CT scans to find things that a simple look cannot reveal. Xrays are usually used first to find fractures and dislocations, but CT scans give more information about injuries to soft tissues and organs. Because of these techniques, doctors can review issues such as spine discs and bone strength which helps build the case for legal action. Not only do they help doctors find the right diagnosis, but they also help explain the events that led to the injury which can have a big impact on the case outcome. To summarize, mixing Xrays with CT scans in forensic work is pretty much indispensable, refining investigative methods and boosting judicial precision in cases of bodily harm (Kirthika et al., 2025; Zhang et al., 2024;) (Figure 8.13).

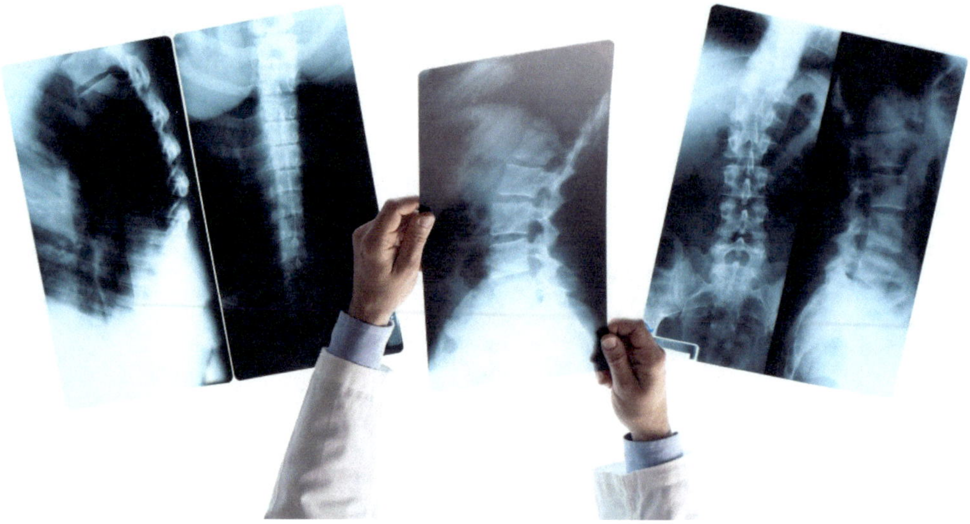

Figure 8.13. X-rays typically serve as the initial tool, quickly exposing things like fractures and dislocations.

Source: https://www.envrad.com/content/uploads/2021/02/doctor-holding-x-rays.jpg.

8.3.4. Autopsy Procedures for Mechanical Injuries

It is not always easy to catch all the details when doing autopsies on mechanical injuries; it usually requires a careful and patient step-by-step process. When looking at the neck which is not always the same in every case, having experts from several backgrounds is very helpful. New research suggests that only using traditional techniques could mean you miss some important information, but using PMCT along with other imaging methods might uncover more. For example, using PMCT and a regular autopsy together appears to increase the chances of detecting injuries which may be very important in legal cases. And since mechanical injuries can sometimes show up as traumatic brain injuries (TBI), there's an added risk of error—which drives home the need for forensic methods to keep evolving to remain both dependable and accurate (Bilotta et al., 2023).

8.3.5. Toxicology and its Relevance in Injury Analysis

The relationship between toxicology and injury analysis is very important for strong forensic investigations. Physical injuries can cause toxins to be present which can influence the outcome of the injury and the body's response. Substances like alcohol or narcotics can make it harder to use motor skills which may result in accidents or fights; at times, they can make things become out of control. Toxins can cause reading injuries to be harder to understand since they might worsen existing problems or change the body's usual reaction to harm which could be deadly. Recent research generally suggests that there's been a subtle but noticeable shift, with forensic experts increasingly weaving toxicology data into their analyses—especially in fields such as forensic genetics and alcohology (Fracasso et al., 2022). To summarize, these trends emphasize, in most cases, how crucial toxicology is when trying to unravel the many layers of mechanical injury cases (Figure 8.14).

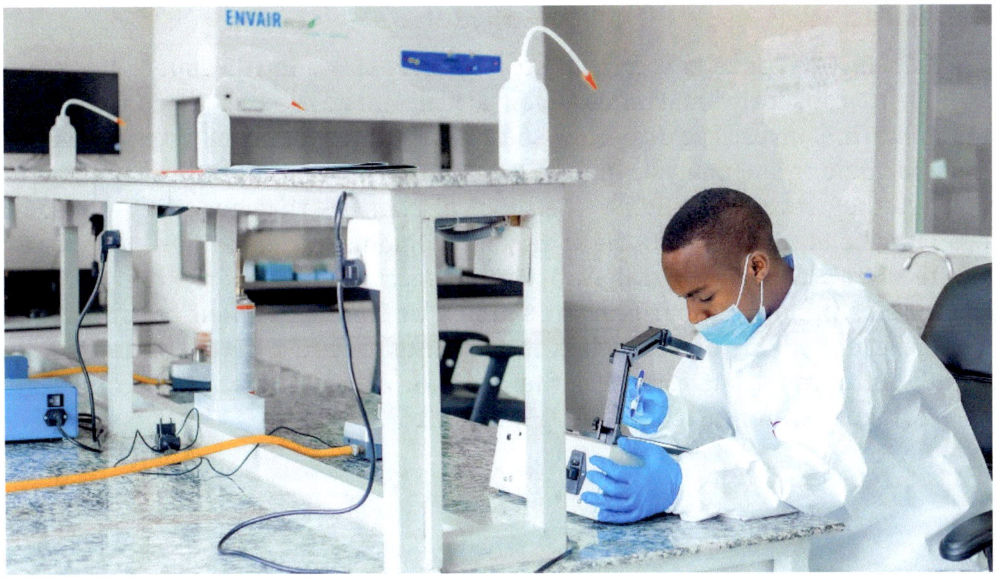

Figure 8.14. Toxicology and injury analysis share a pretty tangled relationship that sits right at the core of solid forensic work.

Source: https://assets.isu.pub/document-structure/240315065246-25ae672d6d8f4fe2e5ac417d0f1c3160/v1/d6cdeb673b6d567310384181833d205d.jpeg.

8.3.6. Expert Testimony in Court Regarding Mechanical Injuries

A mechanical injury case can be decided differently based on what experts say. Many times, courts rely on experts—like engineers or doctors—to help sort out the confusing parts of an incident that the basic facts alone cannot explain. People have pointed out, for instance, that old ideas about pain still mix with today's legal rules, a factor that matters when juries find it tricky to judge subjective injuries (Goldberg, 2017). At times, hindsight bias messes with a juror's view, making them think they knew what was coming simply because they learned about it after the fact Roese et al. (2012). All in all, expert views influence both the way people view the case and the final judgment.

8.3.7. Role of Forensic Pathologists in Injury Assessment

Forensic pathologists have a major part in figuring out how mechanical injuries happened. They try both outdated and new methods and sometimes use them in unexpected ways, to identify what led to the injuries which is essential for setting up timelines and holding people responsible in court. Postmortem imaging, like PMCT, ups the game in spotting broken bones and hidden internal damage; this, in most cases, helps piece together the sequence of events leading to death (Wu et al., 2024). In a similar vein, teaming up with forensic odontologists for dental trauma evaluations can shed extra light on how the injury occurred, subtly boosting the evidentiary weight of the findings (Khan et al., 2024). Combining old and new imaging techniques strengthens the accuracy of the examinations and cements the importance of forensic pathologists for our justice system.

8.3.8. Collection and Preservation of Evidence

Getting and preserving evidence is a critical step in forensics and it's especially important when dealing with injuries caused by machines. Even a little mistake such as contamination or poor handling, can make the investigation show something different from what actually happened. Techniques like periodic tissue analysis give us a surprising peek into both when and how injuries happened because they reveal distinctive histological changes that generally boost the accuracy of the findings (Hadžić et al., 2024). Look at skeletal remains, for example—the work done at the Koboro cave site shows that both straightforward, macroscopic observation and more detailed imaging play big roles in noticing perimortem trauma or signs of violent encounters (Braddick et al., 2024). When these methods mix together, it all points toward a better understanding of injury mechanisms and, quite frankly, underscores the need for consistent, ethical practices in collecting and preserving evidence in forensic science (Figure 8.15).

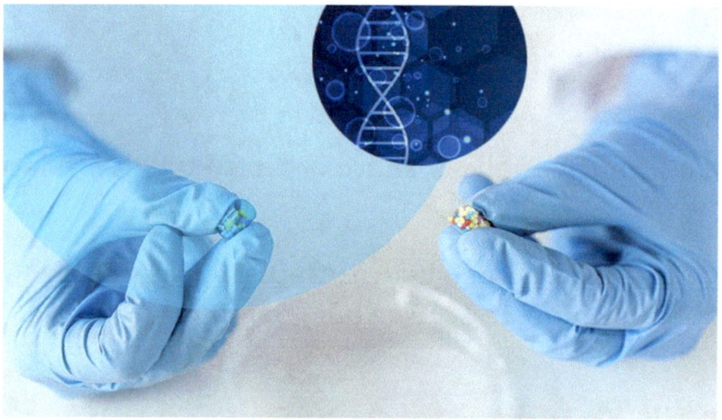

Figure 8.15. Even a tiny slip-up, like contamination or careless handling, can throw off what the investigation ends up showing; in most cases, it means misinterpreting exactly what happened.

Source: https://www.compliancequest.com/wp-content/uploads/2023/01/efficient-oos-and-oot-investigation.jpg.

8.3.9. Challenges in Forensic Analysis of Mechanical Injuries

Forensic work today is not as easy as people might think. How a mechanical injury happens depends on the angle, the object and how much force is involved. As a rule, these unusual events make it difficult to know exactly what happened and why, so experts usually find it hard to testify clearly in court. At the same time, new gadgets such as microfluidic chips are opening up fresh, creative ways to gather and study data, though, in most cases, not every team has the deep technical know-how to make full use of them (Cui et al., 2018). Plus, environmental or situational factors can muddle things even further, making it tough to draw clear conclusions about injuries—just think about the messy aftermath of events like Hurricane Maria (Kishore et al., 2018).

Test Your Knowledge

1. What part does a forensic pathologist play in studying mechanical injuries?
2. What tools are used to find out which way the force came from in a laceration or contusion?

8.4. Legal Implications of Mechanical Injuries

Learning Outcome

1. Know how mechanical injuries play a part in criminal investigations;
2. Be aware of the effects of finding out the cause of death;
3. Explain mechanical injuries in civil litigation;
4. Identify standards of proof in forensic evidence;
5. Learn ethical considerations in forensic analysis;
6. Explain case law related to mechanical injuries;
7. Look at how the evidence presented by forensics can influence the jury's choice;
8. Pinpoint the difficulties of presenting evidence of mechanical injuries in a court of law;
9. Recognize the future directions in which legal issues related to forensic injuries may go.

Mechanical injuries play a major role in forensics because they can change the outcome of a case. Personal injury cases often require attention to every detail and also to the biomechanical aspects which can have surprising effects on the outcome of the case. Generally, research shows that human tissues behave in many unexpected ways, so it is almost necessary to get accurate property assessments when assigning liability. For instance, the tensile behavior of the dura mater can fundamentally reshape how traumatic brain injuries are interpreted, and this nuance often plays a big role in legal judgments (Zwirner et al., 2019). Then again, it doesn't stop there—factors such as age, sex, and the specific context of an incident all add layers of complexity that might alter mechanical responses (Stouffer et al., 2015). In the end, forensic experts must use their knowledge of biomechanics and the law together, since this is often as important as it is difficult.

8.4.1. Role of Mechanical Injuries in Criminal Cases

Often, investigators observe that mechanical injuries can lead to useful findings in a crime and these marks come in many shapes and can tell more than expected. These types of injuries which may look quite different, often reveal details about the accident as if each mark or change is quietly sharing its own story. For instance, when minor shifts in the gum tissues are noticed, they not only point to a specific kind of trauma but also hint at when and how it might have been done (Hadžić et al., 2024) — which is pretty intriguing if you ask me. Looking at dental profiling in veterinary settings, for example, can reveal that even animals leave behind traces that help paint a broader picture of the crime (Viciano et al., 2022). In most cases, a close look at these mechanical injuries doesn't just add another tool to the detective's kit; it also pushes us to mix solid science with hands-on investigation, ultimately making the evidence a lot more trustworthy (Figure 8.16).

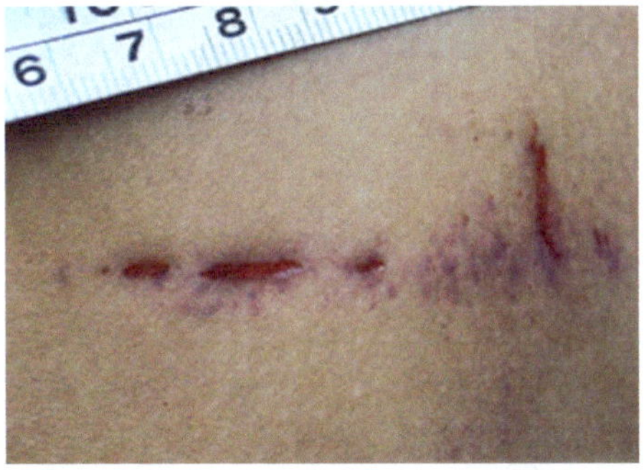

Figure 8.16. Role of mechanical injuries in criminal cases.

Source: https://d45jl3w9libvn.cloudfront.net/jaypee/static/books/9788184482089/Chapters/images/89-1.jpg.

8.4.2. Impact on Determining Cause of Death

Mechanical injuries are not simple which affects forensic work, especially when trying to understand the cause of death. Forensic experts examine different types of injuries and the specifics of each injury can give unexpected hints about the incident. Lately, there's been a rise in cuts from guns and explosions – studies Aenetska et al. (2024) show, in most cases, that even kid mortality rates during wartime are shifting, nudging us to push for updated medical approaches in modern conflict zones. On another note, improved methods for judging how old a hemorrhage is after a traumatic brain injury have, generally speaking, become key in piecing together a death's timeline, as forensic specialists keep trying to lock down the precise cause (Garazdiuk, 2024). Using these new scientific methods in regular forensic work creates a better, but occasionally incomplete, way to understand how mechanical injuries affect how we decide on a person's cause of death.

8.4.3. Mechanical Injuries in Civil Litigation

The relationship between technology and law is very strong now, especially in the handling of digital evidence in civil lawsuits. In 2006, the Federal Rules of Civil Procedure were revised which made electronic data more important and required organizations to review their methods of storing and protecting it. In most cases, these proactive steps not only help companies stay compliant but also ease the risks tied to looming courtroom battles (Wallner et al., 2008). Even so, some specialists are not sure about the reliability of forensic evidence and its use can sometimes result in wrongful convictions. This concern, generally speaking, goes hand in hand with calls to reexamine the criteria for accepting mechanical injuries as valid forensic evidence in civil cases, prompting a more nuanced review (Bidinger et al., 2020). Ultimately, the intricate details of such injuries demand extra care within our legal system if we are to uphold both justice and accuracy in civil litigation (Figure 8.17).

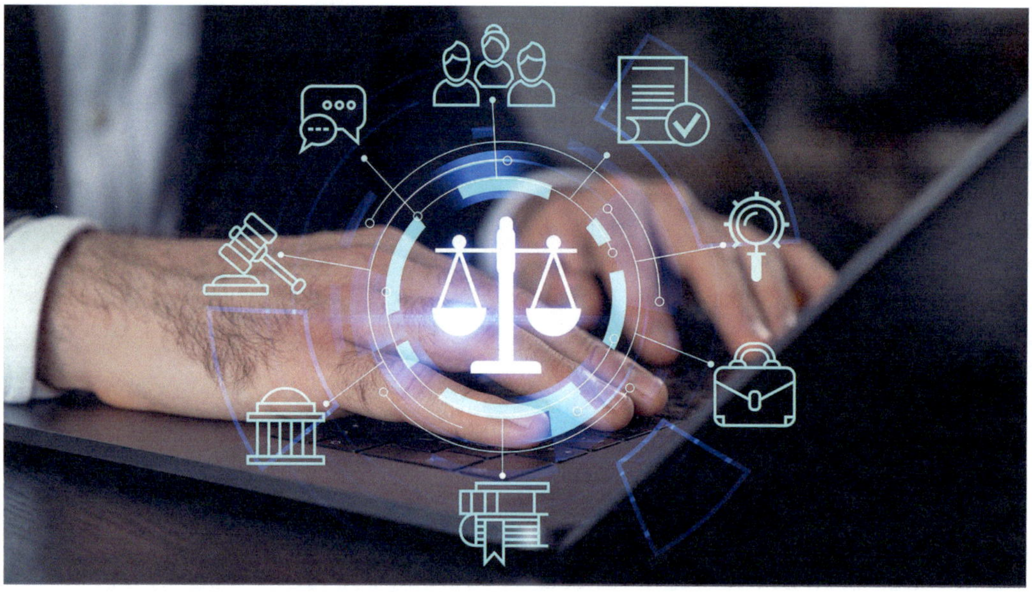

Figure 8.17. Tech and law have become surprisingly intertwined these days, especially when it comes to managing digital records in civil litigation.

Source: https://bolinfirm.com/wp-content/uploads/Top-10-Latest-Trends-in-Civil-Litigation-Bolin-Firm.jpg.

8.4.4. Standards of Proof in Forensic Evidence

Forensic investigators need solid proof for mechanical injuries, mainly when they have to testify in court. What is usually important is figuring out the cause of the injury and the precise time it occurred – details that can change the outcome of most cases. Lately, forensic methods have gotten sharper—digging into cellular and molecular details—to boost the confidence we have in woundage estimates and injury analysis (Li et al., 2018). Still, there are open questions about the broader impact; for instance, we still don't fully get how injuries might affect whole populations, somewhat like other issues raised by environmental contaminants (Senko et al., 2020). Combining these insights into a single framework is very important because it helps legal cases and sets up future research and practice in this area.

8.4.5. Ethical Considerations in Forensic Analysis

Forensic science today combines new tools with traditional techniques and this combination, especially when examining mechanical injuries, brings up ethical issues that need further examination. Nanoparticles, for example, help investigators pick up tiny clues like DNA and gunshot residues; however, they can sometimes cause oxidative DNA damage that might weaken the evidence (Verma et al., 2024).

At the same time, artificial intelligence is getting used to scanning huge facial image databases—a move that seems revolutionary for early diagnostics but also raises some serious worries about privacy and potential government overreach (Kováč et al., 2024). Often, it is very important for forensic work to balance modern technology with ethical responsibility to maintain public trust and justice.

8.4.6. Case Law Related to Mechanical Injuries

There is often a mix between physical evidence and legal concerns in the field of forensics and this mix is not always easy to predict. Looking over many forensic reports, you notice that gun-related injuries generally top the list of fatal incidents (Saghir et al., 2020)—a fact that calls for stronger legal guidelines. Besides more typical injuries, arrows and bows are now being recognized as sources, so our view of these mechanical traumas is always evolving. For example, the way different arrowheads pierce a target can reveal extra details that sometimes sway legal decisions (Beattie et al., 2018). In short, the way courtroom precedents and injury evidence relate shows that using thorough but sometimes messy forensic methods is necessary to maintain legal standards.

8.4.7. Influence of Forensic Findings on Jury Decisions

How clearly the details are shown in evidence and at trial greatly affects the outcome. Clarity matters—a lot. Jurors are asked to understand complicated details of mechanical injuries, but if the forensic reports are not clear, mistakes may happen. If reports are full of surprises and disorder, there is a good chance important details will be overlooked which can result in an unfair decision. Further, Reeder et al. (2024) hint at this by noting that when forensic texts lose their readability, their impact literally fades, and crucial details end up getting overlooked which, in turn, distorts what the jury grasps. New technology such as micro Computed Tomography, now allows forensic scientists to see details they could not before. Generally speaking, such improvements help forensic pathologists nail down injury diagnoses more accurately while also boosting the confidence jurors hold in the evidence—this dual benefit, as noted in Baier et al. (2019), adds heft to the judicial process. In many cases, mixing technical insights with everyday language helps keep the evidence accessible and maintains that all-important fairness in the courtroom (Figure 8.18).

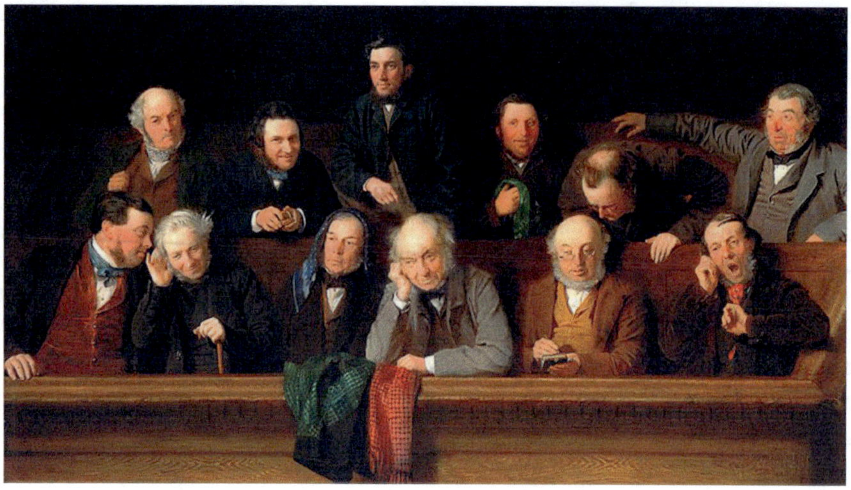

Figure 8.18. Influence of forensic findings on jury decisions.

Source: By John Morgan - The Jury by John Morgan.jpg in Wikipedia (English), Public Domain, https://commons.wikimedia.org/w/index.php?curid=4912282.

8.4.8. Challenges in Presenting Mechanical Injury Evidence in Court

Mechanical injuries can be a big challenge in court, since the evidence needs to be very clear which is not always possible. Forensic experts, wrestling with these messy details, are increasingly leaning on modern tools like micro Computed Tomography (micro-CT) to break down the complexity; studies even show that this method helps pathologists catch injuries that might otherwise slip by unnoticed—think, for example, strangulation marks—and gives juries a better feel for just how severe these wounds can be in cases of assault or homicide (Baier et al., 2019). 3D printing, too, has stepped in with a promising twist by letting us create physical, touchable models of crime scenes, which can, in most cases, make it easier for jurors to wrap their heads around spatial details (Carew et al., 2020). Still, while these new technologies are very exciting, people keep questioning whether they should be used in court and if they can be used reliably. All in all, the main issue isn't learning new technology, but making sure all those in the courtroom trust what they see.

8.4.9. Future Trends in Legal Implications of Forensic Injuries

Because of new technology, forensic science is exploring new areas and legal duties for forensic injuries are changing a lot. Cyber-physical systems (CPS) are now popping up everywhere, which brings many challenges that aren't always straightforward to sort out. Mohamed et al. (2020) points out that the tangled nature and delicate state of these systems mean we need solid security measures and clever investigation tools to get every detail of an incident. Mixing machine learning and deep learning can be interesting and it often helps our analysis, but it can also introduce some risks. Some experts worry that, despite their promise, these tech advances can be fooled by savvy adversaries, hinting at the need for stricter privacy and security standards (Qayyum et al., 2020).

Since forensic methods are always advancing, the rules of law should also keep up. It is generally important that the law is able to respond quickly to the new developments in technology related to forensic injury cases.

Test Your Knowledge

1. Outline the legal importance of noticing blunt force trauma in a homicide investigation.
2. Why should doctors pay attention to documenting injuries caused by mechanical devices in suspected domestic violence cases?

Summary

Dealing with mechanical injuries in forensic cases is not easy and usually requires using classic methods as well as some advanced imaging tools. Recent work shows that using PMCT along with angiography (PMCTA) ups our game in spotting issues like fractures and torn organs, which in turn boosts the quality of forensic exams (Wu et al., 2024). Sometimes the situation gets even more complicated—take children affected by firearm or explosive incidents, for instance; these cases push surgical practices to adjust quickly to meet today's challenges (Pletenetska et al., 2024). When we use forensic information in everyday medical care, it helps us improve treatment decisions and see the complete effects of trauma. So, moving our forensic methods ahead is very important if we want better results in both legal and medical cases.

Generally, connecting the way people talk about accidents with the detailed analysis done by forensic experts is a key point for advancing research on mechanical injuries. Diving into many forensic reports shows that if documents aren't effortlessly clear or easy to read, their reception can take a hit—sometimes even key details end up obscured, as noted in Reeder et al. (2024). Also, using the latest tools like micro Computed Tomography helps us raise the standards and professionalism in our criminal justice system. Some observations even suggest that these approaches smooth out the assessment of injuries from both strangulation and sharp force events, which in turn paves the way for easier weapon identification and heightened diagnostic accuracy, as emphasized in Baier et al. (2019). All in all, these ideas suggest that using simple language and current technology is necessary to address the tough issues of mechanical injuries and to maintain justice.

KEY TERMS FROM THIS CHAPTER

- Abrasions
- Assault
- Bones
- Bruises
- Bullet
- Complication
- Contusions
- Electrical hazards
- Fractures
- Genital lacerations
- Gums
- Gunshot wound
- Injury
- Lacerations
- Mechanical trauma
- Penetrating injuries
- Photovoltaic (PV) systems
- Trauma analysis

Short Answer Questions

1. Differentiate between contusion and abrasion.
2. Lacerations and puncture wounds are not the same.
3. What are the different ways mechanical injuries are grouped by their seriousness?
4. What kind of mechanical injury comes from blunt force trauma?
5. How can a fracture result from a mechanical injury?
6. Describe the pathophysiological process of a contusion.
7. How important are mechanical injuries in deciding the way someone died?
8. Can the way mechanical injuries occur help to tell if a death was accidental or caused by homicide?
9. What causes electric shock to cause harm to the human body?

Critical Thinking Questions

1. **Which of the following is a characteristic feature of a contusion (bruise)?**
   a. Caused by a sharp object
   b. Characterized by swelling and discoloration
   c. Results in a puncture wound
   d. Always leads to a fracture
2. **Which kind of injury is usually linked to blunt force trauma?**
   a. Stab wounds
   b. Contusions
   c. Abrasions
   d. Lacerations
3. **What is the primary difference between lacerations and abrasions?**
   a. Lacerations involve scraping of the skin, while abrasions involve tearing of the skin
   b. Lacerations are caused by blunt force, while abrasions are caused by sharp force
   c. Lacerations involve the tearing of skin, while abrasions involve scraping of the skin
   d. There is no difference
4. **Which of these is correct about sharp force trauma?**
   a. It is caused by blunt objects like fists or hammers
   b. It results in injuries such as stab wounds or incised wounds
   c. It causes contusions and abrasions
   d. It only occurs in gunshot wounds
5. **What can we learn about a case from fractures that are the result of mechanical injury?**
   a. The victim fell from a height
   b. The victim was struck with a blunt object

c. The injuries were self-inflicted

d. All of the above

Answers to Critical Thinking Questions

1. (b); 2. (b); 3. (c): 4. (b): 5. (d)

References

1. Ahn, K. W., Corliss, G., Groffy, R. L., Jeutter, et al. (2014). Replication of known dental characteristics in porcine skin: Emerging technologies for the imaging specialist. Retrieved from: https://core.ac.uk/download/213078616.pdf (accessed on 29 May 2025).

2. Aimar, A., Palermo, A., & Innocenti, B. (2019). The role of 3D printing in medical applications: A state of the art. *Journal of Healthcare Engineering, 2019*, 1–10. https://doi.org/10.1155/2019/5340616.

3. Ansari, N., Dasgupta, J., Umre, S., & Rajput, P. (2024). Harnessing electron microscope for trace evidence analysis. In *IntechOpen eBooks*. https://doi.org/10.5772/intechopen.1004112.

4. Atzrodt, J., Derdau, V., Kerr, W. J., & Reid, M. (2017). Deuterium- and tritium-labelled compounds: Applications in the life sciences. *Angewandte Chemie International Edition, 57*(7), 1758–1784. https://doi.org/10.1002/anie.201704146.

5. Baier, W. (2019). *Applications of Micro-CT in the Criminal Justice System of England and Wales: An Impact Assessment* (Doctoral dissertation, University of Warwick).

6. Barnes, C., Di Maio, V. J. M., Heard, B., Hejna, M., Karger, B., Karger, C., et al. (2015). Determined to die! Ability to act following multiple self-inflicted gunshot wounds to the head. The Cook County Office of Medical Examiner experience (2005–2012) and review of literature. Retrieved from: https://core.ac.uk/download/54522925.pdf (accessed on 29 May 2025).

7. Beattie, E., Fraser, J., MacPhee, N., et al. (2018). A comparison of penetration and damage caused by different types of arrowheads on loose and tight fit clothing. Retrieved from: https://core.ac.uk/download/228178194.pdf (accessed on 29 May 2025).

8. Bidinger, M. S. (2020). Faulty forensics: Bolstering judicial gatekeeping in Georgia courts. Retrieved from: https://digitalcommons.law.uga.edu/cgi/viewcontent.cgi?article=1250&context=glr (accessed on 29 May 2025).

9. Bilotta, C., Perrone, G., Zerbo, S., Salerno, S., Adelfio, V., Viola, I., Lo Re, G., & Argo, A. (2023). The multidisciplinary approach for the diagnosis of laryngohyoid lesions: A systematic literature review and meta-analysis. *La Clinica Terapeutica, 174*(1), 97–108. https://doi.org/10.7417/CT.2023.2504.

10. Bonin, S., D'Errico, S., Medeot, C., Moreschi, C., Ciglieri, S. S., Peruch, M., Concato, M., Azzalini, E., Previderè, C., & Fattorini, P. (2023). Evaluation of a set of miRNAs in 26 cases of fatal traumatic brain injuries. *International Journal of Molecular Sciences, 24*(13), 10836. https://doi.org/10.3390/ijms241310836.

11. Braddick, I., Kubo, D., Matsumura, H., & Schulting, R. J. (2024). Violence-related skeletal trauma in the Epi-Jomon period: A case study from the Koboro cave site in Hokkaido, Japan. *Asian Journal of Paleopathology, 6*, 1–5.

12. Carew, R. M., & Errickson, D. (2020). An overview of 3D printing in forensic science: The tangible third-dimension. *Journal of Forensic Sciences, 65*(5), 1752–1760. https://doi.org/10.1111/1556-4029.14442.

13. Chen, Y. (2021). Current state and progress of research on forensic biomechanics in China. *Forensic Sciences Research, 6*, 1–12. https://doi.org/10.1080/20961790.2021.1879365.

14. Crawford, L. S., Downing, N. R., Famurewa, A. D., Markowitz, J. R., & Han, G. (2024). Genital lacerations following sexual assault and consensual sexual intercourse: A systematic review and meta-analysis. *Journal of Forensic Sciences, 70*, 161–169. https://www.semanticscholar.org/paper/a8298b2035beaa324948777f0bf0aeb401647412 (accessed on 29 May 2025).

15. Cui, P., & Wang, S. (2018). Application of microfluidic chip technology in pharmaceutical analysis: A review. *Journal of Pharmaceutical Analysis, 9*(4), 238–247. https://doi.org/10.1016/j.jpha.2018.12.001.

16. Das, N. G., Das, N., & Sil, A. (2025). Pattern and forensic significance of defense injuries in homicide cases: A cross-sectional study. *Cureus, 17*. https://www.semanticscholar.org/paper/b220d59af690d815386e317b288a0dd397b6051b (accessed on 29 May 2025).

17. Das, S., Dey, A., Pal, A., & Banerjee Roy, N. (2015). Applications of artificial intelligence in machine learning: Review and prospect. *International Journal of Computer Applications, 115*, 31–41. https://doi.org/10.5120/20182-2402.

18. Davceva, N., Basheska, N., & Balažič, J. (2015). Diffuse axonal injury—A distinct clinicopathological entity in closed head injuries. *American Journal of Forensic Medicine & Pathology, 36*(2), 127–133. https://doi.org/10.1097/paf.0000000000000168.

19. Davis, J. R., Lane, H. W., & Stepaniak, P. C. (2025). Loss of signal: Aeromedical lessons learned from the STS-107 Columbia space shuttle mishap. https://core.ac.uk/download/pdf/42730063.pdf (accessed on 29 May 2025).

20. dos Santos, L. M. P., da Cunha, M. R., Reis, C. H. B., Buchaim, D., da Rosa, A. P. B., Tempest, L. M., da Cruz, J. A. P., et al. (2025). Using human tissue surrogates in anatomical modeling for gunshot wounds simulations: An overview about "how to do" experimental terminal ballistics. *Frontiers in Bioengineering and Biotechnology, 13*. https://www.semanticscholar.org/paper/ff8e57ef5a798ea388159e30601ab683f18ecde6 (accessed on 29 May 2025).

21. Drath, J., Jarzęcka-Stąporek, J., Zacharczuk, J., Lisman, D., Cytacka, S., Szargut, M., Bulut, Ö., et al. (2024). Perpetrators from Treblinka: Interdisciplinary investigations of seven single graves with "Trawniki Men." *Heritage Science, 12*. https://doi.org/10.1186/s40494-024-01184-7.

22. Faragó, D., & Kiss, R. M. (2020). Geometric and mechanical characterization of human carpal bones–A preliminary study. *Periodical Polytechnical Civil Engineering, 64*(1), 138–143. https://doi.org/10.3311/PPci.15125.

23. Fracasso, T., Pfeiffer, H., Schmeling, A., & Wirth, I. (2022). From Deutsche Zeitschrift to International Journal of Legal Medicine—100 years of legal medicine through the lens of journal articles: Part 2: Deutsche Zeitschrift für die gesamte gerichtliche Medizin from 1948 to 1969. https://core.ac.uk/download/586719534.pdf (accessed on 29 May 2025).

24. Fracasso, T., Pfeiffer, H., Schmeling, A., & Wirth, I. (2023). From Deutsche Zeitschrift to International Journal of Legal Medicine—100 years of legal medicine through the lens of journal articles: Part 3: Zeitschrift für Rechtsmedizin–Journal of Legal Medicine from 1970

to 1990. https://core.ac.uk/download/586717646.pdf (accessed on 29 May 2025).

25. Garazdiuk, M. (2024). Using the diffuse tomography method for researching the time of hemorrhage formation in the substance of the human brain. *Neonatology, Surgery and Perinatal Medicine*. https://www.semanticscholar.org/paper/b11139decd47b6d92b35029e9aaffcd3c48e2bfd (accessed on 29 May 2025).

26. Goldberg, D. S. (2017). Pain, objectivity and history: Understanding pain stigma. *Medical Humanities, 43*, 238–243. https://doi.org/10.1136/medhum-2016-011133.

27. Grukhovskiy, S., Velenko, P., Bychkov, A., Marchenkov, R., Globa, I. V., Berezovskiy, D. P., & Barinov, E. H. (2024). Forensic analysis of head injuries of a driver in a fatal car injury. *Russian Journal of Forensic Medicine*. https://www.semanticscholar.org/paper/5f108ee42b73fa1cb8873c858f8afdbe972f869a (accessed on 29 May 2025).

28. Hadžić, Z., & Puhar, I. (2024). Forensic assessment of trauma using periodontal tissues evaluation: Possibilities and future perspectives. *Bulletin of the International Association for Paleodontology, 18*(1). https://core.ac.uk/download/613208833.pdf (accessed on 29 May 2025).

29. Jacobsen, C., Bech, B. H., & Lynnerup, N. (2009). A comparative study of cranial, blunt trauma fractures as seen at medicolegal autopsy and by computed tomography. *BMC Medical Imaging, 9*, 18. https://core.ac.uk/download/pdf/8344057.pdf.

30. Jin, G., Nakayama, S., & Tu, M. (2020). Game based learning for safety and security education. https://core.ac.uk/download/628905943.pdf (accessed on 29 May 2025).

31. Khan, A. S., Karki, A., Karki, R. K., & Singh, P. K. (2024). An epidemiological survey of fatal head injuries autopsied at a tertiary care center in Dhulikhel, Nepal. *Med Phoenix, 9*(2), 11–14. https://doi.org/10.3126/medphoenix.v9i2.73406.

32. Khan, M. S., Suhartono, A. W., & Auerkari, E. I. (2024). Clinical implications of dental injury analysis in forensic odontology: A review article. *E-GiGi, 13*(1), 217–224. https://doi.org/10.35790/eg.v13i1.54118.

33. Kirthika, C. P., Senthil Kumar, S., & Venkata Sai, P. M. (2025). MRI study of lumbar and cervical intervertebral disc degeneration–A cross-sectional analysis. *Cuestiones de Fisioterapia*. https://www.semanticscholar.org/paper/ac63aea240e1c2dbc34ec11abe4c094da00ae37d (accessed on 29 May 2025).

34. Kishore, N., Marqués, D., Mahmud, A. S., Kiang, M. V., Rodriguez, I., Fuller, A., Ebner, P. J., et al. (2018). Mortality in Puerto Rico after Hurricane Maria. *New England Journal of Medicine, 379*(2), 162–170. https://doi.org/10.1056/nejmsa1803972.

35. Köcher, L., Beppi, C., Penner, M., Meyer, S., Bögli, S. Y., & Straumann, D. (2024). Concussion leads to opposing sensorimotor effects of habituation deficit and fatigue in zebrafish larvae. *Brain Communications, 6*. https://www.semanticscholar.org/paper/ad5ea1f918175977b39ad2ac389bea0f7b01939e (accessed on 29 May 2025).

36. Kováč, P., Jackuliak, P., Bražinová, A., Varga, I., Aláč, M., Smatana, M., Lovich, D., et al. (2024). Artificial intelligence-driven facial image analysis for the early detection of rare diseases: Legal, ethical, forensic, and cybersecurity considerations. *AI*. https://www.semanticscholar.org/paper/48b479a78ec64873f6078910115f3812c2a5ebf3 (accessed on 29 May 2025).

37. Kroman, A. M. (2007). *Fracture Biomechanics of The Human Skeleton* (PhD dissertation,

University of Tennessee). https://trace.tennessee.edu/utk_graddiss/218 (accessed on 29 May 2025).

38. Layden, J. E., Ghinai, I., Pray, I. W., Kimball, A., Layer, M., Tenforde, M. W., Navon, L., et al. (2019). Pulmonary illness related to e-cigarette use in Illinois and Wisconsin–Final report. *New England Journal of Medicine, 382*(10), 903–916. https://doi.org/10.1056/nejmoa1911614.

39. Li, N., Du, Q., Bai, R., & Sun, J. (2018). Vitality and wound-age estimation in forensic pathology: Review and future prospects. *Forensic Sciences Research, 5*(1), 15–24. https://doi.org/10.1080/20961790.2018.1445441.

40. McNulty, S. L. (2016). *An Analysis of Skeletal Trauma Patterning of Accidental and Intentional Injury* (Master's thesis). https://core.ac.uk/download/268773673.pdf (accessed on 29 May 2025).

41. Messina, A. D., Carotenuto, G., Micciché, R., & Sìneo, L. (2013). Fatal cranial injury in an individual from Messina (Sicily) during the times of the Roman Empire. *Journal of Forensic and Legal Medicine, 20*(8), 1018–1023. https://doi.org/10.1016/j.jflm.2013.09.023.

42. Mohamed, N., Al-Jaroodi, J., & Jawhar, I. (2020). Cyber–physical systems forensics: Today and tomorrow. *Journal of Sensor and Actuator Networks, 9*(3), 37. https://doi.org/10.3390/jsan9030037.

43. Neal, T. M. S., & Grisso, T. (2014). Assessment practices and expert judgment methods in forensic psychology and psychiatry. *Criminal Justice and Behavior, 41*, 1406–1421. https://doi.org/10.1177/0093854814548449.

44. Nogayeva, S., Gooch, J., & Frascione, N. (2021). The forensic investigation of vehicle-pedestrian collisions: A review. *Science & Justice, 61*(2), 112–118. https://doi.org/10.1016/j.scijus.2020.10.006.

45. Nüchtern, J., Sellenschloh, K., Bishop, N., Jauch, S., Briem, D., Hoffmann, M., Lehmann, W., et al. (2013). Biomechanical evaluation of 3 stabilization methods on acromioclavicular joint dislocations. *The American Journal of Sports Medicine, 41*(6), 1387–1394. https://doi.org/10.1177/0363546513484892.

46. Nyagudi, N. M. (2013). *Post-Westgate SWAT: C4ISTAR Architectural Framework for Autonomous Network Integrated Multifaceted Warfighting Solutions Version 1.0: A Peer-Reviewed Monograph.* http://arxiv.org/abs/1401.6379 (accessed on 29 May 2025).

47. Piegari, G. (2018). *New Insights in Veterinary Forensic Medicine and Pathology* [Doctoral dissertation].

48. Pletenetska, A. O., Mykhailychenko, B., Rudenko, Y., & Biliakov, A. (2024). Forensic medical analysis of child mortality due to mechanical trauma in peaceful and wartime: Impact on improving surgical care. *Pediatric Surgery (Ukraine), 4*(85), 8–15. https://doi.org/10.15574/PS.2024.4(85).815.

49. Prometheus Forensic Services Limited, & Smith, S. P. (2015). *The Recognition of Fires Originating from Photovoltaic (PV) Solar Systems.* https://core.ac.uk/download/30713291.pdf (accessed on 29 May 2025).

50. Putri Dianita Ika Meilia, Freeman, M., Herkutanto, & Zeegers, M. P. (2018). A review of the diversity in taxonomy, definitions, scope, and roles in forensic medicine: Implications for evidence-based practice. *Forensic Science, Medicine, and Pathology, 14*, 460–468. https://doi.org/10.1007/s12024-018-0031-6.

51. Qayyum, A., Qadir, J., Bilal, M., & Al-Fuqaha, A. (2020). Secure and robust machine learning for healthcare: A survey. *IEEE Reviews in Biomedical Engineering, 14*, 156–180. https://doi.org/10.1109/rbme.2020.3013489

52. Reeder, T. C. (2024). *An Examination of Scientific and Technical Communication for Forensic Engineering and Forensic Pathology*. https://core.ac.uk/download/604797913.pdf (accessed on 29 May 2025).

53. Roese, N. J., & Vohs, K. D. (2012). Hindsight bias. *Perspectives on Psychological Science, 7*(5), 411–426. https://doi.org/10.1177/1745691612454303.

54. Saghir, R. (Rabia). (2020). Retrospective autopsy-based analysis of nature and prevalence of fatal injuries in Lahore. https://media.neliti.com/media/publications/301998-retrospective-autopsy-based-analysis-of-ce6fc605.pdf (accessed on 29 May 2025).

55. Schweitzer, W., Thali, M. J., & Egger, D. A. (2018). Case-study of a user-driven prosthetic arm design: Bionic hand versus customized body-powered technology in a highly demanding work environment. *Journal of NeuroEngineering and Rehabilitation, 15*. https://doi.org/10.1186/s12984-017-0340-0.

56. Senko, J. F., Nelms, S. E., Reavis, J. L., Witherington, B. E., Godley, B. J., & Wallace, B. P. (2020). Understanding individual and population-level effects of plastic pollution on marine megafauna. *Endangered Species Research, 43*, 234–252. https://doi.org/10.3354/esr01064.

57. Shatalova, Y., Zakupova, T., Galitskiy, F. A., Gülmen, M. K., Kaya, K., & Yavuz, T. K. (2023). Analysis of the pregnancy outcome in severe injury in pregnant women according to forensic examinations for 2008–2017 in Astana. *Deleted Journal, 28*, 41–46. https://doi.org/10.17986/blm.1620.

58. Stouffer, K., Pillitteri, V., Lightman, S., Abrams, M. D., & Hahn, A. (2015). Guide to industrial control systems (ICS) security. https://doi.org/10.6028/nist.sp.800-82r2.

59. Takayama, N., Sasanuma, H., Rifu, K., Nitta, N., Akiyama, I., & Taniguchi, N. (2023). Acoustic radiation force impulse-induced lung hemorrhage: Investigating the relationship with peak rarefactional pressure amplitude and mechanical index in rabbits. *Journal of Medical Ultrasonics (2001), 50*(2), 143–150. https://www.semanticscholar.org/paper/4949f833dcb1666f6402627656167dde00071da6 (accessed on 29 May 2025).

60. Tang, Z., Tu, W., Zhang, G., Chen, Y., Lei, T., & Tan, Y. (2012). Dynamic simulation and preliminary finite element analysis of gunshot wounds to the human mandible. *Injury, 43*(5), 660–665. https://doi.org/10.1016/j.injury.2011.03.012.

61. University of Rhode Island. (2013). *Research & Innovation for 2012–2013*. https://core.ac.uk/download/56696586.pdf (accessed on 29 May 2025).

62. Valcarcel Llerandi, J., Morales Peralta, E., Fernández González, M. del C., & Pérez Borrego, A. (2024). Environmental factors associated with cleft lip and palate in children treated at the William Soler Hospital. *Salud, Ciencia y Technology*. https://www.semanticscholar.org/paper/241d01cc65b29c9430a37fa7efcba079c1cabed9 (accessed on 29 May 2025).

63. Varfolomeiev, Y., Pletenetska, A., & Bondar, S. (2024). Detection of the vital origin of the strangulation mark in mechanical asphyxia as an indicator of the development of forensic medicine. *Forensic-Medical Examination, 1*, 12–20. https://www.semanticscholar.org/paper/5936f650e0c952251b93ebdee49d9c863b3f4133 (accessed on 29 May 2025).

64. Verma, P., Ujjainia, P., Moza, B., & Mukherjee, D. (2024). Nanoparticles as silent witnesses: Significance, challenges and ethical considerations in forensic analysis. *RASAYAN Journal of Chemistry*. https://www.semanticscholar.org/paper/fd7ecfa4fad5650e9c140c2f182254e28798a550 (accessed on 29 May 2025).

65. Viciano, J., López-Lázaro, S., & Tanga, C. (2022). Post-mortem dental profile as a powerful tool in animal forensic investigations–A review. *Animals, 12*(16), 2038. https://doi.org/10.3390/ani12162038.

66. Völlm, B., Clarke, M., Tort Herrando, V., Seppänen, A., Gosek, P., Heitzman, J., & Bulten, E. (2018). European Psychiatric Association (EPA) guidance on forensic psychiatry: Evidence based assessment and treatment of mentally disordered offenders. *European Psychiatry, 51*, 58–73. https://doi.org/10.1016/j.eurpsy.2017.12.007.

67. Walczak, A. (2024). Influence of the maintenance on protective properties of firefighters' helmets under low-impact energy condition. *Journal of Achievements in Materials and Manufacturing Engineering, 126*(2), 49–57. https://doi.org/10.5604/01.3001.0054.9204.

68. Wallner, G. L. (2008). Developing a proactive framework for e-discovery compliance (Master's thesis). Regis University. https://epublications.regis.edu/theses/115 (accessed on 29 May 2025).

69. Wilhelmson, H., & Dell'Unto, N. (2015). Virtual taphonomy: A new method integrating excavation and postprocessing in an archaeological context. *American Journal of Physical Anthropology, 157*(3), 305–321. https://doi.org/10.1002/ajpa.22715.

70. Wu, B., Li, Y., Li, Y., Wu, B., Hu, X. F., Xia, Z. Y., Li, W., He, G. L., & Li, J. J. (2024). A pilot study on forensic imaging of mechanical injuries. *Journal of Forensic Science and Medicine, 10*(4), 304–308. https://doi.org/10.4103/jfsm.jfsm_157_24.

71. Zhang, N., Li, Z., Zhao, Y., Wu, J., Wang, S., & Wang, X. (2024). Advancements in CT three-dimensional reconstruction of rock samples. *International Geomechanics Conference*. https://www.semanticscholar.org/paper/ebb38ece7e1f7c8db5d0f2af485d80d110650123 (accessed on 29 May 2025).

72. Zwirner, J., Scholze, M., Waddell, J. N., Ondruschka, B., & Hammer, N. (2019). Mechanical properties of human dura mater in tension–An analysis at an age range of 2 to 94 years. *Scientific Reports, 9*, 16652. https://doi.org/10.1038/s41598-019-52836-9.

FIREARM INJURIES

9

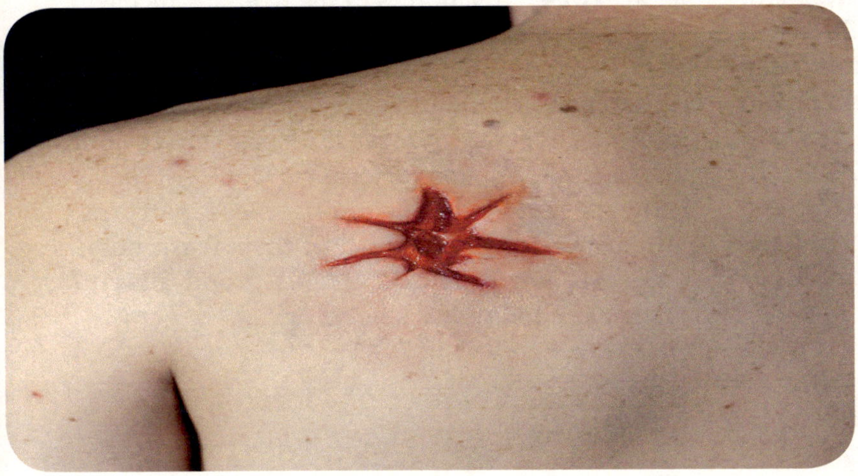

LEARNING OBJECTIVES

After studying this chapter, you will be able to:

1. Identify types of firearm injuries;
2. Understand forensic analysis of firearm injuries;
3. Explain the legal implications of firearm injuries;
4. Discuss prevention and public health strategies.

Introduction

Each week, there are about 10 murder-suicides using firearms which cause the deaths of 1,200 people nationwide. Besides taking a life, gun injuries also cause emotional pain that can stay with families and communities for a very long time. Such a trend points out that there is a public health issue that often needs more immediate attention. Considering the way these events break people and leave lasting mental marks, it is obvious that prevention is the most important thing. In the ongoing debate over gun regulations, viewpoints clash: some insist on tighter controls—citing successful methods from abroad—while others stand firmly by the Second Amendment to protect their rights (Banuelos et al., 2018). So, it is necessary to relate the findings of forensic investigations to policy decisions to handle the current situation and think about lasting solutions.

Definition of Firearm Injuries

Gun injuries create many complications and unexpected challenges. A bullet or other projectile leaving a firearm causes them, so the injuries can be as light as a mark or as serious as death. Research generally finds that injury rates and deaths have been going up, with young men being affected the most. For example, one study in French Guiana found that roughly 60% of these cases occurred at night and were mostly tied to assaults with long-barreled guns (Fremery et al., 2024). A nationwide study in Sweden, on the other hand, noted that many deaths resulted from trauma to the trunk and head, which underscores the need for quick medical care (Nyberger et al., 2024). To summarize, putting these pieces together is key if we're to craft more effective prevention plans and refine our forensic methods (Figure 9.1).

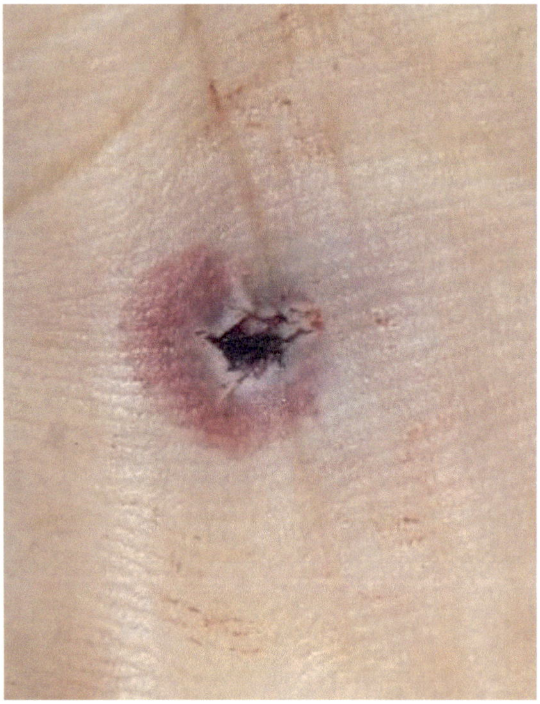

Figure 9.1. Gun injuries are a tangled problem—messy and full of unexpected twists.

Source: https://img.medscapestatic.com/pi/meds/ckb/03/314603tn.jpg.

Importance of Studying Firearm Injuries in Forensics

The consequences of gun injuries are felt by people and also by hospitals and the community. Examining the details, forensic investigations provide new knowledge that can affect how we treat trauma and create public policies. In most cases, a study from French Guiana shows a notable spike in gun-related trauma, with young males taking the brunt of the impact (Fremery et al., 2024); this points to the need for focused, sometimes even personalized, intervention strategies. In South Africa, the data points to these injuries being a major cause of emergency cases which puts pressure on resources and makes it hard for services to cope. Forensic experts, when they examine these patterns, often find messy details, but their work helps improve how resources are used and aims to improve community safety.

Historical Context of Firearm Injuries in Forensic Investigations

Firearm injuries have often been managed differently because of the impact of past conflicts. Take, for example, the digging up of bodies at the Ovčara mass grave—when investigators checked things out, forensic work showed that about 95% of the victims died from gunshot wounds to the head, clearly a part of a planned ethnic cleansing effort (Ekštajn et al., 2021). It shows that forensic investigations are important for identifying people and also for proving organized acts of violence, although the details are usually not neat. Over the years, as techniques have slowly improved—with experts now looking into how projectiles affect various organs—the field has gotten better at piecing together injury patterns and figuring out the manner of death (Humphrey et al., 2017); events like these demonstrate how forensic science runs deep with broader social implications concerning firearm fatalities.

Relevance to Public Health and Safety

Lessen the effects of gun violence on public health by preventing injuries from guns. There is still a lack of complete data on these cases in emergency medicine which suggests more focused studies are needed to improve interventions. One study from last year includes 59 questions about various problems such as intimate partner violence and accidents that were not planned. Some evidence even hints that tougher gun laws generally line up with fewer deaths; this certainly underscores the role of policy in keeping communities safer (Kelley et al., 2020). When these areas are given attention, researchers and policymakers may create a stronger way to address all the problems linked to gun injuries which can lead to a safer society.

9.1. Types of Firearm Injuries

Learning Outcome

1. Understand gunshot wounds;
2. Know penetrating versus perforating injuries;
3. Explain the types of firearms involved;
4. Learn common locations of injuries on the body;
5. Perform immediate medical implications;
6. Know the long-term effects of firearm injuries;
7. Discuss the psychological impact on victims;
8. Describe variability in injury patterns;
9. Pay attention to case studies that explain different kinds of injuries.

There is more to gun injuries than just the statistics—they involve many feelings and situations that change the situation. About 1,200 people in the United States die every year in murder–suicides, usually using guns which demonstrates the impact of gun violence on families and communities. Many times in forensic work, it is not simple to tell if wounds were caused by the victim or by someone else; it is more like a puzzle that needs all the details. Cases where someone takes multiple self-inflicted shots, for instance, bring their own set of hassles—often pushing investigators to dig into the victim's past mental health struggles and the messy circumstances that led up to the event (Barnes et al., 2015). All in all, understanding these types of injuries helps experts with sorting out fatalities and also leads to more talks about how to prevent them and the significant mental impact of easy access to guns.

9.1.1. Gunshot Wounds

Many times, analyzing gunshot wounds is a major challenge in forensics. The way an injury happens can depend on how far the shot was taken and what ammo was used and there is often more to it than meets the eye. In many cases, a postmortem exam shows a wound with an abrasion ring plus subtle signs of life—a sign that, generally speaking, points to a nearby firearm discharge; studies have even tied these clues to lead deposits on animal cadavers (Piegari et al., 2024). Then there are times when the damage gets so messy—like when severe skull destruction masks the usual entry points—that even experienced examiners without specialized training can get thrown off (Wankhade et al., 2024). To summarize, these mixed signals drive home the point that detailed, thoughtful forensic evaluations are key to interpreting evidence correctly and keeping criminal investigations on track (Figure 9.2).

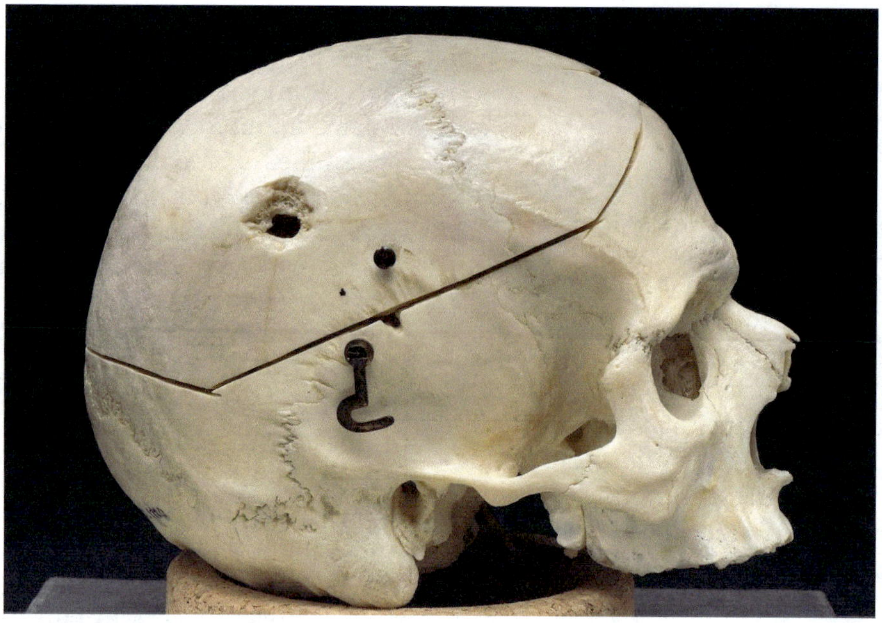

Figure 9.2. Gunshot wound.

Source: By National Institutes of Health, Health & Human Services - National Museum of Health and Medicine. From exhibition "Visible Proofs: Forensic Views of the Body"U.S. National Library of Medicine, 8600 Rockville Pike, Bethesda, MD 20894, Public Domain, https://commons.wikimedia.org/w/index.php?curid=1432903.

9.1.2. Penetrating Versus Perforating Injuries

Firearm cases depend on being able to tell apart penetrating from perforating injuries. When a bullet remains in the body, it causes a penetrating wound which can result in local tissue damage and sometimes bleeding inside, but when it tears through the body, leaving marks at both ends, it is called a perforating injury and tracking its path can be harder. Usually, these differences are very important for making sure the evidence is accurate and the law is clear, even if they seem minor. Recent work even hints that body armor can help cushion the blow in many scenarios, especially in overmatching cases where high-speed rounds defeat the gear (Mabbott et al., 2016). Because forensic medicine is always advancing and using knowledge from several fields, practitioners are using this knowledge more often to solve the mystery of such injuries.

9.1.3. Types of Firearms Involved

Forensic work hinges on knowing different kinds of firearms. The ballistic behavior of handguns, rifles and shotguns can directly shape the injuries caused and the way gunpowder residue is spread. How bad the injuries are can depend on the type and size of the ammo, since each weapon releases its energy differently. Usually, testing is necessary to determine the shooting distance—comparing the residue from the victims with the test residue can help solve many questions during the reconstruction of the crime. Studies generally show that even if a particular model reliably gives consistent results, switching up the ammunition brand might still change things up, which underscores why classifying firearms properly is so important (Hodges et al., 2008; Lewey et al., 2007). To summarize, these little nuances help move an investigation forward, sometimes leading to clearer conclusions about firearm injuries (Figure 9.3).

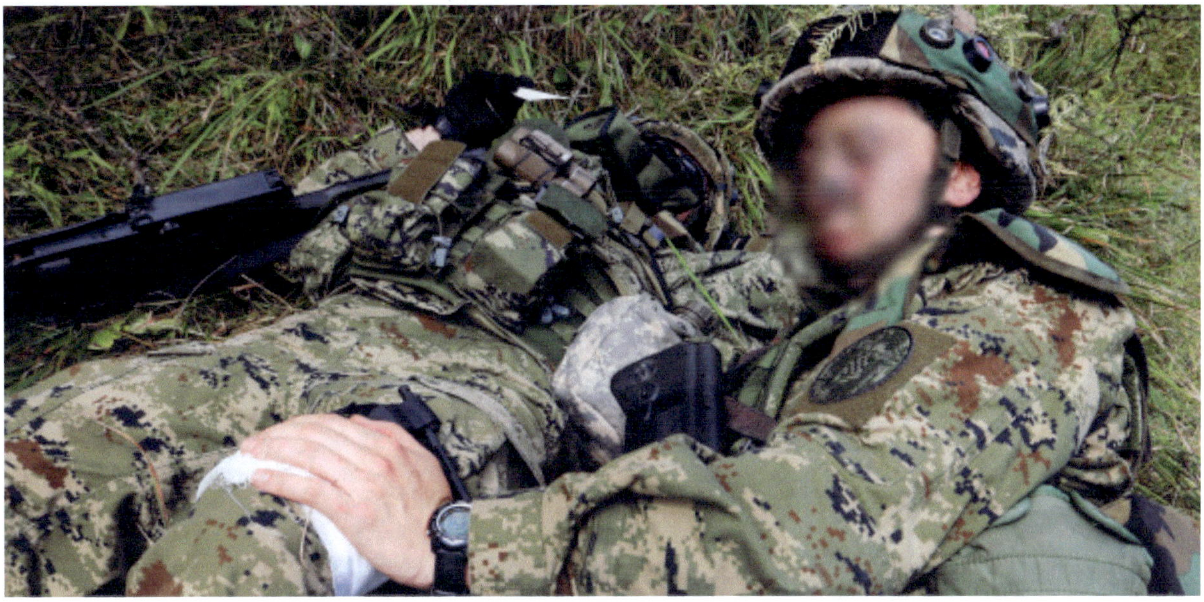

Figure 9.3. Handguns, rifles, shotguns—they each come with their own set of ballistic quirks that can directly affect injury patterns and how gunshot residue ends up spreading.

Source: https://www.defensivestrategies.org/images/tccc.jpg.

9.1.4. Common Locations of Injuries on the Body

Gunshot wounds tell us a lot about what happened. The area that is struck can give important information about the cause. A lot of the time, injuries happen on the abdomen, chest or head and the outcome can be non-fatal or fatal, depending on the weapon and how close the shot was. Understanding where a wound is found helps explain what happened which is very important for a good investigation. If the person has injuries on the upper torso, it is likely they were attacked very close by; lower injuries could mean they were trying to escape or defend themselves. Sometimes, the exact hit spot also gives us a hint of whether the attack was planned or more random, shedding some light on the offender's behavior (Fletcher et al., 2022). Clearly, more research is needed to fill in our understanding of the patterns behind these wounds and to see how weapon choice plays into the whole picture (Black et al., 2019).

9.1.5. Immediate Medical Implications

Being helped fast after a shooting is very important because it reduces the problems that can follow. Because the wounds are so severe, doctors have to act fast and adjust their treatments on the spot when people who are shot arrive. Sometimes things get even trickier: when you dive into the data, you see that a good number of these cases involve damage to the head, neck, or chest, and these injuries generally tend to be linked with higher death rates, especially among younger guys (Fremery et al., 2024). One curious point is that the type of gun—most often a long-barreled one—seems to shape the kind and spread of the injury (Fremery et al., 2024). After the initial care, the forensic part comes in to help and to study the common types of injuries which can gradually improve the way treatment is given. In many cases, grasping what these wounds imply is key to both lifting patient recovery and steering public health efforts against gun violence (Figure 9.4).

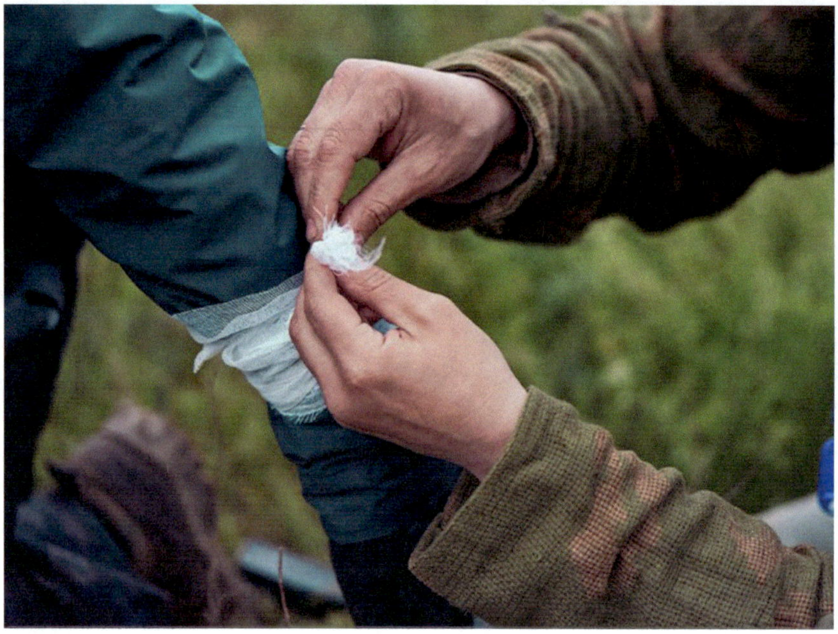

Figure 9.4. Getting help quickly after a shooting is absolutely vital—it cuts down on the complications that often come next.

Source: https://media.post.rvohealth.io/wp-content/uploads/2022/02/Hands-bandaging-a-wounded-arm-thumbnail.jpg.

9.1.6. Long-term Effects of Firearm Injuries

A gunshot wound can cause harm that goes beyond the first injury. Often, survivors have to manage ongoing issues such as pain and mental problems which require them to visit healthcare and rehab regularly. A lot of emergency rooms find that these injuries contribute a large share to their trauma cases. In South Africa, many hospital admissions are due to gunshot injuries which often require major surgery and a long time in the hospital. Such a pattern affects patients and also puts a lot of pressure on healthcare resources, so long-term support plans are often needed. Plus, the body sometimes reacts in unpredictable ways—metabolic and inflammatory shifts may eventually trigger heart problems—so it seems clear that careful follow-up care is essential to handle these lingering effects (Basu et al., 2024).

9.1.7. Psychological Impact on Victims

The effects of gun injuries can be seen in the body and also in the mind for a long time. Many studies have found that a lot of victims develop symptoms similar to post-traumatic stress disorder and these inner scars may stay for a long time. For example, one study found that about 32% of people had sky-high scores on the Impact of Event Scale (IES), which clearly signals severe PTSD and might even throw off how their immune system works (Abbas et al., 2021). It is obvious that studying these psychological effects will help us design strategies that really work. More studies are being done on EM-related firearm injuries which has revealed the importance of better mental health care for those involved. To summarize, taking care of the inner wounds isn't just a side issue; it's an essential part of mounting a truly comprehensive forensic response (Figure 9.5).

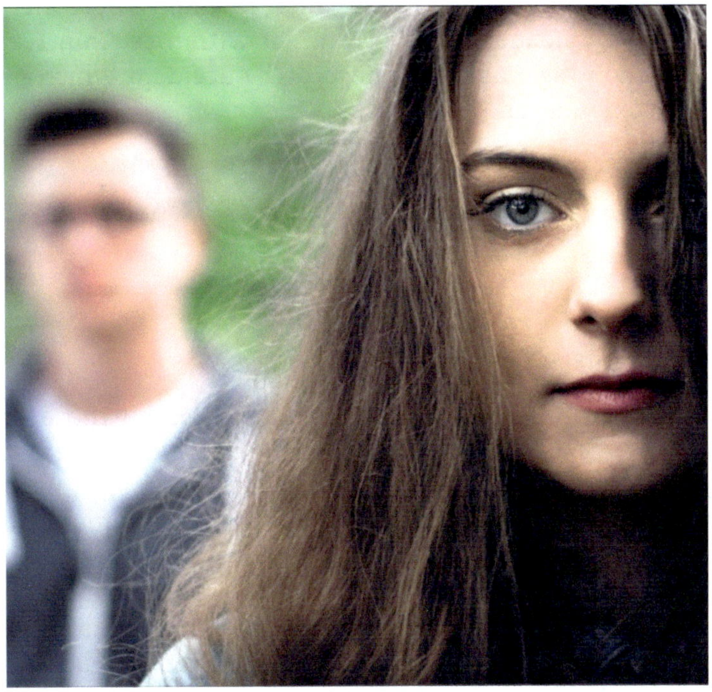

Figure 9.5. Gun injuries don't just leave a physical mark—they can wound the mind in deep, lasting ways.

Source: https://www.goodtherapy.org/blog/blog/wp-content/uploads/2014/06/couple-in-crisis2.jpg.

9.1.8. Variability in Injury Patterns

A gunshot wound investigation usually shows that many different factors cause the injuries to vary greatly. How a gunshot wound appears can change a lot, depending on the distance, kind of bullet and exact place on the body it hits. When shots are fired at close range, the bullet can be seen deforming and the muzzle blast is stronger which helps investigators find clues more easily. It's also important to note that surrounding details can complicate matters; studies have shown that when the data is ambiguous or scarce, even experienced analysts might proceed with extra caution—sometimes misclassifying injuries—resulting in about a 13% error rate in pattern recognition (Taylor et al., 2016). Ultimately, grasping these subtle, intertwined variables is key for accurate forensic interpretation, serving as a reminder of the field's inherent challenges (Branas et al., 2015).

9.1.9. Case Studies Illustrating Different Types of Injuries

Firearm injuries can be complicated and these complications can lead investigators to new and helpful ideas. It is common for case studies to reveal that the injury pattern is affected by the projectile, how fast it travels and the part of the body it hits. High-speed projectiles are known to do major damage to the heart and lungs. Research using fresh porcine organs to mimic human conditions (Humphrey et al., 2017) generally backs this up. Then there are those cases with several self-inflicted gunshot wounds that bring their own set of challenges; they almost always call for a thorough look into everything going on at the time, including personal psychological factors (Barnes et al., 2015). All things considered, being familiar with these injuries gives forensic experts a better chance to tell if a shooting was on purpose or by accident which helps explain the scene and improve the legal outcome in gun death cases.

Test Your Knowledge

1. Define a firearm injury in forensic medicine.
2. Outline the principal types of firearm injuries that are investigated in forensics.

9.2. Forensic Analysis of Firearm Injuries

Learning Outcome

1. Learn autopsy procedures for firearm injuries;
2. Perform ballistics analysis;
3. Explain gunshot residue testing;
4. Discuss documentation and evidence collection;
5. Explain the use of imaging techniques;
6. Determine the range of fire;
7. Identify the type of firearm used;
8. Describe challenges in forensic analysis.

It is not easy to understand firearm injuries when there are unusual social and demographic factors involved locally. In French Guiana, for example, a look back at the records generally speaks of a high rate of such injuries—most incidents involve young males and take place in violent settings, often with long-barreled guns (Fremery et al., 2024). It was also pointed out by the study that having wounds or damage to certain organs usually resulted in more deaths which suggests that public health measures should focus on these problems. At the same time, modern techniques like post-mortem computed tomography (PMCT) are steadily becoming a go-to tool in forensic work. This new approach, surprisingly, matches the traditional autopsy process and can quickly locate entry wounds and bullets inside the body which has greatly improved most forensic investigations. Overall, combining epidemiological research with technological advancements looks to be a good way to learn more about and respond better to, firearm injuries in forensic science.

There are unique problems with firearm injuries that forensic pathologists are especially equipped to solve. They carefully examine the autopsy, looking for any clue that can show the path of the bullet, the gun used and even a possible reason for the crime. In some retrospective studies of firearm deaths (Ricciardi et al., 2024), you see cases where bullet trajectories stray from what's expected, making the work a bit trickier than usual. Nowadays, artificial intelligence has started lending a hand, helping these experts pick out subtle patterns in evidence like blood spatter and the arc of a gunshot trace (Singh et al., 2023). The combination of old-fashioned knowledge and new technology usually makes it easier to understand how a death happened and often helps the legal process to make sure justice is done.

9.2.1. Autopsy Procedures for Firearm Injuries

The number of gunfire injuries is going up which means we should examine how forensic autopsies are performed. A careful look at the wound is usually important, as it provides information about the event as well as the injury.

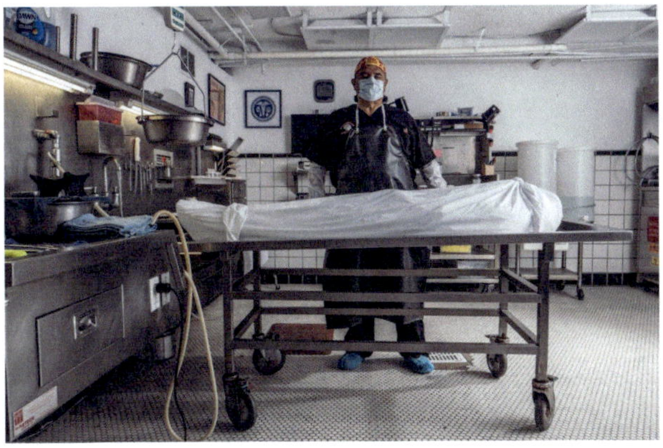

Figure 9.6. Gunfire injuries are on the rise, and that calls for a careful look at how forensic autopsies are done.

Source: https://i.natgeofe.com/n/fadc5d8d-7bfe-445e-93d6-2bb78a20a9f9/mm9412_200717_000522.jpg.

Sometimes, an autopsy ends up checking both what's seen on the outside and what's hidden inside; for example, tracking the bullet's trajectory can lead to bringing in an Xray to spot any projectiles stuck inside and to gauge potential harm to important organs (Shrestha et al., 2024). Studies generally point out that in many fatal cases, the damage isn't limited to a single spot but often hits key areas like the head and the torso together, which makes these investigations trickier (Nyberger et al., 2024). Using both imaging techniques and traditional checks usually makes injury assessments more accurate which helps move forward the investigation and any legal reviews. Overall, these in-depth autopsy procedures are a crucial piece of the puzzle when it comes to understanding gun-related lethality, and they can go a long way toward shaping public health strategies aimed at cutting down these incidents (Figure 9.6).

9.2.2. Ballistics Analysis

Even the most experienced investigators can find it hard to follow the injuries left by firearms. You need to understand ballistics which explains what occurs inside the weapon, the path of the bullet after it leaves and the result of the impact, to begin understanding. Wound ballistics, basically a slice of terminal ballistics, looks at how a bullet wiggles through body tissues; this little detail offers clues that help experts piece together what went down during a shooting incident (Bolton et al., 2016). It has been observed in many cases that how fast and what kind of projectile hits can greatly determine the harm done to organs like the heart and lungs. For example, some tests with pig organ simulants have pointed out damage patterns that change with different bullet velocities; these findings help explain skeletal trauma and even hint at the cause of death (Humphrey et al., 2017). In short, knowing these factors improves forensic work and also points out the need for constant care in handling and examining evidence when guns are part of the case.

9.2.3. Gunshot Residue Testing

It is not always easy to tell how a gun was involved in a crime scene. Here, gunshot residue analysis helps a lot—it allows investigators to see how far the firearm was from the scene by noticing residue patterns on the victim and nearby surfaces. In a lot of labs, the standard is to use the real weapon to get a precise result. Yet, recent studies generally show that using any firearm of the same make and model produces nearly identical residue patterns(Hodges et al., 2008; Lewey et al., 2007). Most of the time, this allows you to use other weapons instead which gives you more options when the original is not available. Such subtle shifts in testing methods could, arguably, influence how forensic evidence is collected and interpreted in cases involving firearm injuries, possibly reshaping outcomes in unexpected ways (Figure 9.7).

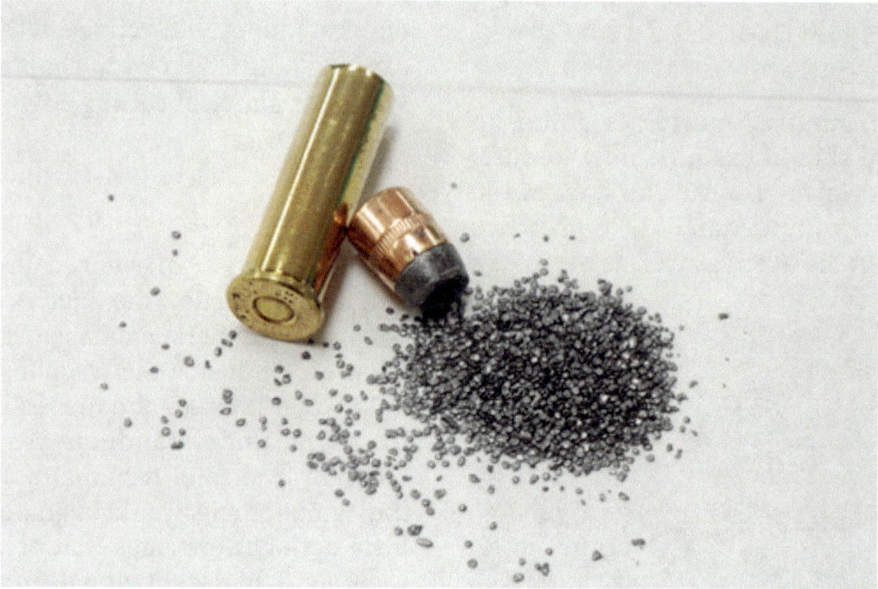

Figure 9.7. Gunshot residue analysis.

Source: https://www.facrimelab.com/wp-content/uploads/2017/04/svc_crim_gsr.jpg.

9.2.4. Documentation and Evidence Collection

When you look into gunshot injuries, you need to document and collect evidence together. Labs are usually in charge of finding out how far a shot was taken, so they analyze the gunshot residue patterns. They say you should use the same gun and ammo from the incident — a rule that's followed even though solid backing for it is kind of thin; one study, for instance, pointed out that switching guns doesn't change distance estimations, but different ammunition brands do show clear differences (Hodges et al., 2008). Because registered nurses may be involved in treating victims or suspects, they can notice and gather important clues in hospitals. Their encounters, which might give up physical marks or pieces of spoken evidence, mean that jotting every detail down is pretty important for keeping the investigation solid (Cordoma et al., 2016). Usually, the success of the forensic process relies on being very meticulous with notes and evidence.

9.2.5. Use of Imaging Techniques (e.g., X-rays, Computer Tomography (CT) Scans)

Forensic science has improved a lot and now imaging methods are changing how gunshot injuries are studied. Experts can now use X-rays and CT scans to look inside a body without performing invasive procedures which allows them to view the effects of a gunshot without disturbing the remains. Virtopsy, which bundles these methods together, might just be shifting the whole postmortem game, especially in places that usually avoid classic autopsies (Lawson et al., 2022). Micro-CT, too, gets in on the act, examining toolmarks in fine detail, and helping to nail down specifics about firearms and their shots (Cordoma et al., 2016). Overall, these advancements not only bump up the accuracy of forensic work but also deal with the messy ethical and practical issues that come with modern practice, generally leading to legal outcomes that folks can count on (Figure 9.8).

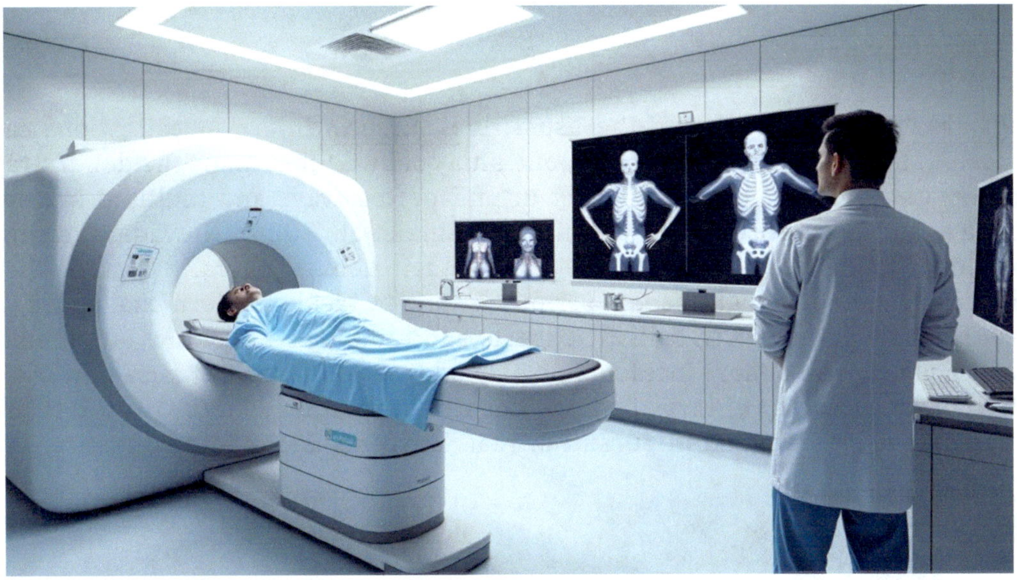

Figure 9.8. Virtopsy.

Source: https://simplyforensic.com/wp-content/uploads/2025/04/Virtual_Autopsy.webp.

9.2.6. Determining the Range of Fire

Examining firearm injuries can give important details about the shooting such as how far away the shooter was. In a lot of cases, the marks on a wound can reveal both the type of firearm and how far away the shooter was when they shot. You might notice, for instance, that gunshot residues (GSR) and even tiny features like an abrasion ring serve as clues to the shooting range; studies have shown that the spread of lead can vary in surprising ways depending on that distance (Piegari et al., 2024). Generally speaking, these subtle details help forensic experts piece together the series of events, even when determining the manner of death is at stake, lending support to the medicolegal angles in most cases (Rani et al., 2023). How these clues appear can be a little random, sometimes appearing in a mix of hints, but they all help the story move forward. In the end, figuring out the exact distance at which a firearm can be used is very important for a complete investigation of firearm injuries.

9.2.7. Identifying the Type of Firearm Used

Forensic investigation of gunshot wounds is very important for solving crimes—law enforcement depends on it greatly. Usually, the first task is to determine the type of weapon used which can direct the investigation and affect legal proceedings. Bullet wounds, because of their caliber and unusual patterns, can give clues about the gun used and they often add more details to the story. Using ballistic tests and looking at trace evidence often allows labs to identify the type of gun used. In many homicide studies, researchers have noted that mixing these forensic approaches generally turns out to be a game-changer in cracking cold cases, especially when the usual evidence just doesn't cut it (Lunn et al., 2012). Oddly enough, even mass grave investigations show that careful forensic scrutiny can sometimes nail down specific firearms, handing prosecutors the kind of solid proof they need to push a case forward (Ekštajn et al., 2021).

9.2.8. Challenges in Forensic Analysis

When things aren't done according to the usual rules, firearm injury investigations can become very complicated. Looking back at past cases, one study showed that many incidents stray far from expected injury patterns—wound paths twist in unexpected ways and multiple injuries pop up, often puzzling even the most seasoned examiners (Failla et al., 2024). Nowadays, techniques like three-dimensional spatial reconstruction are making their debut, generally pushing the idea that traditional forensic methods might need a serious update to tackle modern challenges (Zmiievska et al., 2024). Forensic pathologists, ballistic experts and radiologists are now often teaming up to solve these difficult cases. As more incidents display odd, atypical details, these newer approaches not only sharpen the accuracy of investigations but also stress the need for protocols that flexibly adapt to each unique situation, all in pursuit of real, fair conclusions toward justice (Figure 9.9).

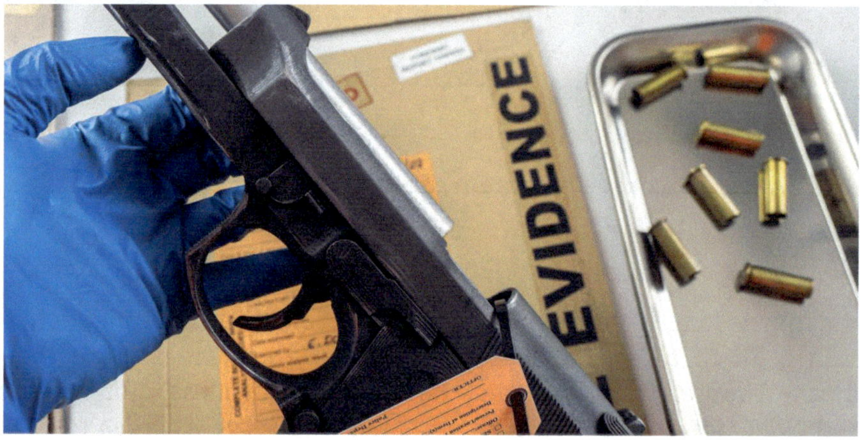

Figure 9.9. Firearm injury investigations can be a real maze, especially when things don't follow the usual rules.

Source: https://magazine.publichealth.jhu.edu/sites/default/files/styles/feature_image_1200_1x_/public/forensic_firearms_header.jpg.

Test Your Knowledge

1. Define gunshot residue (GSR) and explain its forensic value.
2. What is the term range of fire and how do experts find it during autopsy?

9.3. Legal Implications of Firearm Injuries

Learning Outcome

1. Understand the role of forensic evidence in court;
2. Identify standards of proof in firearm injury cases;
3. Be aware of how firearm injuries shape criminal investigations;
4. Explain case law related to firearm injuries;
5. Focus on ethical considerations in forensic testimony;
6. Learn victim rights and advocacy;
7. Describe legislative responses to firearm injuries;
8. Understand the role of expert witnesses;
9. Explain public perception and media influence.

The number of gun injuries in the United States is rising which has caused legal problems, safety concerns and questions about police actions. These events—accounting for roughly 2.6% of trauma hospital stays and hitting marginalized groups the hardest (Salottolo et al., 2024)—force our legal system to wrestle with issues of responsibility and how to stop further harm, generally speaking. It's interesting how tracking a gun from its legal purchase all the way to its role in a crime points to the crucial need for smarter rules designed to curb gun violence effectively (Robinson et al., 2024). At times, the legal process is driven by victims as well as by those who want those who design, make and sell weapons to be held responsible. Because the ways people are injured by firearms keep changing, laws must also change and lawmakers must keep reviewing the rules to ensure the safety of all while supporting individual rights. In short, because things are always changing, legal experts in this field must be ready to learn about new trends and the resulting legal consequences.

9.3.1. Role of Forensic Evidence in Court

Court cases about gun injuries often use forensic evidence to turn vague stories into facts that can be tested. When a fatal shooting occurs, looking at clues like gunshot residue—analyzed through controlled tests using particular firearms and ammo (Hodges et al., 2008)—can reveal, in many instances, how far the shooter was from the victim. At the same time, these scientific techniques help with victim identification; in some mass grave investigations, for example, autopsy reports have repeatedly shown that gunshot wounds were the primary cause of death (Ekštajn et al., 2021). To summarize, these strong pieces of evidence not only fortify the prosecution's argument but also illuminating the underlying intent behind the crime, making the overall chain of events easier to unravel (Figure 9.10).

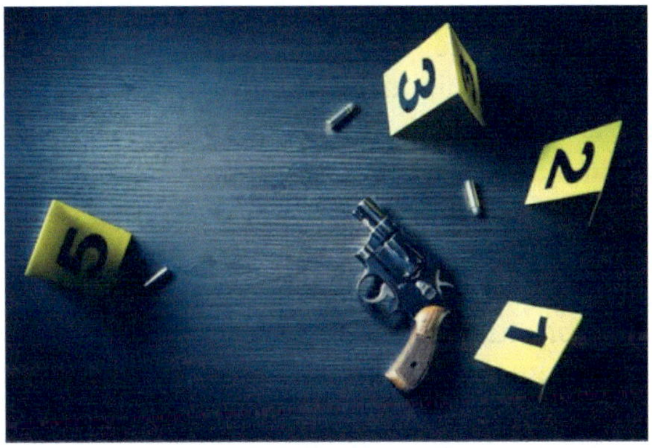

Figure 9.10. Forensic evidence stands as a key factor in court cases about gun injuries, often shifting vague accounts into real, testable facts.

Source: https://cowboylawgroup.com/wp-content/uploads/2024/07/the-woodlands-gun-crimes.webp.

9.3.2. Standards of Proof in Firearm Injury Cases

How much evidence is needed to prove a case is very important in firearm injury cases. Labs shoot the weapon at various distances to see the gunshot residue patterns and then they compare these to the patterns found on the victims or targets. It is usual for labs to test the same firearm and ammo that were involved in the incident, but some people think this rule isn't fully justified. In most cases, studies show that changes in the firearm don't majorly affect distance estimates, but switching ammunition brands can lead to noticeable differences (Hodges et al., 2008). Overall, getting a clear grasp of these points is crucial for legal pros and forensic experts alike, since, at the end of the day, the whole outcome of a case rides on how believable the evidence turns out to be—even with all the messy details that come with firearm injuries (Hodges et al., 2008).

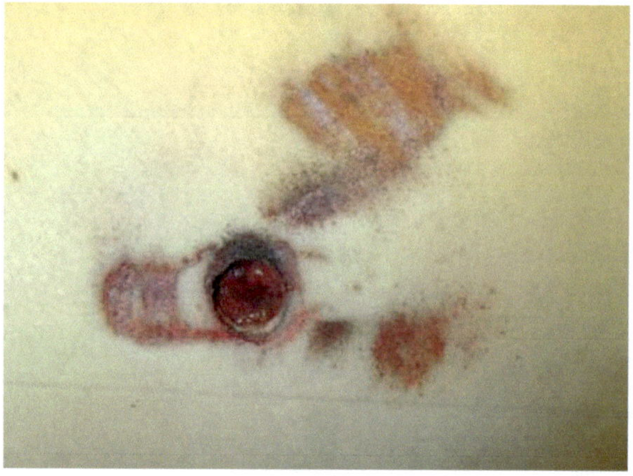

Figure 9.11. Firearm injuries have a puzzling complexity that, in many cases, shifts the course of criminal investigations in unexpected ways.

Source: https://img.medscapestatic.com/pi/meds/ckb/99/13099tn.jpg.

9.3.3. Impact of Firearm Injuries on Criminal Investigations

Firearm injuries are often complex and this can change the direction of many criminal investigations. Figuring out the distance of the shot is usually the first step - experts test the gun to see if the residue matches which leads to further investigation. These residue checks turn out to be key for building timelines and teasing out possible motives, since different ammo brands can lead to small but significant changes in injury patterns, which adds layers to the investigative story (Hodges et al., 2008). Sometimes the kind of weapon used even hints at an offender's behavior, especially in serial homicide cases where the choice may depend on available opportunities or a bit of premeditated planning (Fletcher et al., 2022). By looking at different crime scenes and evidence, forensic experts try to understand the minds of suspects. Generally speaking, this careful—if not always perfect—approach shows that firearm injuries do more than reveal victim circumstances; they also offer a glimpse into the nature of those responsible, firmly establishing this method as a cornerstone of forensic science (Figure 9.11).

9.3.4. Case Law Related to Firearm Injuries

Gun violence has recently caused us to rethink how we see legal injuries. Over the last few years, matters have become more complicated which is clear in how society responds. A study covering 2017–2022 points out that most cases hit men, and about one in three of these incidents ended up with broken bones (Teke et al., 2024). This data makes it clear that these injuries are very serious. It's not just about counting numbers either. It gets even more complicated when you have to tell which guns are legal and which have been changed for illegal reasons. In one strange case, an ordinary air rifle had been modified for illegal use, raising many questions about who's responsible and what exactly counts as a firearm (Mulani et al., 2024). Forensic experts document these errors and this makes it harder to tell where the law ends and science begins. Because of all this, it is often clear that we need policies to help prevent such injuries and to clarify who is responsible in court.

9.3.5. Ethical Considerations in Forensic Testimony

Forensic experts give testimony in court, but they must be very careful about the ethical issues involved. If the people responsible for evidence are not skilled, it could easily be lost or mishandled which could weaken the case. One study, for example, showed that emergency nurses in New Zealand have a rather shallow grasp of forensic details (Donaldson et al., 2020). This result suggests that there is a major problem that could harm the medical care of people with firearm injuries. Most of the time, experts who testify in court have to be both knowledgeable and aware of any chance that evidence could be used wrongly which might lead to convicting the innocent or acquitting the guilty. Additionally, gatherings like conferences and workshops—think of events organized by UK/CLE—help deepen the understanding of these critical ethical issues, ensuring that forensic testimony remains both solid and fair (Office of Continuing Legal Education at the University of Kentucky College of Law, 2002).

9.3.6. Victim Rights and Advocacy

Firearm injuries touch people in ways that can't be fixed only by quick medical attention—it's mainly about supporting the victims. You see, young men seem to carry most of the burden; studies, like one out in French Guiana where over 21% of the victims didn't make it due to limited modern care (Fremery et al., 2024), drive that home. A forensic look at gunshot wounds also shows that the kind and spot of an injury give us big clues about survival, underlining how harsh the reality can be for these folks (Savka et al., 2024). Most of the time, it means we should focus on both treating injuries and working for better policies to stop more of them. When victim voices break through, unsure as it may be at first, they can nudge lawmakers toward changes that might, eventually, ease the long-term fallout from firearm violence (Figure 9.12).

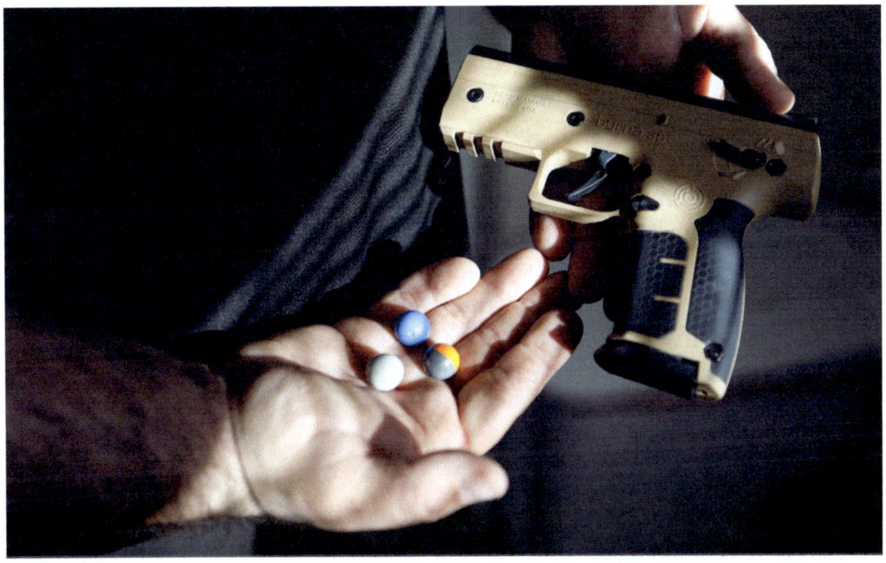

Figure 9.12. Firearm injuries hit people in ways that aren't fixed just by quick medical care—it's more about standing up for those hurt.

Source: https://www.thetrace.org/wp-content/uploads/2023/11/B4A4354-crop-scaled.jpg.

9.3.7. Legislative Responses to Firearm Injuries

Because firearm injuries cause many problems for public health and safety, it seems clear that a multi-faceted approach to legislation is almost necessary. Legislators are more often using concepts from both disease and crime research, instead of following only one traditional approach. For example, boosting police efforts through ballistic intelligence systems can help different regions swap vital details about weapons involved in crimes (Bowen et al., 2016). In most cases, looking into youth gun violence with tactics like the EpiCrim method might actually tackle the root issues, rather than just acting on problems as they pop up (McMillan et al., 2020). While these steps are not perfect, they play a big role in reducing gun injuries and exposing the social and cultural factors behind gun violence.

9.3.8. The Role of Expert Witnesses

Usually, in complex firearm injury cases, the first step is to find how the injury happened and what the outcomes could be and then seasoned experts are called in. Forensic pathologists, ballistic analysts and others with relevant knowledge provide the necessary details to help shape the legal process. One study, for example, looked into some pretty unusual firearm injuries where expert input was crucial for teasing apart odd trajectories and wound patterns (Failla et al., 2024)—a factor that, in most cases, shifted how the evidence was viewed legally. In episodes of violence, even those unfolding in politically charged settings, expert testimonies act as a reminder that thorough, careful forensic checks are key to supporting claims of criminal behavior (Mishalov et al., 2024). Forensic experts use their observations to interpret the evidence and also connect scientific facts to the rules of the law which helps the judicial process. All in all, these experts are crucial for catching the special features that every case presents.

9.3.9. Public Perception and Media Influence

How people feel about gun injuries and the details of the cases are often influenced by stories in the media and the opinions of the public. Sensational news tends to highlight a dramatic shooting which can affect our usual ideas and make us more afraid of gun violence. This effect can lead a misinformed population to assume that gun injuries mainly come from serial murders, overlooking other causes like domestic strife or even accidental discharges (Fletcher et al., 2022). As folks keep hearing these recurring stories, their reactions to police moves and forensic checks shift too—especially when considering the emotional and mental strain brought on by so-called "less-lethal" options like Tasers (Waters et al., 2017). Looking at how these angles are presented helps us see more clearly the effects of gun injuries and proves why correct information is important for policy decisions.

Test Your Knowledge

1. What legal problems can be solved using a ballistic examination of recovered bullets?
2. How important is bullet trajectory analysis in proving cases in a criminal court?

9.4. Prevention and Public Health Strategies

Learning Outcome

1. Know education and awareness programs;
2. Learn community intervention strategies;
3. Explain the role of law enforcement in prevention;
4. Understand gun control policies and their effectiveness;
5. Focus on mental health resources for at-risk individuals;
6. Describe research on firearm injury prevention;
7. Focus on collaboration between agencies and organizations;
8. Know the impact of socioeconomic factors;
9. Explain future directions for prevention efforts.

If you are looking at firearm injuries in a forensic setting, you have to focus on the main causes of violence to prevent them. Some studies suggest that guns are involved in most murder-suicides which is a reason to take steps to reduce their availability. Usually, finding out the causes of repeated violent injuries assists in designing better intervention programs. A statewide study even revealed that many people grappling with violent injuries also face socioeconomic setbacks, hinting at an overall approach that mixes mental health support with improved access to community resources to lower repeat incidents (Kaufman et al., 2016). If these actions are followed, public health efforts can help lower the number of firearm injuries and build safer communities.

9.4.1. Education and Awareness Programs

Firearm injuries are not simple and sharing information about them should be done in a wider and sometimes more unexpected way, for both doctors and ordinary people. Many primary care physicians, for instance, say they don't feel ready to talk about gun safety with their patients; this clearly points to a pressing need for more organized training within graduate medical education (Titus et al., 2021). They should not only mention the risks; they should also provide useful tools for counseling, for example, giving ready-made templates that can be used in electronic health records. Then again, we also have to face the deeper issues – think the regular circulation of unlicensed guns and the fact that children rarely get early lessons about firearm safety, which are both key for long-term prevention (Feola et al., 2020). By building a culture of awareness and a sense of responsibility (sometimes through small, everyday changes), these education efforts can empower both medical professionals and the wider public to cut down on firearm injuries and boost public health outcomes (Figure 9.13).

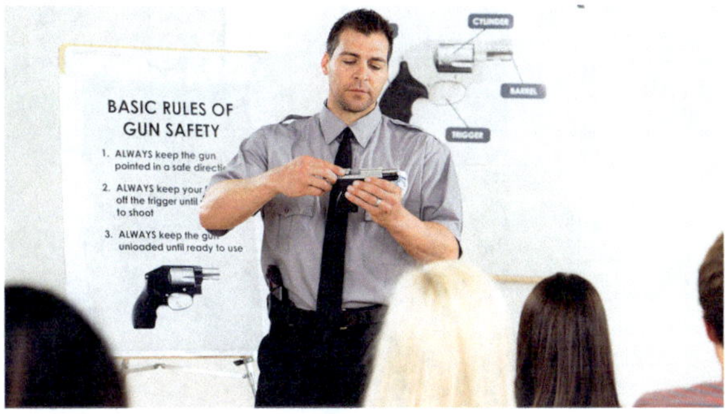

Figure 9.13. Firearm injuries are a complicated issue that call for a broader, sometimes less predictable, way to spread knowledge—both among doctors and everyday folks.

Source: https://www.aamc.org/sites/default/files/gun-safety-class-168857982.jpg.

9.4.2. Community Intervention Strategies

Gun injuries are increasing and people in communities are finding new ways to address the problem. Local groups made up of doctors, nurses and police are now getting involved to investigate what causes gun violence. In many cases, studies in Emergency Medicine have found that injuries linked to domestic violence or youth fights are often missing important links which suggests that the issues often go back to daily challenges. When you mix epidemiology and criminology, some call it EpiCrim and it can point out that urban youth gun incidents often happen because of certain behaviors, so looking at problems locally is very important. Teaming up with people from other parts of the community, they usually develop strategies that address their area's unique issues and aim to reduce gun injuries and improve the community's health.

9.4.3. Role of Law Enforcement in Prevention

Gun injuries create a situation that involves more than medical help—law enforcement is also needed quickly. If officers are active in community-based work and teach the public, there is a chance to decrease these incidents. You could notice police patrolling at-risk spots or working with the community to find out what is causing the violence. We should also focus on gathering information about firearm injuries, because it helps create better and more effective policies. According to research, applying a thorough, evidence-based strategy tends to lower both gun crimes and injuries. And when you consider the mental toll—like PTSD among victims—it becomes clear that law enforcement should also offer some supportive resources alongside their preventive moves (Abbas et al., 2021) (Figure 9.14).

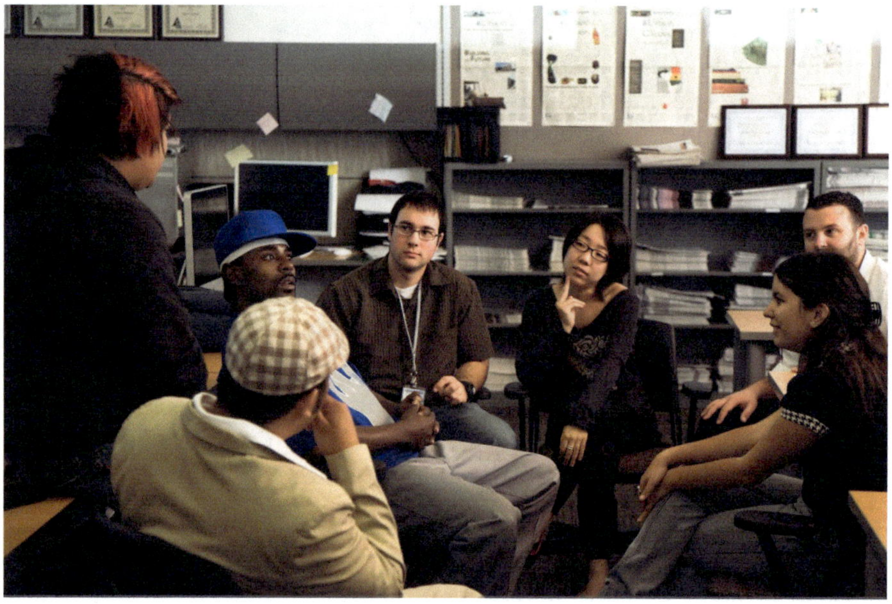

Figure 9.14. Gun injuries present a tangled challenge that goes beyond just rushing someone to the hospital—law enforcement quickly becomes a key player in the mix.

Source: https://www.bmsg.org/wp-content/uploads/2024/09/GettyImages-88752183.jpeg.

9.4.4. Gun Control Policies and Their Effectiveness

It becomes important to look at gun control policies when we see that firearm injuries keep being a problem for public health. Researchers often flag that we're missing critical pieces of the puzzle—gaps that largely stem from long-standing federal funding limits which slow down the kinds of thorough, evidence-based studies needed to draw solid conclusions (Stevenson et al., 2019). If there isn't much reliable evidence, public talks may be superficial and lawmakers struggle to design good rules. Emergency medicine professionals are now paying more attention to problems such as suicide and domestic violence involving guns which could mean our policies should be looked at again. Since gun violence is still a major problem, seeing how current actions are working is very important. Such knowledge can guide new actions to lower injuries and bring policies in line with what is good for our health.

9.4.5. Mental Health Resources for At-risk Individuals

It is complicated how mental well-being and gun injuries are linked which suggests that we should provide more personalized mental health care for at-risk people. Sometimes repeated violent incidents seem tied to deeper mental struggles; in most cases, individuals facing hardships like poverty or homelessness tend to experience this cycle more often (Kaufman et al., 2016). Public stories, as we've heard, reveal that many harassment cases stem from untreated mental issues—this not only troubles the victims but can backfire on the aggressors as well (Every-Palmer et al., 2015). When mental healthcare is part of intervention, it appears to reduce these risks by addressing the emotional causes of the violence. In short, making sure that those who are most vulnerable have ready access to these mental health services remains a key piece of any broader plan to reduce gun injuries and boost community safety (Figure 9.15).

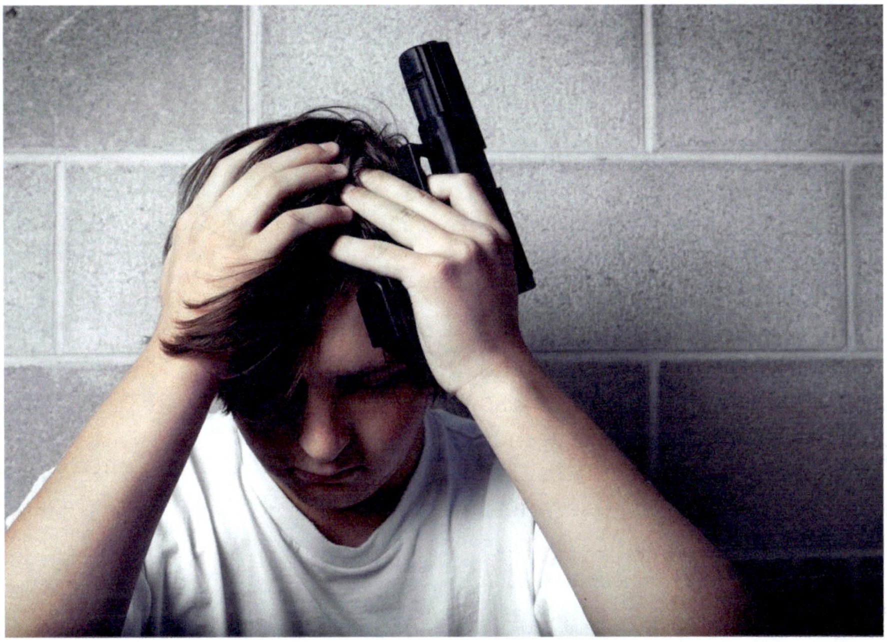

Figure 9.15. Mental well-being and gun injuries link in a complicated, almost tricky, way, hinting that we need more personalized mental health support for those who might be at risk.

Source: https://www.rand.org/content/rand/pubs/commentary/2013/01/can-improved-mental-health-care-prevent-gun-crimes/jcr:content/par/teaser.crop.1200x900.cm.jpeg/1495292493340.jpeg.

9.4.6. Research on Firearm Injury Prevention

Firearm violence is such a big issue that it makes you consider how to prevent accidents every day. One research finds that every year, more than 1,200 Americans are killed in murder-suicide and in most cases, guns are the weapon used. Almost, it seems like these statistics call out the problem of easy access to guns and softly suggest that taking smarter steps could ease the problem. Then there's this other angle: more than 11% of those treated for interpersonal violence end up with further injuries within a two-year span (Kaufman et al., 2016). Because of this, we are encouraged to back tighter gun rules and neighborhood programs that help locally. Most of the time, making people aware and having well-planned policies could be the answer to dealing with gun violence.

9.4.7. Collaboration Between Agencies and Organizations

Firearm injuries are handled in forensics by bringing together groups from different agencies and organizations. When people share important information and resources, it provides a clearer, sometimes complicated, picture of what leads to gun violence. Take the EpiCrim idea, for instance; mixing up epidemiology with criminology can expose risky behaviors in urban youth, and this usually ends up pointing toward the right kind of interventions (McMillan et al., 2023). It is also obvious that pointing out the main Emergency Medicine research questions demonstrates that teamwork between healthcare providers and researchers is possible. When experts from different fields collaborate, they come up with plans that are based on evidence, may seem a bit rough and are designed to deal with urgent matters to improve prevention and control. In short, using different approaches ensures policies are formed using many viewpoints which helps keep communities safer.

9.4.8. Impact of Socioeconomic Factors

Many people regularly deal with the effects of gun violence. When the economy is unstable and money is scarce such violence makes everyday difficulties worse by causing businesses to shrink and reducing trust among people. It's a tough cycle: more gun incidents discourage new investments and push poverty further, as seen in research pointing out that neighborhoods hit hard by gun violence often suffer severe economic downturns (Gurvis et al., 2016). As an example, the Croatian effort to disarm communities proves that reducing violence is partly about making sure everyone has equal economic opportunities. In most cases, when improvements in economic health go hand in hand with disarmament efforts, communities end up feeling a bit safer and more secure, with studies noting that a combined policy approach helps bolster overall well-being (Figure 9.16).

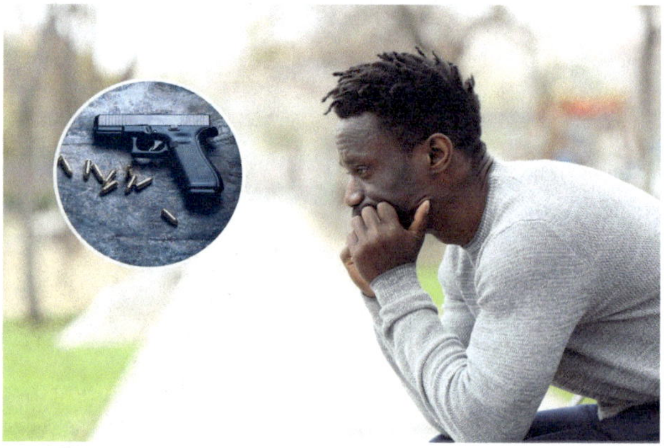

Figure 9.16. Gun violence ties deeply into the everyday struggles many face.

Source: https://d.newsweek.com/en/full/2397663/man-gun.jpg?w=1200&f=c24a96516b66bb5943a5f8641ef290b0.

9.4.9. Future Directions for Prevention Efforts

More and more is being discovered about how alcohol and gun violence are linked and this is leading to new ways to stop harm. Research shows, in most cases, that when people drink, it often goes hand in hand with various gun-related problems (Matthay et al., 2025) – so cutting back on alcohol might just lower the risk of injuries involving firearms. There's also the issue of reaching out to folks for studies; for example, recruiting vulnerable groups like rural adolescents has proven tricky (Weybright et al., 2024), and that makes it all the more important to rethink how we gather data. A number of experts believe that using research that involves the community can get people engaged and lead to solutions that fit the community's real needs. In most places, rules that prevent those with alcohol-related offenses from owning guns have helped reduce both gun homicides and suicides. All in all, a mix of personal actions and larger social changes is important for making prevention strategies that work everywhere.

Test Your Knowledge

1. Is there anything public health can learn from how firearm injuries happen?
2. In what ways can forensic data help improve the care given to trauma patients?

Summary

Thinking about firearm injuries from a forensic standpoint, they touch a wider range of society than most people realize. With the rise in these cases, it is clear that our methods for investigating them and treating patients require major changes and these changes are necessary and urgent. Research generally shows that, even though such injuries happen way less often among women and kids, the resulting drop in individual productivity and the spike in healthcare bills underline the call for better awareness and action (Teke et al., 2024). It may seem strange, but little numbers can still have a big effect on society. At the same time, forensic science isn't staying behind; new tricks like 3-D modeling give investigators a sharper look at injury details, offering a practical, almost indispensable tool in their work (Zmiievska et al., 2024). All in all, using both data and new methods proves that using a wider approach is important for understanding and reducing the effects of firearm injuries. Dealing with firearm injuries is not easy and understanding them is crucial for forensic work and preventing more harm. It all starts with something as small as GSR; these particles usually show traces of lead, barium, and antimony that can link a suspect to the scene, while the very shape of a gunshot wound reveals clues about how far away the shot was fired and what the shooter might have been aiming to do (Piegari et al., 2024). Sometimes, when you dig into injuries from less destructive firearms – particularly in the Arctic – you notice distinct patterns where demographic quirks like age, gender, and even social habits tend to play their part (Yasheva et al., 2024). Reviews of the statistics often highlight that many victims suffer from multiple wounds which makes it clear how complicated these cases can be. All in all, these studies point out that we need to use better forensic tools and examine personal and social factors which will help develop better strategies and policies.

KEY TERMS FROM THIS CHAPTER

Conflict
Handguns
Prevention
Rifles
Emergency medicine
internal bleeding
Psychological damage
Shotguns
Gunshot wound
Policymakers
Public health

Short Answer Questions

1. What is the difference between entry and exit wounds?
2. Describe the characteristic features of a close-range gunshot wound.
3. What is meant by tattooing or stippling in a firearm injury and what does it show?
4. What does an abrasion collar or a grease collar look like and where are they found?
5. What are the differences in how contact wounds and distant gunshot wounds look?
6. What could make an exit wound be larger and more irregular than an entry wound?
7. How does the type of firearm (handgun versus shotgun) affect the injury pattern?

Critical Thinking Questions

1. What is a common sign seen in an entry wound in a gunshot injury?

a. Everted margins
b. Larger than the exit wound
c. Inverted margins with an abrasion collar
d. Surrounded by tissue prolapse

2. Gunshot residue (GSR) is typically found on:

a. The victim only
b. The bullet only
c. The shooter's hands and clothing
d. The gun barrel only

3. Around the area of a gunshot wound, stippling or tattooing happens because of:

a. Flame from the muzzle
b. Contact with the bullet
c. Partially burnt gunpowder
d. Bullet ricochet

4. Which of the following best describes a contact wound?

a. Soot and stippling around the wound
b. Burned skin with a muzzle imprint
c. No powder residue
d. Everted wound margins

5. An exit wound from a firearm is typically:

a. Smaller and more regular than the entry wound
b. Surrounded by an abrasion collar
c. Larger and more irregular than the entry wound
d. Circular with soot deposition

Answers to Critical Thinking Questions

1. (c); 2. (c); 3. (c); 4. (b); 5. (c)

References

1. Abbas, K., Altaf, R., Jogi, M. A., Malik, S., et al. (2021). Medico-legal cases (MLC) presented at a tertiary care center and acute symptoms of post-traumatic stress disorder among the survivors. *Pakistan Journal of Neurological Surgery, 25*(2). https://core.ac.uk/download/478593241.pdf (accessed on 29 May 2025).
2. Alsop, K. (2022). *3-Dimensional Imaging and Analysis of Forensically Relevant Toolmarks Using micro-CT* (PhD thesis, University of Warwick). https://core.ac.uk/download/567877521.pdf
3. Assembly Committee on Public Safety. (2001). *Public Safety 2001: Creating a safer California*. https://core.ac.uk/download/233105876.pdf (accessed on 29 May 2025).
4. Banuelos, K. (2018). Domestic and international firearm laws: Can implementation be used to nationally decrease firearm violence and mass shootings? *Themis: Research Journal of Justice Studies and Forensic Science, 6*(1), Article 12. https://scholarworks.sjsu.edu/themis/vol6/iss1/12 (accessed on 29 May 2025).
5. Barnes, C., Di Maio, J., Heard, K., Hejna, K., Karger, K., et al. (2015). Determined to die! Ability to act following multiple self-inflicted gunshot wounds to the head: The Cook County Office of Medical Examiner experience (2005–2012) and review of literature. https://core.ac.uk/download/54522925.pdf (accessed on 29 May 2025).
6. Basu, C., Cannon, P. L., Awgulewitsch, C. P., Galindo, C. L., Gamazon, E., & Hatzopoulos, A. (2024). Transcriptome analysis of cardiac endothelial cells after myocardial infarction reveals temporal changes and long-term deficits. *Scientific Reports, 14*. https://www.semanticscholar.org/paper/b4cda738ee0f009f74fc881b2d9a0be592c292d0 (accessed on 29 May 2025).
7. Black, O. B. (2019). Physical and chemical trace evidence from 3d-printed firearms, and use of a quadcopter for targeted sampling of gaseous mercury in the atmosphere. https://core.ac.uk/download/335347944.pdf (accessed on 29 May 2025).
8. Bolton-King, R., & Schulze, J. (2016). Firearms and ballistics. https://core.ac.uk/download/80691312.pdf (accessed on 29 May 2025).
9. Bowen, E., & Poole, H. (2016). Examination of firearms and forensics in Europe and across territories: Final report.
10. Branas, C. C., Kastanaki, A. E., Michalodimitrakis, M., Tzougas, J., Kranioti, E. F., Theodorakis, P. N., Carr, B. G., et al. (2015). The impact of economic austerity and prosperity events on suicide in Greece: A 30-year interrupted time-series analysis. *BMJ Open, 5*, e005619. https://doi.org/10.1136/bmjopen-2014-005619.
11. Cordoma, J. V. (2016). Exploring and understanding the factors that may influence the outlook of registered nurses regarding potential criminal evidence identification, collection and preservation on patients presented to them. https://core.ac.uk/download/151531092.pdf (accessed on 29 May 2025).
12. Donaldson, A. E. (2020). New Zealand emergency nurses' knowledge about forensic science

and its application to practice. *International Emergency Nursing, 53*, 100854. https://doi.org/10.1016/j.ienj.2020.100854.

13. Ekštajn, H., Kružić, I., & Bašić, Ž. (2021). Forensic investigation of a mass grave at Ovčara, near Vukovar, of victims killed by the Serbian army in 1991. https://core.ac.uk/download/481997335.pdf.
14. Every-Palmer, S., Barry-Walsh, J., & Pathé, M. (2015). Harassment, stalking, threats and attacks targeting New Zealand politicians: A mental health issue. *The Australian and New Zealand Journal of Psychiatry, 49*(7), 634–641. https://doi.org/10.1177/0004867415583700.
15. Failla, A. V. M., Licciardello, G., Cocimano, G., Di Mauro, L., Chisari, M., Sessa, F., Salerno, M., & Esposito, M. (2024). Diagnostic challenges in uncommon firearm injury cases: A multidisciplinary approach. *Diagnostics (Basel, Switzerland), 15*(1), 31. https://doi.org/10.3390/diagnostics15010031.
16. Feola, A., Mastroianni, V., Scamardella, I. A., Zangani, P., Della Pietra, B., & Campobasso, C. P. (2021). Isolated right atrial rupture from blunt chest trauma in motor vehicle collisions: Mechanisms of injury and outcomes. *The American Journal of Forensic Medicine and Pathology, 42*(1), 67–69. https://doi.org/10.1097/PAF.0000000000000591.
17. Fletcher, E. (2022). *Weapons of Choice: A Statistical Comparison Between Different Weapons and Resulting Injuries, Opportunist Weapon Selection and Forensic Awareness*. https://core.ac.uk/download/533941028.pdf (accessed on 29 May 2025).
18. Fremery, A., Beguinot, E., Franchi, A., Douchet, M., Tertre, V., Hamiche, K., Adenis, A., et al. (2024). Epidemiologic analysis and mortality outcome of firearm injuries in French Guiana (2016–2019). *European Journal of Trauma and Emergency Surgery, 50*, 1649–1659. https://www.semanticscholar.org/paper/7f390ca8480c7e50085f458905ffbc72c741a00b (accessed on 29 May 2025).
19. Gurvis, A., Bai, B., Mohr, E., & Irvin-Erickson, Y. (2016). The effect of gun violence on local economies. https://core.ac.uk/download/141922665.pdf (accessed on 29 May 2025).
20. Hodges, S. K. (2008). *Forensic Gunshot Residue Distance Determination Testing Using Identical Make and Model Handguns and Different Ammunitions* (Master's thesis). https://dc.etsu.edu/etd/1915 (accessed on 29 May 2025).
21. Humphrey, C. (2017). *Characterization of Soft Tissue and Skeletal Bullet Wound Trauma and Three-Dimensional Anatomical Modelling* (Unpublished thesis).
22. Kaufman, E., Rising, K., Wiebe, D. J., Ebler, D. J., Crandall, M. L., & Delgado, M. K. (2016). Recurrent violent injury: Magnitude, risk factors, and opportunities for intervention from a statewide analysis. *The American Journal of Emergency Medicine, 34*(9), 1823–1830. https://doi.org/10.1016/j.ajem.2016.06.051.
23. Kelley, A. (2020). Examining how stricter firearm laws lower mortality rates in the United States. https://core.ac.uk/download/352952738.pdf (accessed on 29 May 2025).
24. Lawson, N. E. (2022). *Autopsy V. Virtuosi: A New Approach for Postmortem Forensic Examination* (Undergraduate thesis). https://scholarworks.bgsu.edu/honorsprojects/851 (accessed on 29 May 2025).
25. Lewey, H. (2007). Examining significant differences of gunshot residue patterns using same make and model of firearms in forensic distance determination tests. https://core.ac.uk/download/214065644.pdf (accessed on 29 May 2025).

26. Lunn, M. M. (2012). Cold case homicides: An examination of clearance factors. https://core.ac.uk/download/217364561.pdf (accessed on 29 May 2025).

27. Mabbott, A. J. (2016). The overmatching of UK police body armor. https://core.ac.uk/download/74410011.pdf (accessed on 29 May 2025).

28. Matthay, E., Gobaud, A., Branas, C. C., Keyes, K. M., Roy, B., & Cerdá, M. (2025). Assessing links between alcohol exposure and firearm violence: A scoping review update. *Alcohol Research: Current Reviews, 45.* https://www.semanticscholar.org/paper/67e6809e71f6e31a37ef2d9e0ea27b6c5b43e1dc (accessed on 29 May 2025).

29. McMillan, J. A. (2020). *Epidemiology and Criminology: Managing Youth Firearm Homicide Violence in Urban Areas* (Doctoral dissertation). Walden University. https://scholarworks.waldenu.edu/dissertations/7941 (accessed on 29 May 2025).

30. McMillan, J. A. (2023). Epidemiology and criminology: Managing youth firearm homicide violence in urban areas. https://core.ac.uk/download/560926889.pdf (accessed on 29 May 2025).

31. Mishalov, V., Voroshilov, K., Petrochak, O., Khyzhniak, V., & Morgun, A. (2024). Cases of sexual violence in the temporarily occupied territories of the Kyiv region in 2022–Criminal consequences of Russian aggression. *Forensic-Medical Examination.* https://www.semanticscholar.org/paper/1eea02b27ffd9482a1682785cad303b4398e0c28 (accessed on 29 May 2025).

32. Mulani, K., Kadam, M., Patil, S., Gosavi, N., & Ghumatkar, S. (2024). Forensic firearm identification of an ingeniously modified air rifle-firearm. *The Egyptian Journal of Forensic Sciences and Applied Toxicology.* https://www.semanticscholar.org/paper/9169d8918a47a3ad4ec82f69b10985d67f68f403 (accessed on 29 May 2025).

33. Nyberger, K., Strömmer, L., Bennedich Kahn, L., & Wahlgren, C. (2024). Firearm mortality in Sweden 2012-2022: An analysis of injuries based on clinical data and autopsy findings. *British Journal of Surgery.* https://www.semanticscholar.org/paper/0fdd4da89e6b1bfb32bace99306e1eff6c2187a4 (accessed on 29 May 2025).

34. Office of Continuing Legal Education at the University of Kentucky College of Law. (2002). *Scientific, Technical, And Forensic Evidence.* https://core.ac.uk/download/232583377.pdf (accessed on 29 May 2025).

35. Piegari, G., D'Aquino, I., Salanti, G. V., Romano, V., Miletti, G., Sannino, E., Di Napoli, E., et al. (2024). Pathological changes and sodium rhodizonate test as tools for investigating gunshot wounds in veterinary forensic pathology. *Animals, 14.* https://www.semanticscholar.org/paper/a05fa616de967e655825d0e39ca88e2801e04f4b (accessed on 29 May 2025).

36. Rani, S., & Arun, M. (2023). Distant-range abdominal shotgun injury. *Medical Journal of Dr. D.Y. Patil Vidyapeeth, 16,* 102–104. https://www.semanticscholar.org/paper/63d46dd9f9e25980857c9ba4a8dff769e2373d72 (accessed on 29 May 2025).

37. Ricciardi, G., Licciardello, G., Cocimano, G., Mauro, L., Chisari, M. G., Sessa, F., Salerno, M., et al. (2024). Diagnostic challenges in uncommon firearm injury cases: A multidisciplinary approach. *Diagnostics, 15*(1), 31. https://doi.org/10.3390/diagnostics15010031.

38. Robinson, S. L., McCort, C. D., Smirniotis, C., Wintemute, G., & Laqueur, H. S. (2024). Purchaser, firearm, and retailer characteristics associated with crime gun recovery: A longitudinal

analysis of firearms sold in California from 1996 to 2021. *Injury Epidemiology, 11*. https://www.semanticscholar.org/paper/755b26a547c615c7fb422513abf23bff7c8c4912 (accessed on 29 May 2025).

39. Salottolo, K. M., Sliter, R. J., Marshall, G., Palacio Lascano, C., Quan, G., Hamilton, D., Madayag, R. M., et al. (2024). A join point analysis examining trends in firearm injuries at six US trauma centers from 2016 to 2022. *Injury Epidemiology, 11*. https://www.semanticscholar.org/paper/fb4df31be906afc9ad3a195394833510152b890f (accessed on 29 May 2025).

40. Savka, I., & Zmievska, Y. (2024). Forensic-medical analysis of gunshot injuries according to expert cases. *Forensic-Medical Examination*. https://www.semanticscholar.org/paper/974c4d868d2fc4b30aef3294bee45aa1224ee2c5 (accessed on 29 May 2025).

41. Shrestha, K., Shrestha, N., Yadav, S., & Yadav, D. (2024). Localization of a bullet in a firearm injury victim using X-ray imaging during autopsy: A case report. *JNMA: Journal of the Nepal Medical Association, 62*, 780–784. https://www.semanticscholar.org/paper/3c0d3ed00199b994f32720c14b3f676254b323f0 (accessed on 29 May 2025).

42. Singh, W. U., & Singh, K. P. (2023). The transformative role of artificial intelligence in forensic medicine and toxicology. *Journal of Medical Society, 37*, 101–102. https://doi.org/10.4103/jms.jms_54_24.

43. Stevenson, D. (2019). The urgent need for legal scholarship on firearm policy. https://core.ac.uk/download/328163401.pdf (accessed on 29 May 2025).

44. Taylor, M., Laber, T., Kish, P. E., Owens, G., & Osborne, N. K. P. (2016). The reliability of pattern classification in bloodstain pattern analysis, Part 1: Bloodstain patterns on rigid non-absorbent surfaces. *Journal of Forensic Sciences, 61*(3), 922–927. https://doi.org/10.1111/1556-4029.13091.

45. Teke, H., Imat, A., & Arslan, H. (2024). Evaluation of cases applying to forensic medicine polyclinic due to firearm injuries: Ordu example. *Novel Forensic Research*. https://www.semanticscholar.org/paper/a475b5639cb838296f104b19a0fcbd4127a251d5 (accessed on 29 May 2025).

46. Titus, S., Huo, L., Godwin, J., Shah, S., Cox, T. R., Ogola, G., & Ahmed, K. (2021). Primary care physician and resident perceptions of gun safety counseling. *Baylor University Medical Center Proceedings, 35*, 405–409. https://www.semanticscholar.org/paper/a63f2d110cd7be5bcd260ee8c45f63503da1cfa3 (accessed on 29 May 2025).

47. Wankhade, T., & Kumar, B. (2024). Misinterpretation of a gunshot injury by a non-forensic medicine expert: A case report of misguidance in a criminal investigation involving the unusual firearm injury 'Kronlein Shot'. *Cureus, 16*. https://www.semanticscholar.org/paper/b84cd92bcbe679b31b3d223d9f7dcccd8091af7a (accessed on 29 May 2025).

48. Waters, Y. (2017). The psychological impact of taser utilization in police officers [Doctoral dissertation, Walden University]. Walden Dissertations and Doctoral Studies. https://scholarworks.waldenu.edu/dissertations/3420 (accessed on 29 May 2025).

49. Weybright, E. H., Hall, A., Ellyson, A. M., Varrella, G., Kuklinski, M., Gause, E., & Schleimer, J. (2024). Strategies for recruiting adolescents in rural areas in firearm injury research. *Injury Prevention, 30*, 246–250. https://www.semanticscholar.org/paper/e02e4462abe47957bffae81d77e539b9c6e7a971 (accessed on 29 May 2025).

50. Yasheva, S. Y., Barachevskiy, Y., Baranov, A. V., Maslyakov, V. V., Mordovskiy, E., & Kuzin, S. G. (2024). Clinical assessment of injuries inflicted using firearms of limited destruction to residents of the Arctic Zone of the Arkhangelsk region, 2006–2022. *Disaster Medicine.* https://www.semanticscholar.org/paper/3e2a5d58e17a695ca4d4a8ad36723b6d2e573cf9 (accessed on 29 May 2025).

51. Zmiievska, Y., & Savka, I. (2024). Three-dimensional modeling of firearm injuries in forensic medicine. *Galician Medical Journal.* https://www.semanticscholar.org/paper/85a3b3dfdcccf491cce236a99559008ed00460e4 (accessed on 29 May 2025).

TRANSPORTATION INJURIES

10

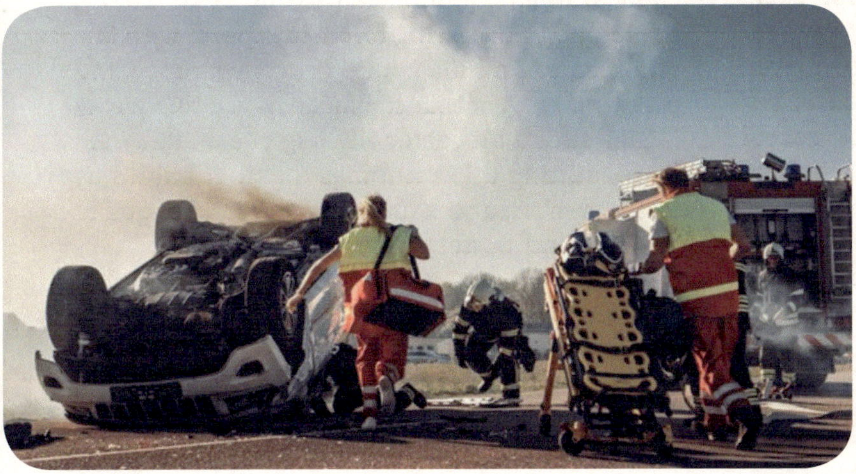

LEARNING OBJECTIVES

After studying this chapter, you will be able to:

1. Explain types of transportation injuries;
2. Understand forensic investigation techniques;
3. Know the legal implications of transportation injuries;
4. Learn prevention and safety measures.

Introduction

Forensic investigations often include transportation incidents which provide hints about how injuries happened and what they mean in court. Being able to recognize these injuries and their frequency can help forensic experts, mainly in homicide cases where car accident marks might turn out to be key evidence. One study, for example, looked back at defense injuries and uncovered some interesting details about the context and style of assaults; even the type of weapon used seemed to affect the wound patterns observed (Das et al., 2025). In another analysis, researchers dug into the demographics and circumstances of knee injuries in certain groups, revealing that these issues are largely linked to road traffic accidents (Matadi et al., 2025). All in all, carefully studying transportation injuries in a forensic way allows investigators to reconstruct crime scenes and also shows how to prevent these injuries from occurring.

Definition of Transportation Injuries

Investigating injuries caused by transportation accidents requires examining what kinds of harm can happen and how they occur. Mishaps with transportation can cause cuts, bruises, broken bones and wounds that break the skin and these can happen in both car crashes and when someone collides with an unmoving item. Many experts pay close attention to finding patterns in the injuries which can indicate the cause and sometimes the type of tool used. For example, when injuries bear unusual marks that one might see from a screwdriver, it stresses the need for a deep, detailed exam; such atypical wounds can sometimes reveal crucial clues about what went down at a crime scene (Albaladejo et al., 2024). In most cases, even catching the diagnostic signs of gunshot injuries – including those caused by ricochets – shows just how intertwined injury analysis and overall forensic investigations are when it comes to understanding the actions behind transportation-related harm (Figure 10.1).

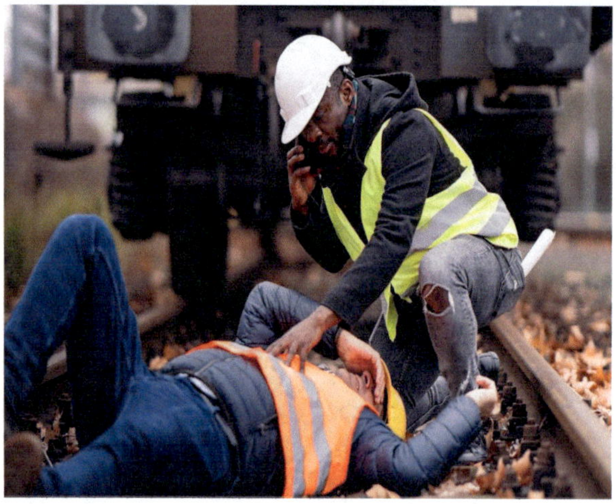

Figure 10.1. Transportation injuries.

Source: https://www.hlmlawfirm.com/wp-content/uploads/2023/04/Transportation-Accidents-Were-the-Leading-Causes-of-Worker-Deaths-in-2021.jpeg.

Importance of Forensics in Transportation Injuries

Because transportation accidents are not simple, it takes a careful forensic investigation to examine all the details. Forensics helps to find out the extent of injuries and what caused the accident to take place. Newer methods, like those used to figure out reserves for Reported But Not Settled (RBNS) claims, generally show that predictive models can tie damage severity right to financial impacts (Kwong et al., 2018). Sometimes, partnering forensic experts with law enforcement builds a kind of transparency and community trust that can make navigating tricky legal issues a bit easier (Kwong et al., 2018). All in all, putting these findings together allows us to learn more and usually results in changes to policies and better transportation rules.

Overview of Common Types of Transportation Injuries

There is a wide variety of accident types in transportation injuries which makes it difficult for forensic experts. Everyone sees car accidents and they can lead to anything from a small muscle injury to a serious head injury. Many pedestrians and cyclists also get into accidents and these often cause more serious harm to those who are less protected. Air and sea accidents can also happen and they are usually complicated by weather conditions and the confusion of many injured people. In most cases, figuring all this out isn't a neat process; forensic experts are busy sorting through the injuries, trying to pin down how each one happened, and lending a hand to law enforcement in getting to the bottom of transportation mishaps (Sust et al., 2021; Trisnadi et al., 2021).

Role of Forensic Science in Investigating Transportation Injuries

Forensic experts look into the details of injuries caused by transportation accidents which can be very unusual and messy. Experts do not use a simple checklist; they look over the victims and the scene of the accident and sometimes find details like the speed of the vehicle or where the impact occurred which usually help to solve the case. Take forensic dentistry, for example; it not only helps nail down a victim's identity but can also reveal trauma signs that tie back to incident-related injuries, showing off its many roles in investigations (Sanzyapova, 2025). New imaging techniques—like 3D Computed Tomography—step in as well, letting investigators measure skeletal remains with impressive precision, even helping with things like estimating sex and unraveling the dynamics of the injuries (Bhatti et al., 2025). All these points prove that mixing approaches from different areas is necessary for handling and solving cases after mass shootings. In most cases, these diverse approaches work hand in hand, painting a fuller picture from a jumble of clues, and sometimes even a small typo or pause in thought reminds us that uncovering the truth isn't always perfect (Figure 10.2).

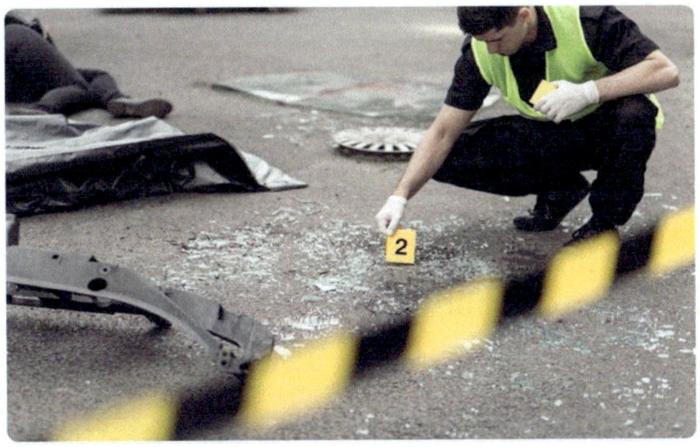

Figure 10.2. Role of forensic science in investigating transportation injuries.

Source: https://d1g9yur4m4naub.cloudfront.net/image-handler/picture/2021/11/shutterstock_301329224.jpg.

Historical Context of Transportation Injuries in Forensics

Transportation injuries have reshaped forensic work in unexpected ways. Cars were new on the roads and the increase in injuries made experts think of new ways to analyze traffic accidents which influenced later improvements. These days, new types of personal rides such as electric scooters and hoverboards, often make it difficult for forensic teams to see any clear patterns. In most cases, road mishaps have sadly become one of the top killers, especially among younger folks, which naturally ramps up the urgency to take a closer look (Kotsyubynska et al., 2023). And then there are drones—unmanned aerial vehicles—that add another twist to collision analysis, sparking a clear call for stricter safety checks and updated legal guidelines (Perz, 2024). Since transportation technology is always advancing, forensic practices must also keep changing to deal with new threats which is very important for public safety.

Significance of Understanding Transportation Injuries

Many transportation accidents are complicated which means investigators have to look deeper than just the surface. Rather than just listing causes, analyzing these incidents involves looking at many factors and every accident appears to have its own story to tell. People in forensics are debating whether new technology such as self-driving cars, could be linked to an increase in road-related deaths and injuries and these discussions usually highlight the need for further research. It's also interesting that these transportation injuries sometimes crop up alongside bigger issues like human trafficking, underlining that forensic science isn't just for solving crimes—it can also help nudge preventative measures along (Sust et al., 2021). Learning all about transportation accidents may help create policies that keep people safe and reduce the number of casualties. Revealing the different aspects of a case can help forensic experts do their job better, even though each new piece may not always be easy to predict.

10.1. Types of Transportation Injuries

Learning Outcome

1. Understand motor vehicle accidents;
2. Explain bicycle-related injuries;
3. Know pedestrian injuries;
4. Learn about aviation accidents;
5. Discuss maritime injuries;
6. Identify train-related injuries;
7. Describe off-road vehicle injuries;
8. Explain public transportation injuries;
9. Focus on recreational vehicle injuries.

Transportation problems are not always the same and can happen in many different ways. A variety of things such as the location of the incident, the type of ride and how passengers act, usually results in a messy situation. Car accidents are especially damaging because the impact and speed involved are very strong. Because of crowded urban streets, pedestrians and cyclists face a higher risk since the way vehicles interact with them may not always be safe. Usually, investigators have to do a lot of detailed work and also reach out to the community to prevent more cases. Generally speaking, studies Kwong et al. (2018); Postle et al. (2007) indicate that legal and social factors also have a say in road safety, and grasping all these different pieces can help improve public protection.

10.1.1. Motor Vehicle Accidents

There has been a rise in motor vehicle accidents and this worries people because it can affect public health, forensic work and legal responsibilities. Many times, these accidents are caused by a combination of driver errors, vehicle problems and unusual things in the environment, so we have to examine each one closely. Technology, too, is shaking things up; autonomous vehicles (AVs) are now in the picture, promising safer roads while throwing in fresh troubles about who's at fault when things go wrong. It is generally believed that AVs may help reduce road deaths, but ethical problems about fast decisions still arise. In many urban spots, the uptick in motorcycle use ties in with more fatal crashes, a reminder that transportation innovation and public safety are forever tangled in a delicate dance (Asekhame et al., 2013). At the end of the day, wrestling with these issues is key if we're going to cook up smarter, more effective ways to prevent accidents and pull apart their causes during investigations (Figure 10.3).

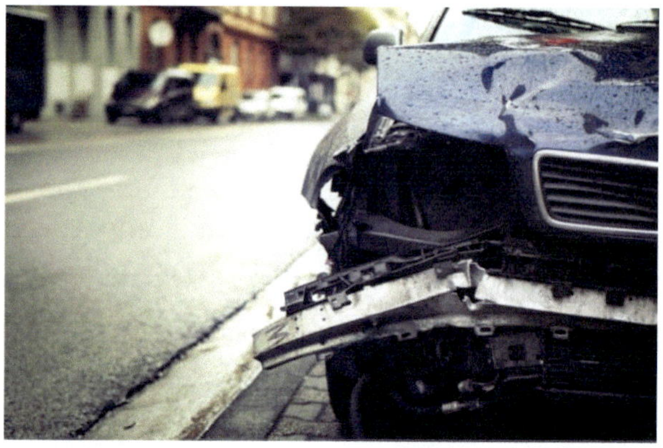

Figure 10.3. Motor vehicle accidents have been on the rise lately, and they stir up concerns that hit not just public health but also forensic investigations and legal responsibility.

Source: https://blog.ipleaders.in/wp-content/uploads/2020/12/Brainerd-Car-Accident-Lawyers.jpg.

10.1.2. Bicycle-related Injuries

Many cities encourage cycling as a clean alternative to driving, but a big increase in bike accidents makes people wonder if more should be done. A lot of the time, these accidents happen because the roads are not well-built and cyclists lack the simple safety equipment they require. It is common for research to show that making small changes to bike paths can reduce the number of accidents a lot, sometimes in unexpected ways. One idea, for instance, involves pairing electric bicycles with child seating options to boost both accessibility and safety, especially for families (Molero et al., 2021). Also, examining who is hurt can point out larger public health issues and suggest that specific solutions might help. Ultimately, when urban planners and policymakers put safety first—even if the changes seem small at first—the risks of cycling can drop, nudging us toward a transportation system that feels both healthier and more sustainable overall (Figure 10.4).

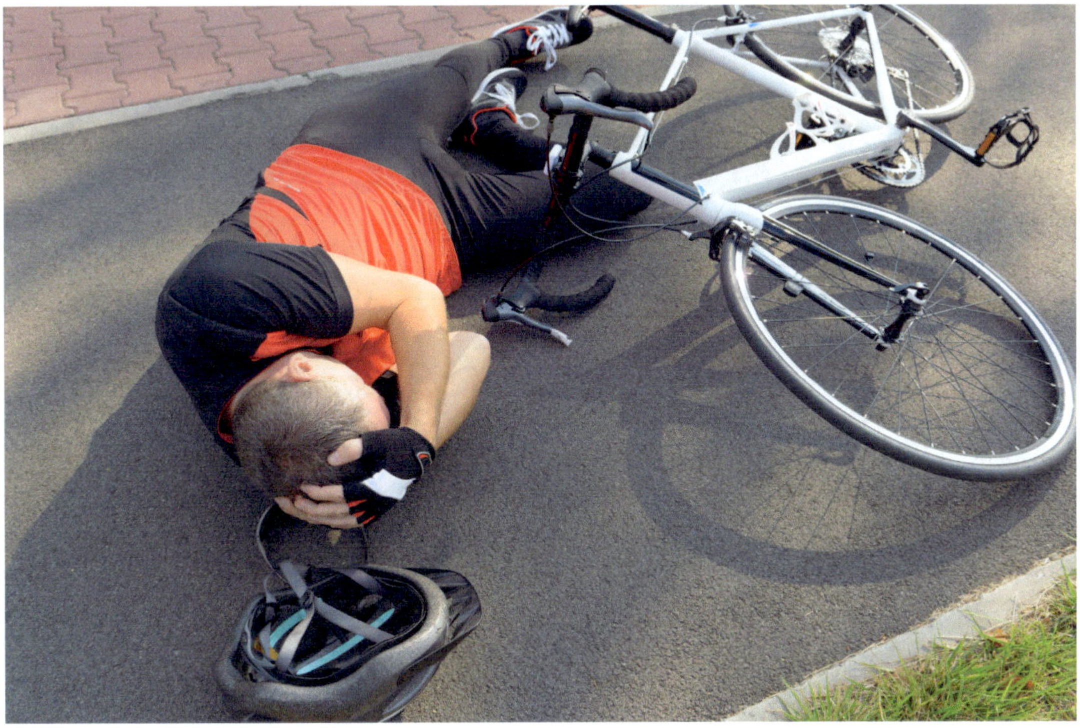

Figure 10.4. Bicycle-related injuries.

Source: https://www.visitcompletecare.com/attachment/shutterstock_328014935-1/.

10.1.3. Pedestrian Injuries

There has been a lot of attention on pedestrian injuries in cities lately because accidents appear to be increasing. Experts today must handle a range of difficulties; they must examine the damage and also work out what happened during each incident. Tools like the FORTIS forensic system come into their own here, helping score injuries more precisely while giving road transportation experts some much-needed support when plain words just don't cut it (Bobrov et al., 2017). Recently, studies have generally noted that the financial fallout from bodily injury claims leans heavily on how accurately disability severity is assessed, which can push claim costs up or down for insurers (Bobrov et al., 2017). In short, as forensic methods keep evolving, our grasp on pedestrian injuries gets a little firmer, nudging legal outcomes and overall road safety in a better direction (Figure 10.5).

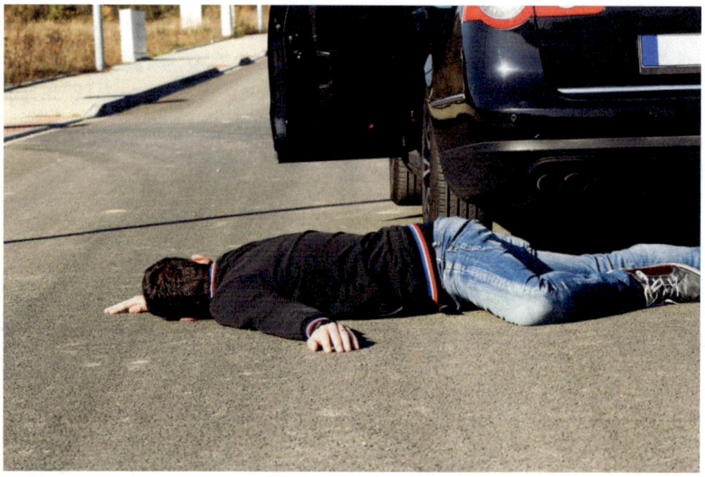

Figure 10.5. Pedestrian injuries.

Source: https://nicoletlaw.com/wp-content/uploads/2024/10/What-Are-Common-Pedestrian-Accident-Injuries.jpg.

10.1.4. Aviation Accidents

Investigations following aviation accidents usually find new information about errors by people and problems with equipment which usually result in improved safety. A good example is the Space Shuttle Columbia disaster which brought about changes in aeromedical practices after a thorough study of the human remains and the scene. As some reports mention, these probes look for more than the immediate reasons for an accident; they also identify any larger, concealed problems in the system.

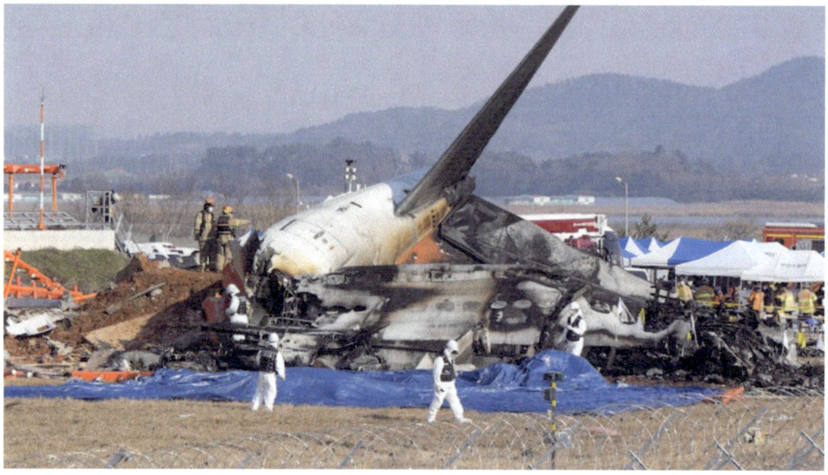

Figure 10.6. Aviation accidents.

Source: https://bsmedia.business-standard.com/_media/bs/img/article/2024-12/30/full/1735533540-9583.jpg?im=FeatureCrop,size=(826,465).

Thorough examinations of these accidents have pointed out that forensic science is crucial for understanding the details of crashes which has often led to new ideas about safety and ways to prevent further accidents. By piecing together evidence from various fields, forensic analyses—however unusual they might sometimes seem—play a big part in our ongoing push toward safer travel (Figure 10.6).

10.1.5. Maritime Injuries

Maritime jobs are not easy, as they bring many risks to workers and these risks are hard to identify and document when injuries happen. Accidents at sea are more likely because of the vessel's size, rough conditions and the mood on board and these factors can sometimes mix unexpectedly. There might be cases of slips, falls or accidents with heavy machinery and these often need thorough forensic examination for court cases and claims. The problem doesn't end with the damage; in a lot of cases, it leads to messy lawsuits about who should be held responsible. It's pretty important to wrap your head around how maritime disaster management works - several studies even compare how injury prevention and response differ internationally (Minguez, 2017). By folding in forensic science during investigations, experts can usually figure out what went wrong, which in turn helps update safety rules for maritime workers, filling a notable gap in current occupational safety research (Sust et al., 2021) (Figure 10.7).

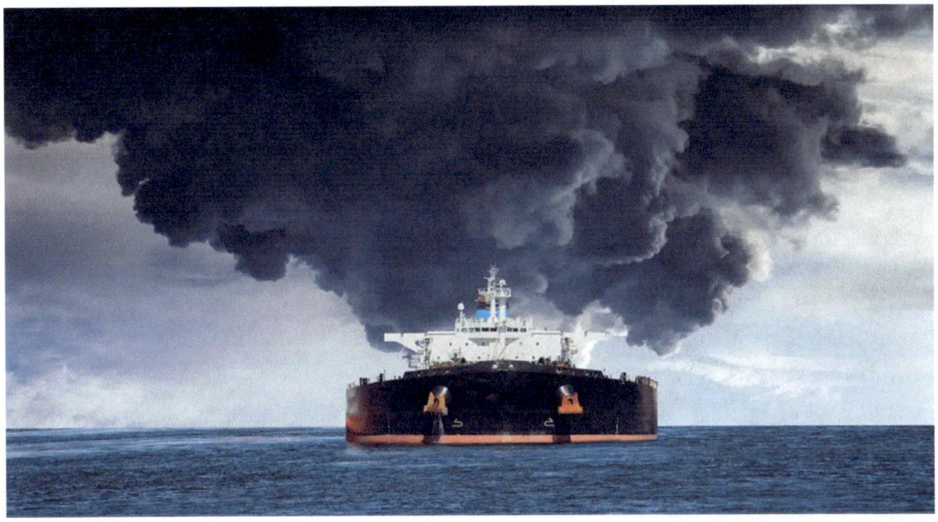

Figure 10.7. Maritime injuries.

Source: https://barrilleauxlaw.com/wp-content/uploads/2018/11/largeshipatseastockphoto.jpg.webp.

10.1.6. Train-related Injuries

Dealing with train accidents in forensics has always been tough, mainly because of the people who are usually involved. Most research indicates that around 1% of autopsied deaths in rail accidents are caused by trains which is often surprising. One study even found that most victims are men, with a noticeable peak among manual laborers in their 50s; both age and the type of work seem to add up to the overall risk (Kumar et al., 2017). Sometimes these unfortunate events happen in risky situations—like when someone is crossing the tracks or maybe even under the influence—hinting that behavior plays a key role, too (Kumar et al., 2017). Many of the injuries are deep cuts and scrapes, most often on the head and arms which shows how strong these accidents are. It is very important to understand these trends if we want to improve rail safety prevention.

10.1.7. Off-road Vehicle Injuries

When off-road vehicles have accidents, they draw attention which can lead to a closer look at transportation issues under forensic analysis. About 681 patients in New Brunswick were involved in incidents over eight years and most were men aged around 38 years. It seems that all-terrain vehicles were involved in many of the accidents and alcohol was a factor as well; 54.2% of those tested had been drinking. Many off-road accidents and sudden rollovers caused serious injuries, with a median severity score of 13 which usually means things could be very serious. This points to the pressing need for better preventative measures to keep public health and safety in check (Priest et al., 2025). In most cases, a layered strategy might work best to tackle these risks, and the off-road sector's decarbonization challenges, for instance, might offer a surprising model for other parts of transportation (Tripathi et al., 2025) (Figure 10.8).

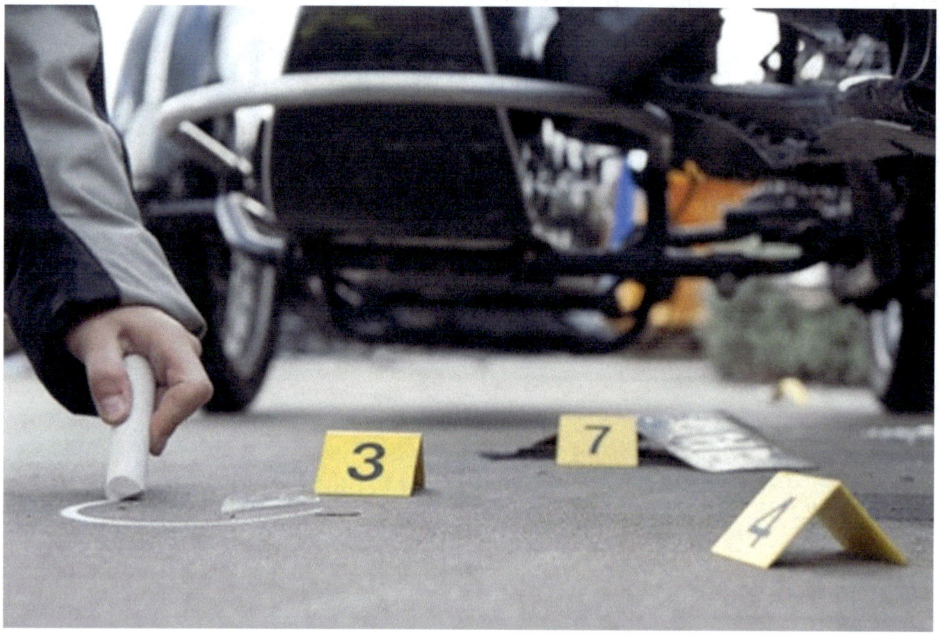

Figure 10.8. Off-road vehicle mishaps grab our attention, spotlighting issues in transportation that sometimes get examined under a forensic lens.

Source: https://clue4evidence.com/wp-content/uploads/2024/05/service-15-1.jpg.

10.1.8. Public Transportation Injuries

More people are using public transport as cities grow which makes injuries from these systems a major concern. Sometimes, injuries happen by accident, like a vehicle accident, a fall or even from being in a crowded place and these can be difficult for the first responders too. Investigators also play a key role, trying to uncover the reason for the accident and who was involved which can lead to safety improvements in the future. Advances in self-driving technology which are often praised for making roads safer, also have their own set of problems that should be examined. These innovations, researchers say, could help reduce traffic-related deaths, however, they also introduce new challenges to maintain secure operations. Understanding how folks view and interact with transportation systems is another piece of the puzzle, one that can guide designs to make user safety a top priority (Sust et al., 2021).

10.1.9. Recreational Vehicle Injuries

There has been a rise in RVs on the roads these days and this seems to be related to a rise in accidents and injuries, so accident investigators are now paying closer attention. Because of their size and the way they drive, these big vehicles are not like most cars. Their tall design means that when they take a sharp turn or make a sudden move, rollovers become a real possibility (Warnica et al., 2015). Driving an RV is not as easy as it might seem and often, how they work can cause drivers to make errors that cause problems later. Some research has shown that knowing how these vehicles react—especially in high-energy accidents like cycling accidents—is very important. If these risks aren't looked into and fixed, it could mean worse injuries not only for the people inside RVs but for everyone sharing the road (Otieno et al., 2015). More people knowing about these risks and better rules could help reduce these dangers.

Test Your Knowledge

1. What kind of injury is usually seen in a pedestrian who is dragged by a vehicle?
2. What are primary impact injuries, and give one example.
3. Define secondary impact injury in a road traffic accident.

10.2. Forensic Investigation Techniques in Transportation Injuries

Learning Outcome

1. Understand scene analysis and documentation;
2. Perform collection of physical evidence;
3. Discuss the use of accident reconstruction;
4. Explain the role of forensic pathology;
5. Focus on toxicology in transportation injuries;
6. Learn digital forensics in vehicle accidents;
7. Witness interviews and statements;
8. Know the use of surveillance footage;
9. Explain collaboration with law enforcement.

Investigators need to handle transportation injuries carefully, using evidence to determine the cause of the incident. Experts do not rely on a set checklist; they use both accident reconstruction and digital forensics to find out the speed of the vehicle and the angle at impact. With these methods, the complicated events become clearer and, usually, point to who is responsible. All kinds of testimonies, police reports and other similar sources are combined to give a clearer picture, though it may seem a bit out of order. Previous studies Kwong et al. (2018); Postle et al. (2007), which generally point out the value of sticking to a careful process, remind us that following set forensic procedures is key. In short, following standard forensic methods helps verify facts, increases legal responsibility and boosts the public's trust in justice.

10.2.1. Scene Analysis and Documentation

Transportation injury scenes need to be documented carefully, since it is not a simple process. Frequently, using traditional methods for data collection, forensic experts may end up with differences that cause them to make wrong conclusions. 3D scanning and photogrammetry are now available and they are making accident scene reconstruction more accurate. This way of looking at data increases trust in it and reveals all the possible reasons behind the accident. Forensic analysts can now create detailed images of events which are much better than police sketches and reports and help with the investigation. In general, as research is moving ahead, it seems sensible to consider integrative fixes—say, a centralized database for traffic accidents—to dig deeper into what causes these tragic events (Kamnik et al., 2022; Postle et al., 2007) (Figure 10.9).

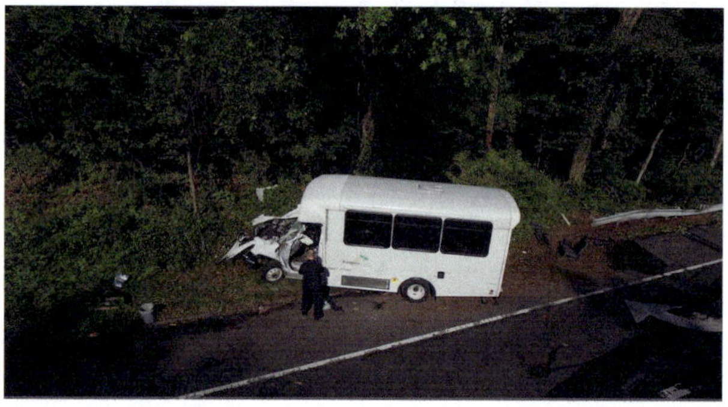

Figure 10.9. Documenting transportation injury scenes calls for a keen grasp of exact methods—it's not as cut and dry as one might think.

Source: https://images.ctfassets.net/go54bjdzbrgi/4ECJyFHfNuCqQo8Akg2AI4/644cecbcefc374bbdc19f3df3f4bb838/forensics-law-enforcement-accident-scene-reconstruction-pix4d-pix4dmapper-profile-2.jpg?w=1200&fm=jpg&q=80.

10.2.2. Collection of Physical Evidence

Collecting physical evidence is key in transportation injury cases. A flexible way to record evidence helps the investigation be trusted and the findings be accepted by the court. New systems, including mobile forensic documentation, make it easier to store evidence in a uniform way which improves analysis. In most cases, the literature points out a lack of detailed discussion on applying forensic science in diverse settings, suggesting more research is needed on merging fresh recording methods (Baggili et al., 2006). Further, looking at the bigger picture can reveal hidden trends that enrich both our methods and the field as a whole (Sust et al., 2021).

10.2.3. Use of Accident Reconstruction

It's important to look into transportation injuries more than just figuring out the cause, since we want to prevent them from happening again. At this point, accident reconstruction begins; experts use different modern techniques to assemble the details of the crash to learn what caused it. Sometimes, this is more about finding those little problems that you wouldn't notice right away such as shaky roads or odd things about the car. Techniques such as 3D scanning and photogrammetry sometimes patch up the gaps left by older, traditional ways of gathering data, giving a clearer, if not always perfect, picture of the accident scene (Kamnik et al., 2022). Since road mishaps tend to hit our most vulnerable folks—think pedestrians—harder than others, a thorough forensic check becomes even more essential in reducing fatalities and fine-tuning safety measures (Nogayeva et al., 2020). To summarize, when you bring these careful investigations together, there's a strong potential for boosting traffic safety and cutting down on injuries (Figure 10.10).

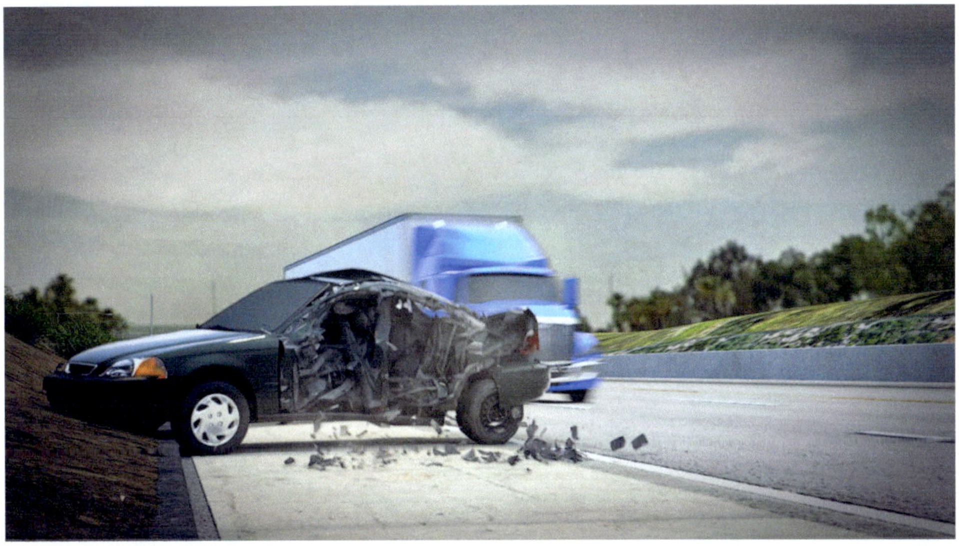

Figure 10.10. Accident reconstruction jumps in here; experts use all sorts of modern methods to piece together crash events so that they can sort out the story behind a collision.

Source: https://courtroomanimation.com/wp-content/uploads/2023/01/image1-1-1024x575.jpg.

10.2.4. Role of Forensic Pathology

Transport injuries are not simple; they often need a detailed investigation by forensic pathology which studies how the injuries occurred. Rather than using a simple checklist, this area looks at how injuries happen and puts together the events of accidents which can bring up surprising clues. Take, for example, findings that suggest vehicles like three-wheelers usually lead to injuries focused on the head and spine (Colombage et al., 2018). And then there's the case of bruising on livestock during transport—this subtle sign of stress before any clear harm shows just how far-reaching these analyses can be (Gallo et al., 2009). In most cases, forensic pathology supports police investigations and helps create safer measures, especially for understanding transportation accidents.

10.2.5. Toxicology in Transportation Injuries

Many clues can be found in toxicology after a road accident. Many times, tests pick up drugs in a person's system, whether they are illegal or prescribed and these drugs can affect the person's response during an accident. At times, things that reduce mental focus or control of the body make drivers take risks which can increase the likelihood of an accident. Alcohol often makes it hard to think clearly and move properly which is hard to overlook. Research generally shows that quite a few victims had signs of substance use, hinting that checking for these chemicals should be a regular part of accident investigations (Talpur et al., 2021). Looking at these substance traces can also help shape public health efforts and education programs aimed at reducing such preventable disasters (Chaudhari et al., 2016) (Figure 10.11).

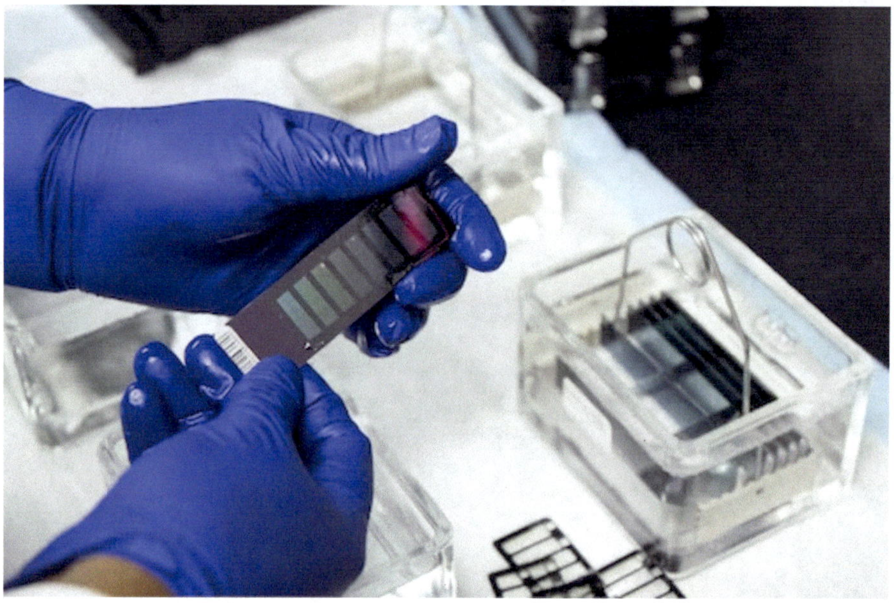

Figure 10.11. Road accidents hide some real clues when you look into toxicology.

Source: https://www.all-about-forensic-science.com/images/the-role-of-forensic-evidence-in-car-accident-investigations.png.

10.2.6. Digital Forensics in Vehicle Accidents

Advanced technology in modern cars is changing the way legal issues related to accidents are handled; evidence collection and analysis are now much different. Vehicles now collect a lot of information which can act like a third witness in legal cases when people's memories are unreliable. This all comes from the smart systems built right into today's vehicles that pick up key details in the crucial moments before a crash, making it tougher for drivers to simply argue their side without that hard data (Postle et al., 2010). Self-driving cars which are appearing on roads more and more, cause even more controversy since they promise to be safer but also introduce new issues about who is responsible in accidents, leading to further research on their connection to traffic deaths. All in all, digital forensics is good at assembling accident evidence, yet it raises many questions about who should get access to and control over the data collected from cars.

10.2.7. Witness Interviews and Statements

Talking to people who witnessed the accident is very important in transportation injury cases. Eyewitness statements about what a vehicle did or how a driver acted can sometimes change the whole understanding of what happened. Stories that are detailed, even with a few mistakes, often match the physical evidence and often make the case stronger. In most instances, when first responders quickly chat with witnesses, it often seems to line up with better legal outcomes; the Alaska State Troopers observed this trend in several incidents, including transportation citations (Postle et al., 2007, 2010). To summarize, mixing in these firsthand recollections isn't just key for resolving legal matters, it also deepens our grasp of how injuries actually occur in real life (Figure 10.12).

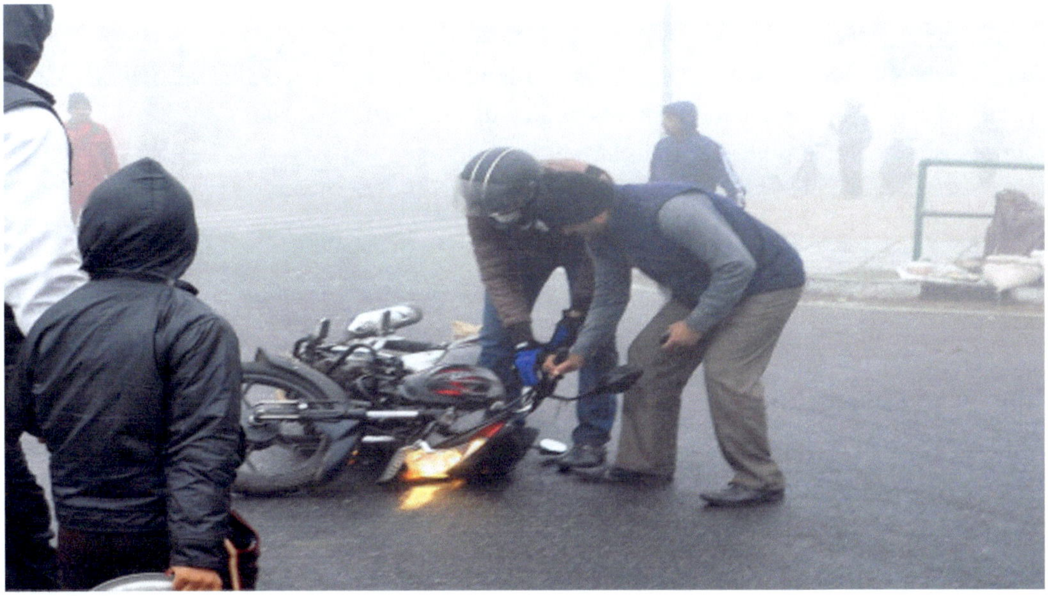

Figure 10.12. Transportation injury cases rely a lot on talking to people who saw what happened.

Source: https://static.toiimg.com/thumb/msid-67391640,width-1280,height-720,resizemode-4/67391640.jpg.

10.2.8. Use of Surveillance Footage

Advanced technology is now playing a big role in how forensic investigations deal with injuries related to transport. The footage from cameras every day is not just background noise, but it gives important details about incidents and helps explain what took place. Investigators can, through video analysis, usually figure out the sequence of events that caused the accident and discover hidden factors. Interestingly, this way of working echoes a change that began in the mid-20th century; back then, transport mishaps began to be seen as subjects for scientific study, which in turn spurred the creation of more precise forensic tools designed to uncover the full context of these events (Siegel et al., 2006). Using surveillance video has helped solve crimes and civil disputes, as seen in the case of Kathy Mabr and has often brought new understanding about the events.

10.2.9. Collaboration with Law Enforcement

Police collaboration is very important when investigating transportation injuries. Many times, forensic experts and law enforcement find that working together leads to new discoveries and reveals hidden details about each injury. The police use what they have learned and share to collect evidence at accident scenes that will stand up in court. At times, when several fields team up, they can come up with new ways to prevent road risks based on data. It is often clear that transportation injuries are linked to bigger health issues which is why safety laws should be included in the approach. To summarize, this kind of teamwork not only smooths out investigations but also builds community awareness and nudges people toward safer roads (Morrison et al., 2004.

Test Your Knowledge

1. What is the purpose of studying injury patterns in investigating traffic accidents?
2. Define trace evidence in the context of transportation injuries.

10.3. Legal Implications of Transportation Injuries

Learning Outcome

1. Explain liability in transportation accidents;
2. Understand the role of forensic evidence in court;
3. Know insurance claims and transportation injuries;
4. Identify criminal charges related to transportation injuries;
5. Learn civil lawsuits and compensation;
6. Look at how transportation laws influence the field of forensics;
7. Describe ethical considerations in forensic investigations;
8. Learn case studies of notable transportation injury cases;
9. Discuss future legal trends in transportation injuries.

Transportation injuries often get mixed up with legal matters because of liability, insurance and many regulations. It is not easy to find out what went wrong in accidents, especially with self-driving cars now available. Most of the time, these systems might save lives on the road, but they raise new questions about who is responsible when problems happen. Even though investigating can feel like putting together a puzzle, forensic evidence is still very important in finding out the truth. Take veterinary forensics, for instance; this emerging area doesn't just stick to human injuries but also dives into cases with animals, which can further complicate the debate over liability and shake up courtroom outcomes (Viciano et al., 2022). In short, dealing with transportation injuries in the law involves exploring new technologies and how forensic science keeps changing.

10.3.1. Liability in Transportation Accidents

Responsibility for accidents in transportation is not as clear now because of new technology and the rise of AVs. Even though new systems are designed to enhance road safety and efficiency, they have caused many people to wonder who should take responsibility when something goes wrong. Usually, drivers were responsible for anything that went wrong, but with AVs, some of the blame can now be given to manufacturers and software developers. Research usually finds that although AV tech may decrease the number of crashes, it also introduces new risks and ethical problems that we haven't faced before. Moreover, the fast-paced development of AI in unmanned vehicles forces us to take another look at our liability laws, making sure they fit today's complex transport scenes (Chen et al., 2025). In short, our legal framework has got to evolve alongside these technological shifts if we're going to keep public safety in check (Figure 10.13).

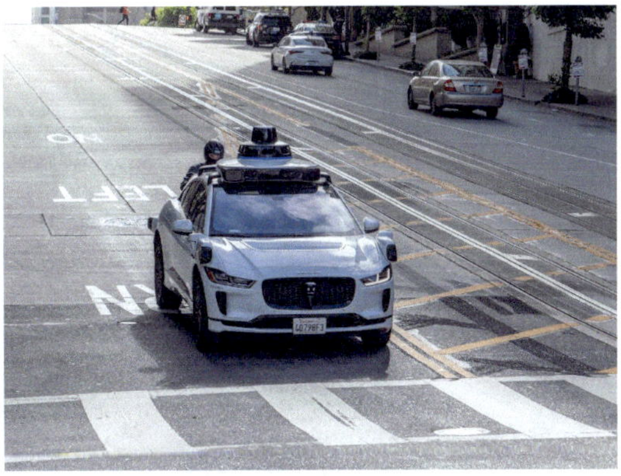

Figure 10.13. Liability in transportation mishaps isn't as straightforward these days—tech is advancing and autonomous vehicles (AVs) are starting to change the game.

Source: https://t4america.org/wp-content/uploads/2023/08/Waymo-AV-San-Francisco.jpeg.

10.3.2. Role of Forensic Evidence in Court

The presence of forensic evidence in court can make a big difference and affect how the case is decided. For cases involving transportation injuries, this evidence supports the person's claims and also helps show the whole picture of what happened. You may find that experts carefully examine all the information which highlights how hard it is to find the "forensic truth" in legal terms. Forensic evidence and strict legal rules sometimes clash and how things are presented in court can make or break a case. When you take a closer look at how every case seems to carry its own set of complications—and consider the sheer effort decision-makers put in—it becomes clear that forensic evidence acts as a tool for clarity while also having the potential to stir up controversy (Klinkner et al., 2008).

10.3.3. Insurance Claims and Transportation Injuries

These injuries often mean you have to deal with insurance companies as well as the physical effects. If an accident happens, you immediately find yourself dealing with many documents and have to carefully examine the situation; sometimes, forensic experts are called in to help determine who is responsible and how much was damaged. Most of the time, insurers use forensic evidence to decide if a claim is real and to decide on a fair compensation. Because accidents can involve drivers, pedestrians and occasionally other people, it becomes very difficult to identify who is at fault. Sometimes, claims become very tense, especially if the injuries are severe and the medical records are checked again for accuracy. Every so often, agencies such as the Arizona Department of Public Safety help by gathering information, even if it is not perfect, to support fair dispute settlement. To summarize, the way these claims are managed can have a huge impact on someone's recovery journey, generally speaking (Figure 10.14).

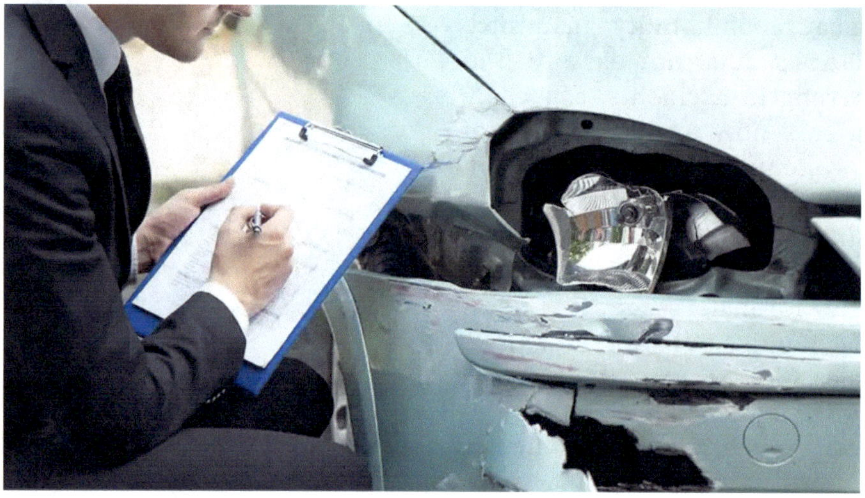

Figure 10.14. Insurance claims and transportation injuries.

Source: https://www.reliancegeneral.co.in/siteassets/rgiclassets/images/blogs-images/the-role-of-car-insurance-in-road-accidents2.webp.

10.3.4. Criminal Charges Related to Transportation Injuries

Mistakes in transportation and associated legal problems can turn lives upside down for those involved in the accident and for those who are later charged. Road accidents can cause charges such as reckless driving, DUI or, in the saddest cases, manslaughter. You could see that gathering evidence such as examining skid marks or damage to the vehicles, is often the main factor in figuring out who is responsible. Lately, tech shifts (especially those tied to smart cities) have nudged accountability and proof gathering into new territory. In many cases, digital evidence from modern information and communications tech can open up investigative pathways that were simply out of reach before (Losavio et al., 2018). To summarize, a mixed, cross-disciplinary approach is generally key for legal experts trying to untangle the multifaceted issues of transportation offenses and modern evidentiary standards (Puerto et al., 2021).

10.3.5. Civil Lawsuits and Compensation

Transportation injury cases in civil law are not only about paying expenses; they also help encourage others to be more careful. People going to court are not only seeking compensation for their expenses and lost earnings – they are also pointing out the systemic factors that might have caused the accident.

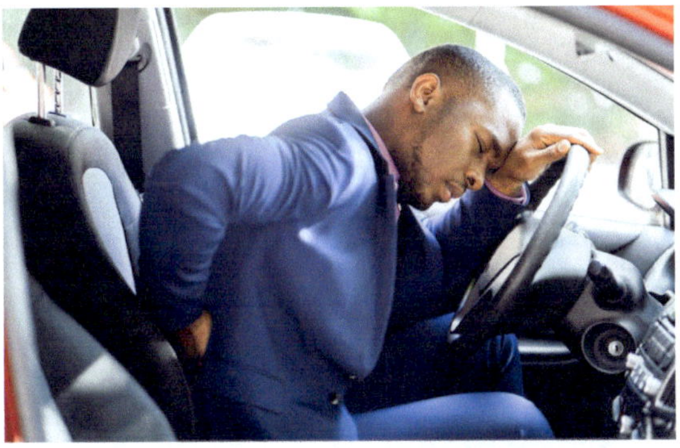

Figure 10.15. Civil lawsuits tied to transportation injuries aren't just about covering bills; they've become a way to nudge everyone toward better accountability and safer practices.

Source: https://www.sgplaw.com/wp-content/uploads/2024/08/shutterstock_1831302199.jpg.

In many cases, the investigation looks into the actions of several players such as manufacturers and transit companies and encourages them to follow safety rules and act more ethically. In many instances, the rulings can even ripple out to shape future regulations; we're noticing this trend now in fast-changing fields such as AI, where questions of liability are evolving rapidly (Nersessian et al., 2021). To summarize, civil lawsuits tend to spark reform, opening up new routes for improvements that ultimately boost public safety and welfare (Luo et al., 2023) (Figure 10.15).

10.3.6. Impact of Transportation Laws on Forensics

How transportation rules are followed and what forensic work shows often affects outcomes in road injury cases. Laws are always being updated and this tends to push forensic experts to use different methods for collecting and examining evidence. Because of vehicle safety guidelines, accident reporting rules and who is blamed for accidents, forensic evidence is often used in legal cases. Having a standard approach for dealing with accident scenes can make the evidence appear stronger. There is not yet much research on the specific role of forensic science in transportation laws, especially as new problems like human trafficking and crime prevention appear. Addressing these research gaps might open the door to new techniques that more closely tie forensic practices with legal proceedings (Jude et al., 2015; Sust et al., 2021).

10.3.7. Ethical Considerations in Forensic Investigations

Ethical problems can make investigations into transportation-related forensic cases very messy. The first thing is to respect those who have passed away; this means finding a balance between cultural habits and religious customs and helping victims and their families. It's not always a neat process, either, because ensuring fair identification means giving even unidentified individuals equal care—a must, especially in spots where resources are scarce and unidentified remains appear more often (Reid et al., 2025). At the same time, using advanced tools such as DNA analysis leads to new worries about privacy and consent which are not always easy to define. In most cases, as forensic methods keep shifting, sticking to strict oversight and being open about how data is handled becomes important—this helps ward off misuse, builds public trust, and keeps ethical standards solid in our criminal justice system (Smith et al., 2024).

10.3.8. Case Studies of Notable Transportation Injury Cases

Transportation injury cases reveal many things about the underlying social and economic factors. A closer look at the numbers reveals that most drowning deaths—particularly in low- and middle-income places—often tie back to things like living too near water or cramped living conditions; oddly enough, these factors sometimes pop up in urban transit situations too (Cenderadewi et al., 2020). In most cases, the uptick in deadly injuries in the United States, which seems to track the opioid crisis's rise, highlights how unpredictable transportation safety can be when it mingles with broader public health challenges (Lundstrom et al., 2023). Looking at these cases, it is obvious that dealing with transportation injuries means using both safety measures and approaches to improve socio-economics to fully understand them.

10.3.9. Future Legal Trends in Transportation Injuries

With new technologies, laws must also evolve and this is especially necessary when road accidents become more complicated.

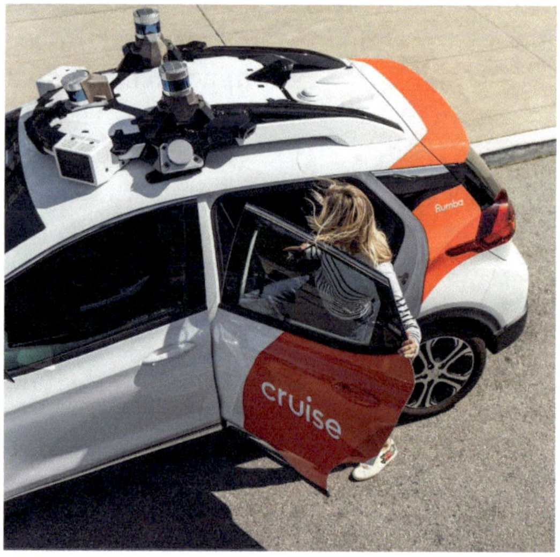

Figure 10.16. Autonomous Vehicles (AVs) seem to promise safer rides and fewer tragic outcomes, yet they also kick off a whole host of debates about who's on the hook when something goes wrong.

Source: https://www.freep.com/gcdn/authoring/authoring-images/2024/08/22/PDTF/74909680007-ridehail-rider-entry.png?width=1733&height=1156&fit=crop&format=pjpg&auto=webp.

Although AVs are expected to make rides safer and reduce accidents, they also start a lot of discussions about who is responsible if something bad happens. Most research shows that these vehicles may lower the number of accidents, but they raise new problems about safety checks and the ethics involved in making quick decisions during emergencies. Forensic science is now being used to analyze transportation accidents and also to consider the effects these accidents have on society and the economy. There's still a notable gap in figuring out how these investigative methods might speed up legal processes and ease the fallout from road injuries (Sust et al., 2021). To summarize, as tech shifts and laws wobble a bit, preparing for these new legal twists is, in most cases, the key to protecting the public interest (Figure 10.16).

Test Your Knowledge

1. What is the legal significance of determining the role of the victim (driver, passenger, or pedestrian) in transportation injuries?
2. What information from forensics is used to determine if an RTA was caused by an accident, suicide or homicide?

10.4. Prevention and Safety Measures

Learning Outcome

1. Understand the importance of safety regulations;
2. Describe how education helps prevent injuries from transportation;
3. Know technological advancements in vehicle safety;
4. Focus on community initiatives for safer transportation;
5. Identify government policies on transportation safety;
6. Know the impact of public awareness campaigns;
7. Discuss the role of engineering in accident prevention;
8. Evaluate current safety measures;
9. Explain future directions for transportation safety.

Reviewing how people are hurt in transportation quickly shows that more prevention and clearer safety steps are required. Studies generally show that injuries to the head and face – a problem you often see in sports like mixed martial arts – hint at larger issues with everyday safety standards, including those in transportation (Parekh et al., 2025). The rise in such accidents often points out that current protections are not enough and that more education about risk management is needed. Look at how voluntary safety systems evolved; they originally started with household appliances, showing that when consumer awareness is boosted and safety tests are carried out, things tend to get safer – and it seems similar ideas might work well for transport contexts (Parry, 2025). By enforcing strict safety measures and regular monitoring, the number of injuries during travel can be reduced which is good for people on the move. In short, using education, technology and strong regulations together is necessary to secure public health.

10.4.1. Importance of Safety Regulations

Technology for transportation is moving fast and safety rules are much more important than we often realize. Such rules ensure safety and also gently encourage new ideas, for example, self-driving cars becoming more common. Most studies indicate that although autonomous tech reduces the risk of traffic accidents, it creates new safety and security issues. In some places, like Benin City where commercial motorcycle rides have been banned, these measures can shape behavior and even shift crime trends, further muddling the whole scene around transport injuries (Asekhame et al., 2013). Ultimately, strict safety standards help lower risks and boost public trust in new transport tech; this, in most cases, is absolutely key when it comes to dealing with injuries and fatalities, which forensic experts closely watch (Figure 10.17).

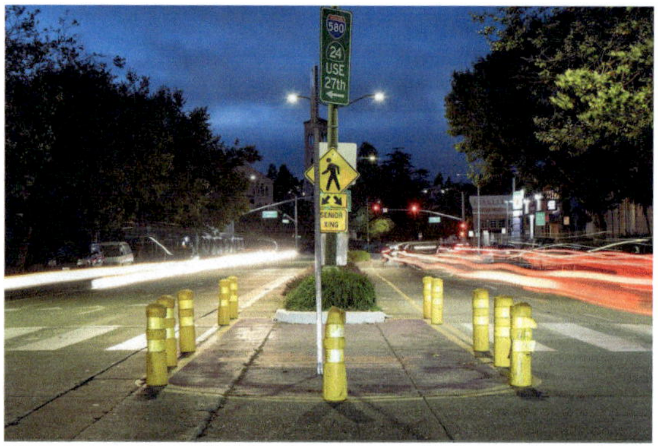

Figure 10.17. Transportation technology is sprinting ahead, and safety rules mean a lot more than we sometimes give them credit for.

Source: https://oaklandside.org/wp-content/uploads/2022/07/large-27th-Street-Resign-5.jpg.

10.4.2. Role of Education in Preventing Transportation Injuries

Lately, there are more transportation injuries, so new ways to teach safety are needed. Instead of using a rigid lesson plan, switching between lessons on safe driving, caring for pedestrians and the dangers of substance misuse can lower the number of road accidents. In many cases, community projects that team up with local law enforcement—engaging people directly and talking frankly about potential dangers—end up making roads safer (Kwong et al., 2018). Also, adding drug-free lessons into school curriculums serves as an important step in preventing impaired driving, linking substance prevention directly with traffic safety (Zimbardi et al., 2005). When people are taught to be aware and responsible, education encourages society to pay more attention to safety which over time leads to fewer transportation injuries. All in all, combining these educational techniques is a major way to improve public health in transportation.

10.4.3. Technological Advancements in Vehicle Safety

Vehicle safety has taken a wild turn recently, thanks to tech leaps like self-driving cars and smart computer systems (AI). Some people say that traffic is moving more smoothly and accidents could decrease a lot now. Most studies reveal that a lot of what enables self-driving cars is advanced AI handling issues such as accidents and jams in innovative ways. Yet, introducing these new vehicles isn't a walk in the park; there's a whole host of fresh challenges, especially when it comes to letting machines make split-second decisions that could affect lives (Chen et al., 2025). As the systems get more complicated and a bit disorganized, it's obvious that we must study them more carefully and make tougher rules to manage all the risks. To summarize, pushing for safer roads isn't just about rolling out the latest gadgets; it's also about navigating the tangled web of ethical and regulatory issues that naturally come along for the ride (Figure 10.18).

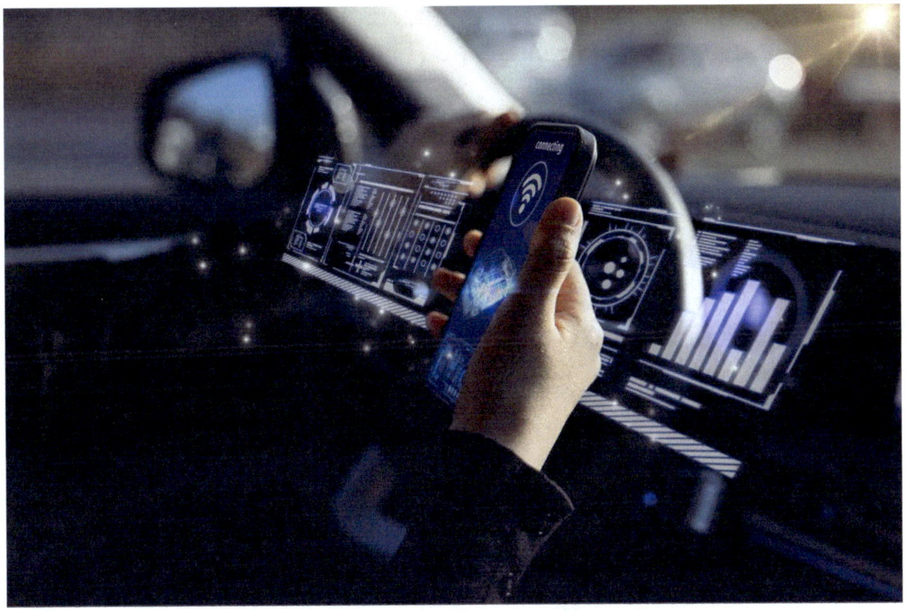

Figure 10.18. Vehicle safety has taken a wild turn recently, thanks to tech leaps like self-driving cars and smart computer systems (AI).

Source: https://etimg.etb2bimg.com/photo/119115133.cms.

10.4.4. Community Initiatives for Safer Transportation

Road injuries need people to take action in ways they may not have thought of before. A few people make programs to educate drivers on safe habits and remind everyone that pedestrians have rights which appears to help communities come together without much planning. They not only encourage people to be accountable—they also help citizens suggest ways to improve the safety of streets. At times, town officials and nonprofit groups team up to make quick improvements such as putting up better signs or making crosswalks stand out more. In many cases, such mix-and-match strategies have led to noticeable drops in both injuries and deaths, kind of proving that when people come together, the small steps add up (even if they sometimes feel a bit rough around the edges). The steady success of these projects shows that collective action, however imperfect, helps build a safer environment for every road user (Missouri University of Science and Technology. INSPIRE - University Transportation Center, 2020; Tennessee, 2014).

10.4.5. Government Policies on Transportation Safety

Both new technologies and new rules can sometimes combine to create both problems and opportunities in transportation safety. AVs have just appeared, leading the government to make changes so people stay safe and new ideas are encouraged. It is thought by some researchers that these cars can make roads safer and cut down on accidents by reducing traffic jams and mistakes from drivers. Still, the benefits are possible only if strong regulations handle both the standard and ethical/technical concerns related to AVs. Usually, for guidelines to work, lawmakers, manufacturers and the public need to talk and cooperate to encourage safety tech and reduce risks. It is also possible to notice similar ideas in safety plans from different places such as the Iowa Department of Public Safety's plan for improving transportation safety. To summarize, smart government action remains a key ingredient in crafting a safer transport landscape (Figure 10.19).

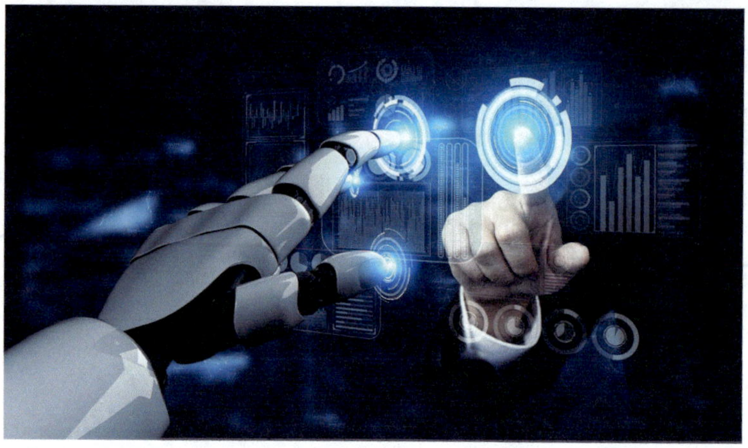

Figure 10.19. Emerging technologies and shifting rules often mix together in ways that spark both challenges and unexpected chances in the world of transportation safety.

Source: https://indian-retailer.s3.ap-south-1.amazonaws.com/s3fs-public/2022-04/future-artificial-intelligence-robot-cyborg.jpg.

10.4.6. Impact of Public Awareness Campaigns

Telling the public about road safety is important for making our communities safer and reducing injuries. They start by warning against things like texting while driving, drinking alcohol and not wearing a seatbelt which encourages people to reconsider their actions on the road. By mixing facts with real examples such efforts aim to create a bond that inspires people to reflect on their travel habits and the outcomes of not being careful. Sometimes, offering simple tips to stay safe in public places helps attract the interest of people and leaders in the community, who want to make their neighborhoods safer. Generally speaking, when informed citizens meet proactive engagement, they end up making a real difference in addressing transportation mishaps in forensics (St. Cloud State University, 2008; Vasileios et al., 2021).

10.4.7. Role of Engineering in Accident Prevention

New tech is often used in road safety, often by combining engineering and advanced technology. Instead of strictly copying a plan, people have realized that modifying how we build things can help lower accident rates. Smart AI routines power autonomous vehicles which make traffic flow better and decrease the chances of human mistakes causing crashes. Research usually finds that when drivers adjust their actions and respond better to road changes, these cars can greatly reduce traffic-related deaths. Still, it's worth noting that rolling out such systems sometimes stumbles into new security issues that demand careful attention to keep everything safe (Asekhame et al., 2013). Also, engineers are involved in giving their opinions on policies, ensuring both safety and the speed of progress in technology are considered. In general, using both advanced technology and traditional engineering plays a big role in preventing accidents on our roads.

10.4.8. Evaluation of Current Safety Measures

Transportation safety is changing in new ways now. A mix of new technology and hands-on methods is becoming more popular than a strict plan. Take game-like training, for example—it's not your old routine; people actually seem to remember about 82% of what they learn this way compared to older methods (Jin et al., 2020). Another example is autonomous vehicles which could make traffic less congested and reduce human error, but they introduce new security problems that we haven't solved yet. In short, as we look back at today's safety, it is obvious that we should focus on new car designs as well as improved ways to teach users how to use them safely.

10.4.9. Future Directions for Transportation Safety

Things are moving fast in transportation and safety is now involved in many issues and exciting possibilities. Autonomous vehicles are introduced here—they could lead to less traffic accidents and more efficient traffic. According to recent studies, these vehicles use many AI advances to reduce accidents for drivers and ease the pressure on the environment. At the same time, this technology can bring about ethical and security issues that have to be carefully reviewed and planned out. On top of that, the growing use of augmented reality in our travel systems adds another twist; sometimes it becomes tricky for investigators to tell the real deal from digital enhancements which might, well, jeopardize forensic work (Antony et al., 2018). Essentially, moving forward in transportation safety isn't just about tech upgrades—it also means building solid rules and ethical guidelines that keep public trust and safety in check (Figure 10.20).

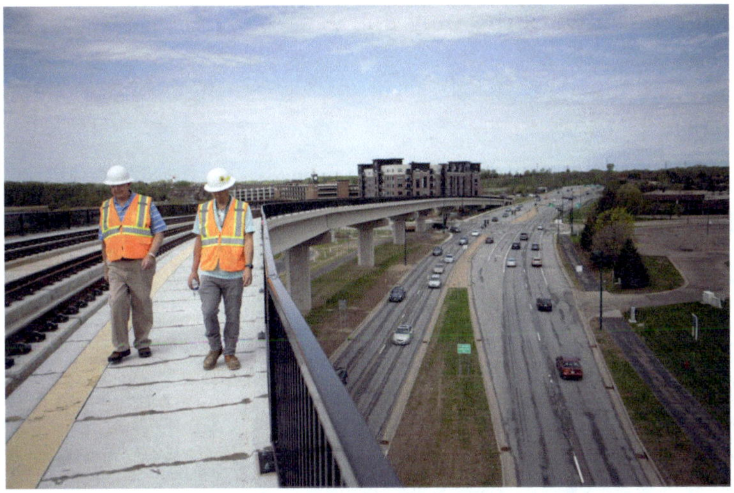

Figure 10.20. Transportation is changing fast and safety now gets tangled in many challenges and bright prospects.

Source: https://minnesotareformer.com/wp-content/uploads/2023/01/IMG_7422-1536x1024.jpg.

Test Your Knowledge

1. What part do helmets play in reducing head injuries from motorcycle accidents?
2. In what ways do seat belts lessen the seriousness of injuries in car accidents?

Summary

Transportation injury research shows that technology is driving a shift and self-driving cars are a major part of it. They are expected to make roads safer and cause fewer accidents, but when they are introduced, many issues need careful attention and detailed study. Digital evidence, too, isn't sticking to the old script; augmented reality is quietly reshuffling the field, pushing forensic investigators to tweak and sometimes completely rethink their standard approaches (Antony et al., 2018). We should always look at both the benefits and drawbacks of new technology to make sure we guide future forensic practices in the right way. If experts keep studying different fields and are ready to change their mindset, it is likely that transportation injuries can be made safer and forensic work can be improved.

Forensic science is often mentioned whenever transport injuries are discussed—it's now obvious that accident investigation relies on these techniques. If you check it out, you realize that forensic experts now use both old and new technologies which makes their work both quicker and more accurate. AI is now being used in traffic systems which can offer many new possibilities, but also brings some issues that cannot be ignored. For example, autonomous vehicles are promoted as helping to reduce traffic and improve safety, but they also involve ethical and technical problems, mainly because human actions and system errors can clash. There's also a bit of a research hiccup when it comes to using forensic tactics to tackle issues like human trafficking in road-related incidents; this gap calls for more of those interdisciplinary conversations (Sust et al., 2021). Basically, as forensic methods improve and are used more, road injuries can be reduced and public safety can increase, even though it's not always the only answer.

KEY TERMS FROM THIS CHAPTER

- Awareness
- Education
- Mindset
- Personal responsibility
- Substance misuse
- Transportation
- Curriculums
- Household appliances
- Pedestrian care
- Safety protocols
- Technology

Short Answer Questions

1. What does a bumper fracture involve and which victims usually have it?
2. What is meant by a dashboard injury?
3. What are two common injuries that often occur in motorcyclists who get into a crash?
4. Explain the term run-over injury with one example.
5. Why does it matter in forensics to identify a seat belt sign on someone who has died?
6. Mention a type of injury that is often experienced by cyclists in RTAs.
7. Tell apart injuries caused by impact from those that happen after a fall.
8. How do the rules about speeding help to prevent injuries in road accidents?

Critical Thinking Questions

1. Of the listed injuries which is the one seen most often in pedestrians struck by a moving vehicle?

a. Whiplash injury
b. Bumper fracture
c. Dash-board injury
d. Steering wheel injury

2. Whiplash injury typically occurs in:

a. Pedestrians struck from behind
b. Front-seat passengers in a frontal collision
c. Drivers in a rear-end collision
d. Cyclists struck from the side

3. In road traffic accidents which of these is regarded as a primary impact injury?

a. Skull fracture from hitting the road
b. Bumper fracture to the tibia
c. Rib fracture from hitting the steering wheel
d. Internal bleeding from seat belt injury

4. A person who is thrown forward in a car crash hits the windshield with their head. This is an example of:

a. Secondary impact injury
b. Primary impact injury
c. Tertiary injury
d. Exit wound injury

5. What kind of injury is common for a motorcyclist who falls from their motorcycle?

a. Fracture-dislocation of the cervical spine
b. Crush injuries to the lower limbs

c. Seat belt abrasions

d. Steering wheel imprint

Answers to Critical Thinking Questions

1. (b) 2. (c) 3. (b) 4. (a) 5. (a)

References

1. Ali Talpur, M. G., Qayyum, S. A., Mangi, A., Ram, H., Qadri, N. A., & Nahyoon, A. W. A. (2021). Forensic evaluation of the patterns of fatal injuries among pedestrians in road traffic accidents in Hyderabad, Pakistan. *JMMC, 11*(2), 62–67. https://doi.org/10.62118/jmmc.v11i2.159.
2. Antony, B., & Cusack, B. (2018). Is working with what we have enough? https://core.ac.uk/download/210552483.pdf (accessed on 29 May 2025).
3. Asekhame, F. F., & Oisamoje, M. D. (2013). Ban on commercial motorcycle operations in Benin City, Nigeria: An appraisal of the benefits and business opportunities. https://core.ac.uk/download/234681418.pdf (accessed on 29 May 2025).
4. Ayuso, M., & Santolino, M. (2025). Prediction of individual automobile RBNS claim reserves in the context of Solvency II. https://core.ac.uk/download/pdf/6301618.pdf (accessed on 29 May 2025).
5. Baggili, I. (2006). Paper session II: Forensic scene documentation using mobile technology. https://core.ac.uk/download/217167398.pdf (accessed on 29 May 2025).
6. Bhatti, M. O. A., Parrey, M., Ali, M. I., Shoro, A. R., Alenazi, A. A., & Alruwaili, R. A. (2025). Gender-based morphometric analysis of the human orbital aperture profile using 3D reconstruction computed tomography: A cross-sectional retrospective study. *Journal of Clinical and Diagnostic Research*. https://www.semanticscholar.org/paper/e322d793603e151e41076512de86563e8521088a (accessed on 29 May 2025).
7. Bobrov, N., & Mandelík, J. (2017). Parametrization of injuries by the FORTIS system and its utilization at solving traffic accidents with pedestrians by the police. https://core.ac.uk/download/235050410.pdf (accessed on 29 May 2025).
8. Boucher, J. P., & Santolino, M. (2025). Modelling the disability severity score in motor insurance claims: An application to the Spanish case. *CORE*. https://core.ac.uk/download/pdf/6301621.pdf (accessed on 29 May 2025).
9. Cenderadewi, M., Franklin, R. C., & Devine, S. (2020). Socio-ecological nature of drowning in low- and middle-income countries: A review to inform health promotion approaches. *International Journal of Aquatic Research and Education, 12*(2), Article 6. https://doi.org/10.25035/ijare.12.02.06.
10. Chaudhari, V. A., & Mohite, S. C. (2016). Socio-demographic and clinical profile of sudden natural deaths in South Mumbai, India. https://core.ac.uk/download/544391290.pdf (accessed on 29 May 2025).
11. Chen, L., Dan, R., Hossin, M. A., et al. (2025). Integrating artificial intelligence in unmanned vehicles: Navigating uncertainties, risks, and the path forward for the fourth industrial revolution. https://core.ac.uk/download/647829878.pdf (accessed on 29 May 2025).

12. Chisholm, S. B., Pishe, T., & Chandra, K. (2025). A multi-year review of major off-road vehicle injuries and deaths in New Brunswick. *Cureus, 17*. https://www.semanticscholar.org/paper/aef4b1d116dd7c8dcd0923559542b142413422ea (accessed on 29 May 2025).

13. Colombage, M., Senerath, M. K. D., Bandaranayake Herath, N. V., Piyarathna, A., et al. (2018). Injury patterns and causes of death among occupants of three-wheelers succumbed to their injuries from road traffic accidents in Sri Lanka. https://core.ac.uk/download/483635584.pdf (accessed on 29 May 2025).

14. Das, N. G., Das, N., & Sil, A. (2025). Pattern and forensic significance of defense injuries in homicide cases: A cross-sectional study. *Cureus, 17*. https://www.semanticscholar.org/paper/b220d59af690d815386e317b288a0dd397b6051b (accessed on 29 May 2025).

15. Davis, J. R., Lane, H. W., & Stepaniak, P. C. (2025). Loss of signal: Aeromedical lessons learned from the STS-107 Columbia space shuttle mishap. https://core.ac.uk/download/pdf/42730063.pdf (accessed on 29 May 2025).

16. Di, X., Gless, S., & Silverman, E. (2022). Ca(r)veat emptor: Crowdsourcing data to challenge the testimony of in-car technology. https://core.ac.uk/download/533955218.pdf (accessed on 29 May 2025).

17. Gallo, C. B., Kemp, B., Metz, J. H. M., Strappini, et al. (2009). Origin and assessment of bruises in beef cattle at slaughter. https://core.ac.uk/download/pdf/29253737.pdf (accessed on 29 May 2025).

18. Gusentsov, A. O. (2024). Algorithm for comprehensive assessment and determination of educational conditions ricochet-induced gunshot injuries. *Military Medicine*. https://www.semanticscholar.org/paper/82608cd3ad559cd5526273db1acae4ea3598db2b (accessed on 29 May 2025).

19. Jin, G. (Ge), Nakayama, S. (Shoji), & Tu, M. (Manghui). (2020). Game based learning for safety and security education. *CORE*. https://core.ac.uk/download/628905943.pdf (accessed on 29 May 2025).

20. Jude, D. (2015). Veterinary practices, reactions and laws: Analyzing the difference in rural and urban practices. https://core.ac.uk/download/217256949.pdf (accessed on 29 May 2025).

21. Kamnik, R., Laković, S., & Topolšek, D. (2022). Modern technologies and methods of data collection in the function of making better traffic analysis of forensic traffic experts. *Environmental Engineering–Inženjerstvo Okoliša, 9*(1, 2). https://core.ac.uk/download/552154050.pdf.

22. Karlos, V., & Larcher, M. (2021). A guide to key information on the protection of public spaces. https://core.ac.uk/download/642867548.pdf (accessed on 29 May 2025).

23. Klinkner, M. (2009). Forensic science expertise for international criminal proceedings: An old problem, a new context and a pragmatic resolution. *The International Journal of Evidence & Proof, 13*(2), 102–129. https://doi.org/10.1350/ijep.2008.12.1.284.

24. Kotsyubynska, Y., Kozan, N., Kharevych, V. M., Lyampel, V. I., & Mickanyuk, O. Y. (2023). Forensic-medical evaluation of injuries received during operation of personal mobility devices: The state of the problem (review). *Art of Medicine*. https://www.semanticscholar.org/paper/aa52b1fdf248e53358e4d47d116e1cce2779747b (accessed on 29 May 2025).

25. Kumar, P. R. (2017). A study of deaths due to railway fatalities at a tertiary care hospital

mortuary 2015-16. *International Journal of Research in Medical Sciences, 6*(1), 264–267. https://doi.org/10.18203/2320-6012.ijrms20175731.

26. Kwong, L. (2018). Increasing police accountability and improving use of force policies in the United States. *Themis: Research Journal of Justice Studies and Forensic Science, 6*(1), Article 11. https://scholarworks.sjsu.edu/themis/vol6/iss1/11 (accessed on 29 May 2025).
27. Losavio, M., Chow, K. P., Koltay, A., & James, J. I. (2018). The internet of things and the smart city: Legal challenges with digital forensics, privacy, and security. *Security and Privacy, 1*. https://doi.org/10.1002/spy2.23.
28. Lundstrom, E. W. (2023). The application of time series analysis to injury epidemiology data. https://core.ac.uk/download/568065467.pdf (accessed on 29 May 2025).
29. Luo, J., Zheng, Z., & Yu, R. L. (2023). Analysis of medical malpractice liability disputes related to novel antineoplastic drugs and research on risk prevention and control strategies. *PLoS ONE, 18*, e0286623. https://doi.org/10.1371/journal.pone.0286623.
30. Matadi, B. M., & Abouzahir, H. (2025). Retrospective study of work-related knee injuries: Analysis of 86 cases among the personnel of the General Directorate of National Security received by the Medico-Legal Institute of Casablanca. *Moroccan Forensic & Law*. https://www.semanticscholar.org/paper/35fd37cce0b8589014d9573cc35523c30bddedad (accessed on 29 May 2025).
31. Mejia Minguez, C. M. (2017). Implementation of a maritime disaster management system in the Dominican Republic—Focused on search and rescue. https://core.ac.uk/download/366846363.pdf (accessed on 29 May 2025).
32. Missouri University of Science and Technology, INSPIRE–University Transportation Center. (2020). INSPIRE newsletter spring 2020. https://core.ac.uk/download/328036442.pdf (accessed on 29 May 2025).
33. Molero, G. D., Poveda-Reyes, S., Malviya, A. K., García-Jiménez, E., Leva, M. C., & Santarremigia, F. E. (2021). Computational solutions based on Bayesian networks to hierarchize and to predict factors influencing gender fairness in the transport system: Four use cases. *Sustainability, 13*(20), 11372. https://doi.org/10.3390/su132011372.
34. Morrison, A., Ellsberg, M., & Bott, S. (2004). Addressing gender-based violence in the Latin American and Caribbean region: A critical review of interventions. https://core.ac.uk/download/pdf/6372976.pdf (accessed on 29 May 2025).
35. Nersessian, D., & Mancha, R. (2021). From automation to autonomy: Legal and ethical responsibility gaps in artificial intelligence innovation. *Michigan Technology Law Review*. https://doi.org/10.36645/mtlr.27.1.from.
36. Nogayeva, S., Gooch, J., & Frascione, N. (2021). The forensic investigation of vehicle-pedestrian collisions: A review. *Science & Justice, 61*(2), 112–118. https://doi.org/10.1016/j.scijus.2020.10.006.
37. Otieno, G. A., & Loosen, A. E. (2016). An analysis of key environmental and social risks in the development of concentrated solar power projects. *AIP Conference Proceedings, 1734*(1), 160012. https://doi.org/10.1063/1.4949253.
38. Parekh, E., Stead, T. S., Elahi, J., & Ganti, L. (2025). Craniofacial injuries in mixed martial arts: An analysis of incidence, risk factors, and prevention strategies. *The Journal of Craniofacial*

Surgery. Advance online publication. https://doi.org/10.1097/SCS.0000000000011330.

39. Parry, A. I. (2025). Making homemakers responsible for safety: Housework, laundry equipment, and the unequal burdens of accident prevention, c. 1910–80. *Technology and Culture*. https://www.semanticscholar.org/paper/871ff05f7739e9ea45db0f40c14d3d4a4ba23dd3 (accessed on 29 May 2025).
40. Perz, R. (2024). The multidimensional threats of unmanned aerial systems: Exploring biomechanical, technical, operational, and legal solutions for ensuring safety and security. *Archives of Transport*. https://www.semanticscholar.org/paper/7e1e0640cb35ffdc385c774134fb5435ec45018c (accessed on 29 May 2025).
41. Postle, G., Rivera, M., Rosay, A. B., TePas, K., et al. (2010). Investigation and prosecution of sexual assault, domestic violence, and stalking. https://core.ac.uk/download/162575881.pdf (accessed on 29 May 2025).
42. Postle, G., Rosay, A. B., TePas, K., Wood, et al. (2007). Descriptive analysis of sexual assault incidents reported to Alaska State Troopers: 2003–2004. https://core.ac.uk/download/162576335.pdf (accessed on 29 May 2025).
43. Reid, K., Suwalowska, H., Martin, L. J., & Heathfield, L. (2025). Ethical considerations in the routine identification of human remains in forensic mortuaries. *Welcome Open Research*. https://www.semanticscholar.org/paper/91c0dc5beb099ba83315408cfab3b43ddb9d39f1 (accessed on 29 May 2025).
44. Reyes Albaladejo, F., Soriano, B. J., & Gitto, L. (2024). Analysis of unique atypical screwdriver injuries. *Journal of Forensic Sciences*. https://www.semanticscholar.org/paper/2a6bc4842563c08cae54bb06ab0e5bfc54105e11 (accessed on 29 May 2025).
45. Salado Puerto, M., Abboud, D., Baraybar, J. P., Carracedo, Á., Fonseca, S., Goodwin, W., Guyomarc'h, P., et al. (2021). The search process: Integrating the investigation and identification of missing and unidentified persons. *Forensic Science International Synergy, 3*, 100154. https://doi.org/10.1016/j.fsisyn.2021.100154.
46. Sanzyapova, R. R. (2025). The role of dentistry in forensic medicine: Identification of human remains. *Patient-Oriented Medicine and Pharmacy*. https://www.semanticscholar.org/paper/d8db5ae62d74c13d619c3b0324e081b54abd3399 (accessed on 29 May 2025).
47. Siegel, G. (2006). Technologies of accident: Forensic media, crash analysis, and the redefinition of progress. https://core.ac.uk/download/210602430.pdf (accessed on 29 May 2025).
48. Smith, J. H., & Singh, M. (2024). Forensic DNA profiling: Legal and ethical considerations. *Journal of Scientific Research and Reports*. https://www.semanticscholar.org/paper/30d2411eb968e68b332f37a253d3eb7fbd0ba08f (accessed on 29 May 2025).
49. Söderberg, M., & Santolino, M. (2025). The influence of decision-maker effort and case complexity on appealed rulings subject to multi-categorical selection. https://core.ac.uk/download/pdf/6273744.pdf (accessed on 29 May 2025).
50. St. Cloud State University. (2008). *The Chronicle*. https://core.ac.uk/download/555614578.pdf (accessed on 29 May 2025).
51. Sust, L. (2021). Forensic science in combat of human trafficking. https://core.ac.uk/download/529714117.pdf (accessed on 29 May 2025).
52. Tennessee Department of Finance & Administration. (2014). *Office of Criminal Justice Programs*

Annual Report 2012–2013. https://core.ac.uk/download/588405704.pdf (accessed on 29 May 2025).

53. Tripathi, S., Kolodziej, C. P., Gohlke, D., Burnham, A., Zhou, Y., & Longman, D. (2025). Fleet-level energy and emissions analysis of the US off-road sector with VISION: Off-Road. *SAE Technical Paper Series*. https://www.semanticscholar.org/paper/f4cb537b4d88b030f94ee2f159da2ec2034c7b69 (accessed on 29 May 2025).
54. Trisnadi, S. (2021). The role of forensic medicine in the criminal evidence process. https://core.ac.uk/download/490626377.pdf (accessed on 29 May 2025).
55. Valsala, K., Sreedevi, C. S., & Sreelekshmi, J. (2017). Analysis of railway track deaths—An autopsy-based study. *International Journal of Research in Medical Sciences, 5*(3), 935–939. https://doi.org/10.18203/2320-6012.ijrms20170639.
56. Viciano, J., López-Lázaro, S., & Tanga, C. (2022). Post-mortem dental profile as a powerful tool in animal forensic investigations—A review. *Animals, 12*(16), 2038. https://doi.org/10.3390/ani12162038.
57. Warnica, M. J. (2015). Biomechanical assessment of cycling helmets: The influence of head form and impact velocity based on cycling collisions associated with injury claims. https://core.ac.uk/download/144148076.pdf (accessed on 29 May 2025).
58. Zimbardi, G. (2005). *Workplace Substance Use, The Risk of Occupational Injury, And Testing* (Master's thesis, University of Pittsburgh).

THERMAL INJURIES

11

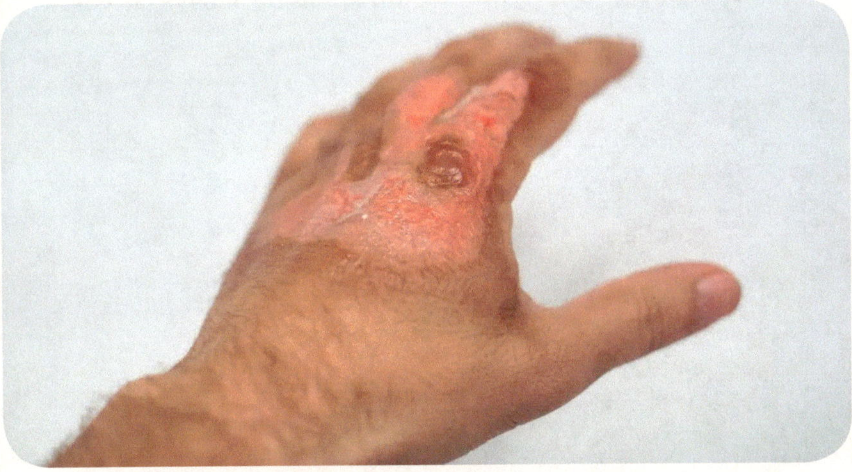

LEARNING OBJECTIVES

After studying this chapter, you will be able to:

1. Identify types of thermal injuries;
2. Explain the mechanisms of injury;
3. Learn forensic analysis of thermal injuries;
4. Focus on psychological and social implications.

Introduction

Thermal injuries require us to think carefully about how they affect forensics. They are not only a problem for patients – they also become major issues in the courts and discussions about public health. In most situations, as injuries increase among those without stable housing, it becomes important to look at their housing situation which may affect the outcomes. For example, some recent studies show that folks without reliable shelter face burn injuries at noticeably higher rates which end up hurting both their health and their ability to get proper care (Lee et al., 2025). Because of the variety of social challenges and injuries, crime scene investigators ought to consider the entire background. To summarize, grasping these intertwined issues is pretty crucial for effective scene analysis and for coming up with preventive strategies that dig into the underlying social roots of these injuries (Das et al., 2025).

Definition of Thermal Injuries

It can be very difficult for forensic experts to solve thermal injuries. Any contact with extreme heat, for example a flame, hot liquid or a hot surface, can cause a burn. Sometimes, you only see a hit on the very top layer of skin—that's what's commonly called a first-degree burn—but in other cases, the damage goes much deeper, upsetting tissues and even organs (these are the second- or third-degree kinds). Those with severe burns are more likely to develop infections or problems in several organs which can make their recovery harder. In the majority of cases, the story goes on after the burn happens. Investigators have to piece together a broader picture, thinking about things like motive or the possibility of foul play (Albaladejo et al., 2024; Santos et al., 2024). All this goes to show that understanding these injuries isn't just about the clinical details—it's also about uncovering the background of the incident, which can be just as important in legal settings (Figure 11.1).

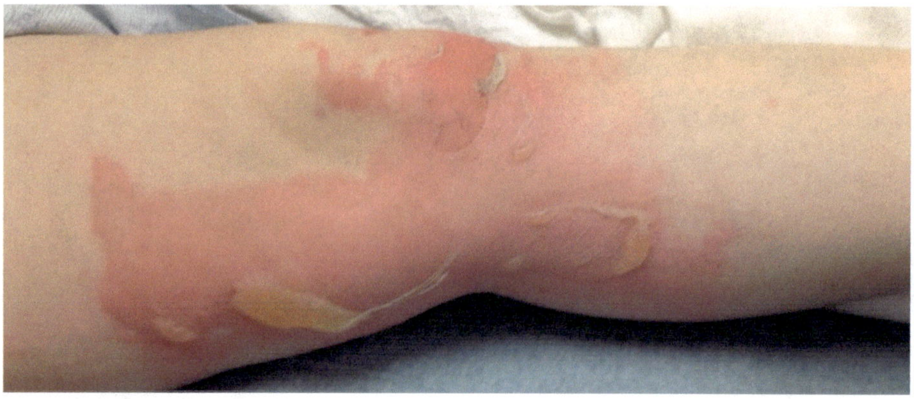

Figure 11.1. Thermal injuries.

Source: https://d148x66490prkv.cloudfront.net/hmp_ln/2024-03/Screenshot%202024-03-22%20at%208.25.24%E2%80%AFAM.png.

Importance of Studying Thermal Injuries in Forensics

Forensic science relies on understanding how heat affects the body's chemistry and biology which often helps solve the confusing aspects of deaths by fire. Volatile organic compounds (VOCs) that the body releases under extreme heat sometimes act as subtle messengers; in many cases, these clues hint at not only when death set in but also if someone might have clung to life a little longer (Drabińska et al., 2021). Experts can sometimes determine from the patterns of burns if a fire was an accident or was set on purpose which often has a big effect on legal investigations. There's also a growing body of work on chemicals in bodily fluids, often linked to inflammation or cell damage from severe thermal exposure, that seems to sharpen the overall accuracy of forensic assessments (Pellati et al., 2018). All things considered, understanding thermal injuries helps explain why and how a death occurred which in turn strengthens the work of forensic experts in our justice system.

Overview of Types of Thermal Injuries

Heat-related trauma can look different each time which can be unexpected for those investigating the case. Burns are commonly put into three main types – superficial, partial thickness and full thickness – but the differences between them can sometimes be unclear. Burns that just affect the top layer of skin are called superficial and they leave red, sore patches that usually do not blister even though they are quite uncomfortable.

Sometimes, partial thickness burns are deep enough to cause blisters and more intense pain because the nerves are involved which is observed by investigators. Full thickness burns destroy all layers of the skin and usually make the skin look charred or white, so they usually need advanced medical treatment to recover. Generally speaking, knowing these differences is vital in forensic work since the precise identification of burn type can influence legal outcomes and investigative strategies—a point further underscored by the growing use of advanced imaging technologies in trauma scene reconstruction (Rodríguez-Gonzálvez et al., 2016; Lawler et al., 2023).

Historical Context of Thermal Injuries in Forensic Science

Thermal injuries in forensic science have developed a lot and the progress has not always been smooth. In the past, investigating burns and heat injuries was very simple which often meant there was a lot of doubt about how people died. Nowadays, forensic experts use chemicals as well as biological information which usually gives their work more accuracy, even if it can be a bit messy. Take microbial studies, for example; these efforts can help gauge how long a body has been changing after death (Aáudia-Ferreira et al., 2023), neatly linking environmental conditions to the burn marks observed. In many cases, the need to unravel arson mysteries and pin down injury patterns has nudged forensic approaches in unexpected directions (Kumar et al., 2023). All in all, these changes underline that even though history is important, new approaches keep changing our view of thermal injuries.

Relevance to Criminal Investigations

Now, forensic science and legal oversight work together to highlight how thermal injuries are examined in criminal cases. Technology is helping investigators by providing many tools to investigate fire-related deaths. Most defense lawyers are open about challenging old methods—they keep arguing that we need stronger evidence in court. Fire investigators, it turns out, must keep tweaking their approaches so that what they find stands firm in legal debates (May et al., 2010). Also, Forensic Analysis – From Death to Justice introduces new ideas by discussing thermal injury assessments and other forensic methods. These kinds of contributions—sometimes repeated and always evolving—play a pretty critical role in helping experts keep the science solid and the path to justice clear (Figure 11.2).

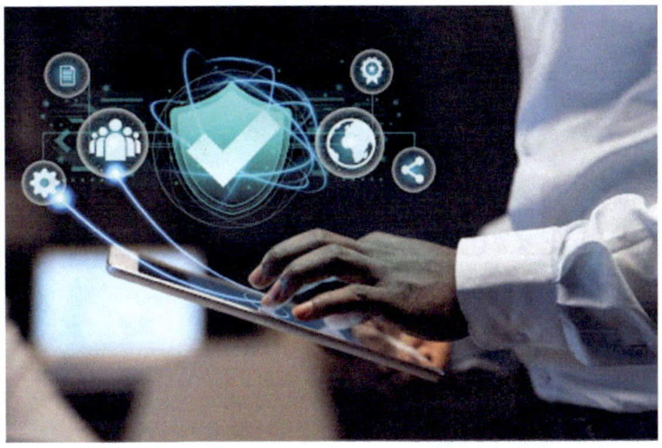

Figure 11.2. Technology is pushing boundaries and, quite frankly, handing investigators many tools to dig into the messy details behind fire-related deaths.

Source: https://blogger.googleusercontent.com/img/b/R29vZ2xl/AVvXsEj0h-p-o_fXCQV8j-r4VV0wMCBLw65DqZL7U3aNBGfQNxGy6KiC3duL7EOnjZXg-HIT6hNynhVJKHTu62Wks1RxdGoCMa7uGdtK1ynWtUqhux_r4W4q11AVWgFLreE59UOq50PMr kyBw5yZOjnkrzsXcAgfaUG8EqDlZNfcq4NR7NM_71qa5I6umnEQyPpd/w447-h296/top%201.5.jpeg.

Methodology for Analyzing Thermal Injuries

When looking into thermal injuries, it is important to follow a set procedure, since getting the details right is very important. Experts usually begin by looking at the tissue under a microscope to see how deep, how large and in what way the burns are. You can also use imaging, for example thermography, to see how heat moves and where injuries appear, without touching the tissue. Nowadays, some investigators are also exploring molecular markers; for example, microRNAs appear quite promising when it comes to gauging burn vitality and even helping determine the time of death in suspected homicide cases (Rocchi et al., 2020). Incidentally, deep learning in image analysis has also been showing some promise by spotting burn patterns with improved accuracy (Egger et al., 2022). In short, using several techniques together helps us better understand thermal injuries and provides the needed evidence for legal purposes.

11.1. Types of Thermal Injuries

Learning Outcome

1. Identify first, second, and third degrees of burns;
2. Know the causes and characteristics of scalds;
3. Focus on frostbite;
4. Explain electrocution;
5. Discuss radiation burns;
6. Pay attention to the usual causes and the effects of chemical burns;
7. Define thermal trauma;
8. Give a comparative analysis of injury types;
9. Learn case studies illustrating different types.

Since thermal injuries often give hints about events at the crime scene, they are very important for investigators. Most of the time, first-degree burns are only on the top layer of skin and disappear quickly, but second-degree burns go deeper and may form blisters and third-degree burns reach all the skin layers and normally require surgery. You might also bump into flash burns – these pop up in explosive situations and have peculiar patterns that can hint at both the heat's source and its intensity (Layden et al., 2019). Experts typically study each burn type, looking not just at the injury itself but also at the messy details of how it formed, which helps them reconstruct the incident (Gardner et al., 2018).

11.1.1. Burns: First, Second, and Third Degree

Looking at burn damage is very important in forensics, since it helps decide how to treat the injury and how to handle the case legally. Burns are divided into three categories to indicate the depth of damage to the tissue. First-degree burns are only on the top layer of skin, so they make the skin red and sore like a bad sunburn. A second-degree burn goes through the outer layer of skin into the dermis which leads to blisters and a lot of pain; because the risk of infection increases, these burns usually need a doctor's care. Third-degree burns reach all the way to the deepest layers of the skin and may also harm the tissues below, so the area often becomes hard and leathery and can lose sensation due to nerve damage. In most cases, knowing these differences is key—especially when fires release toxic fumes, since fatalities tend to come more from inhaling dangerous emissions than from the burns alone (Fonollosa et al., 2018; Lu et al., 2014). Forensic experts lean on this info to work out what happened and how the thermal injuries play into the bigger picture (Figure 11.3).

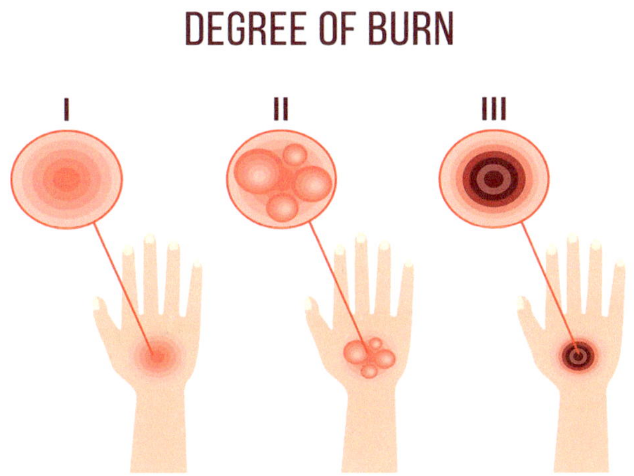

Figure 11.3. First, second, and third degrees of burns.

Source: https://dam.northwell.edu/m/7f5824f9c94bbfdc/Drupal-TheWell_burn-types-symptom-treatment_GettyImages-1283890203.jpg.

11.1.2. Scalds: Causes and Characteristics

Scald injuries which happen when hot water or steam touches the skin, are often not noticed, but they can be important for forensic investigations. They take place when skin touches a liquid that is extremely hot and the seriousness of the injury is generally related to how hot the liquid was and the length of the exposure. Many times, the skin of young children and older adults which is not as strong, suffers more. Such burns may be a key sign that someone is abusing or neglecting the child.

Sometimes scalds pop up alongside other injuries—say, those seen during domestic violence incidents (Doukas, 2022)—which adds a whole other layer to interpreting the situation. And generally speaking, research shows that severe burns come with high mortality rates, stressing the point that we need better prevention and more in-depth studies to tackle this public health challenge (Mobayen et al., 2021) (Figure 11.4).

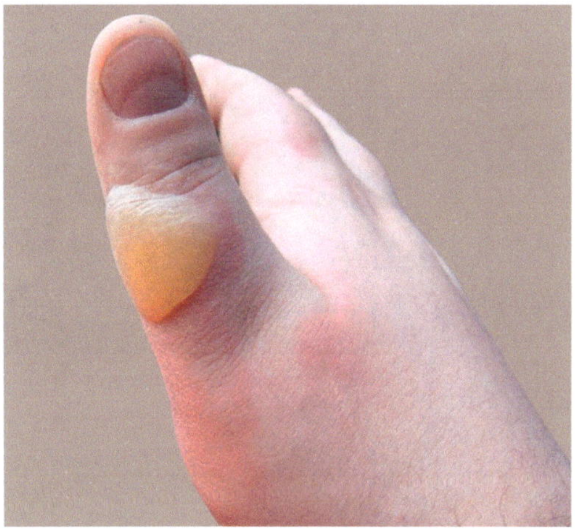

Figure 11.4. Scald injuries.

Source: By The original uploader was Snickerdo at English Wikipedia. - Transferred from en.wikipedia to Commons., CC BY-SA 3.0, https://commons.wikimedia.org/w/index.php?curid=3358773.

11.1.3. Frostbite: Definition and Effects

The body can suffer a lot from extreme cold and frostbite is a common problem that results. If the skin and tissues underneath are frozen because of prolonged exposure to very cold temperatures, the damage may be permanent unless you treat it quickly. At first the area may look red and swollen, but soon it turns into a hard, pale area as the cells die. A wound like this can disrupt blood flow, nerve function and also influence the way the body handles its metabolism. Quickly getting a proper diagnosis and fast treatment is often important to avoid pain that lasts or the need for amputation. In forensics, experts can use knowledge of frostbite to work out the order of events in a person's exposure to extreme weather. It's also worth noting that frostbite often goes hand-in-hand with hypothermia; the two conditions can, quite frankly, worsen each other and complicate both treatment and recovery (Broussard, 2016; Savioli et al., 2023) (Figure 11.5).

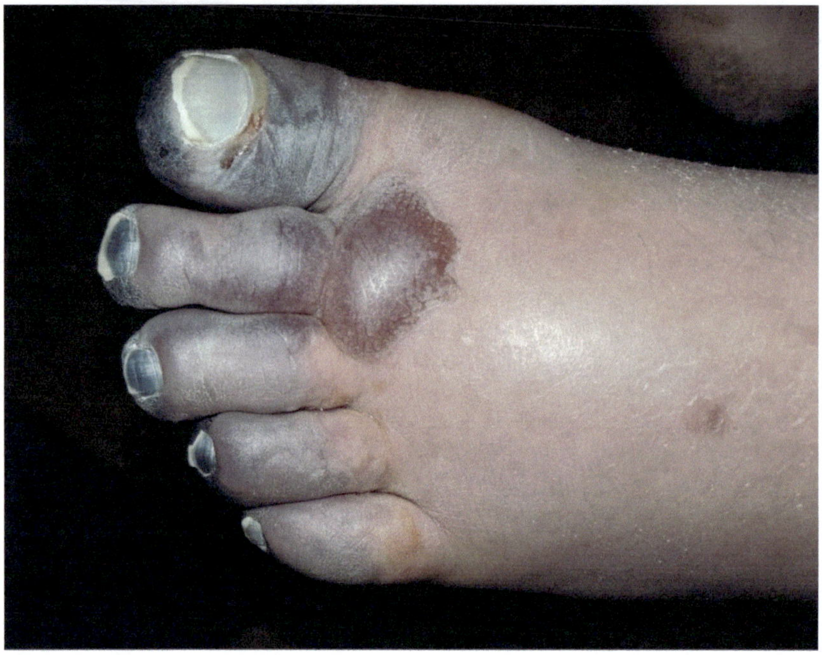

Figure 11.5. Frostbite.

Source: https://upload.wikimedia.org/wikipedia/commons/c/c2/Left_foot_third_degree_frostbite.png.

11.1.4. Electrocution: Mechanisms and Injuries

Understanding the mixing of electricity with a person's body is important in many electrocution investigations. Most of the time, where the current goes, how long it stays and how much power it has determine the injuries from a zap. Electricity often turns into heat in the body and this can make burns worse and add more damage. Research often shows different types of tissue harm, ranging from muscle decay to the sudden collapse of blood vessels, meaning that autopsies have to be thorough to sort out what went wrong (Zissler et al., 2020). Cases involving lightning, for example, also remind us that electrical injuries are seldom one-dimensional; they pull together clues from both the medical side and the surrounding setting, as seen in the investigation of two lightning strike fatalities in South Africa (Hunt et al., 2020). In short, combining these different ideas seems to help us understand electrocution better and keep improving forensic methods.

11.1.5. Radiation Burns: Sources and Impacts

Thermal injuries can be different from the usual burns. Sometimes they come from radiation – which is a serious risk in many clinical settings – and patients often suffer these injuries after being exposed to diagnostic or therapeutic radiation (the same kind used in imaging tests and cancer treatments), especially when proper shielding isn't in place or when the exposure lasts too long (Baker et al., 2024). MRI facilities have experienced a significant number of skin burns which is a common type of incident observed there. It seems that the kinds and causes of burns can change with the seasons which suggests that we might need to adapt our prevention strategies more than we usually do. Studies, in most cases, point out that radiation burns have unique effects on patient care and that a detailed grasp of exposure risks is necessary to boost safety protocols (Qayyum et al., 2024). In any event, keeping these factors in mind is crucial—not only for advancing forensic investigations but also for ensuring patient safety (Figure 11.6).

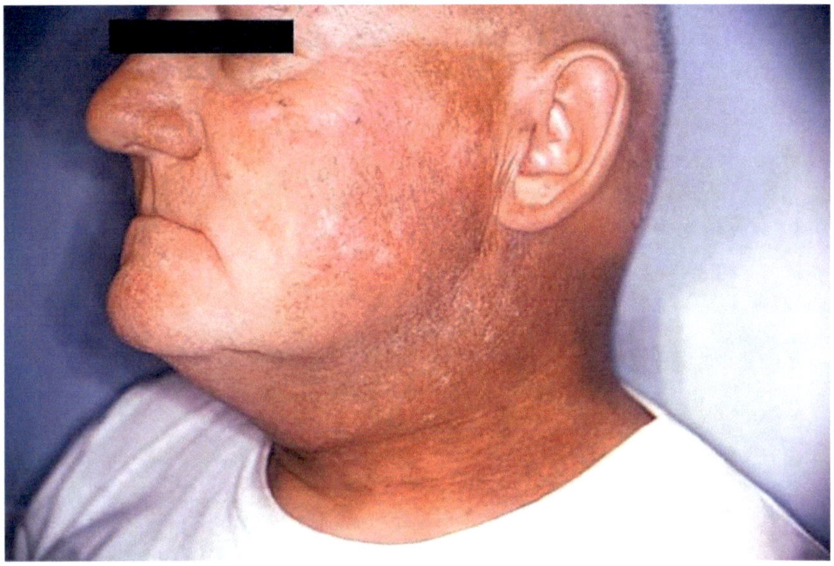

Figure 11.6. Radiation burns.

Source: https://i0.wp.com/cdn-prod.medicalnewstoday.com/content/images/articles/323/323155/radiation-dermatitis-image-credit-cdc-robert-e-sumpter-1967.jpg?w=1155&h=1549.

11.1.6. Chemical Burns: Common Agents and Effects

In forensic analysis of thermal injuries, chemical burns are important since different agents can cause very severe reactions in living tissue. Many substances, for example rough acids and strong alkalis, can destroy proteins, kill tissue and cause inflammation which usually makes it harder to determine and treat the injury. Neutrophils, for example, seem to work in two ways; recent reports even note that they sometimes ramp up inflammation by releasing reactive oxygen species (ROS) (Sikora et al., 2023), a detail that matters in tracking how chemical burns develop. On top of the bodily damage, chemical exposure often ripples out into the environment, sometimes contaminating soil and water – a problem that can eventually show up in human health through food chains (Joseph et al., 2023). All in all, experts need to know the details of these agents because this helps them determine the extent of the injuries and their cause which guides both the legal and medical actions taken.

11.1.7. Thermal Trauma: Definition and Implications

Thermal trauma is not only an injury from extreme heat or cold; it can also be a confusing problem that doctors and lawyers find hard to deal with. When a person is in extreme heat or cold, the injury may seem minor like a burn or it might be very serious and harm the tissues. Because of this, it becomes more difficult for clinicians to assess the situation and may lead to confusion in legal cases when something suspicious is suspected. In most cases, having emergency staff who know how to spot and document these injuries accurately is a must, because any slip in reporting can derail legal proceedings and affect victims' rights (Cattaneo et al., 2023). There's also an interesting overlap when forensic archaeology and anthropology share their insights, pushing home the need for standard ways to gather evidence from remains scorched by fire or heated beyond normal levels (Alfsdotter, 2021). Overall, mixing insights from different fields tends to open up the investigation, improving both justice and the care given to those caught in the aftermath of thermal injuries (Figure 11.7).

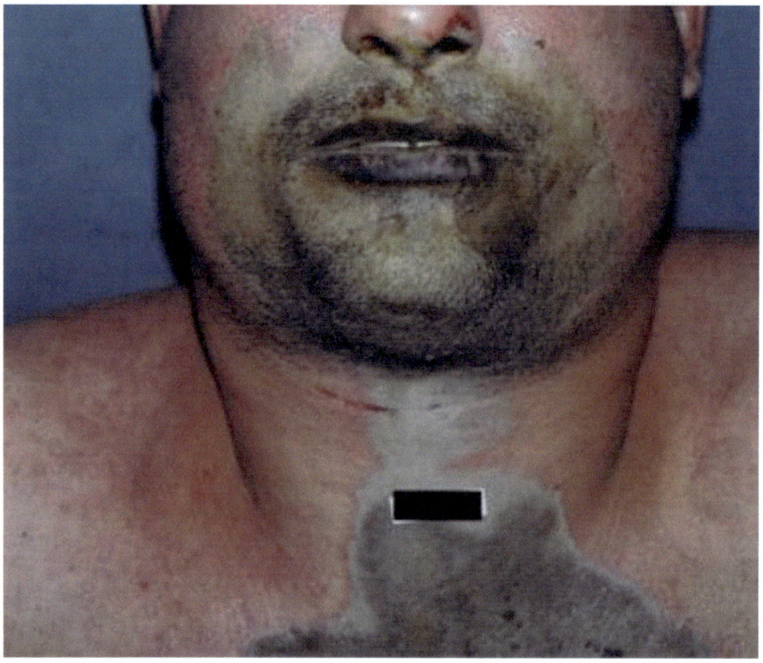

Figure 11.7. Thermal trauma isn't just a simple injury from extreme temperatures—it's a messy, complicated issue that pops up in ways that can stump both doctors and legal teams.

Source: https://img.medscapestatic.com/pi/meds/ckb/52/13152tn.jpg.

11.1.8. Comparative Analysis of Injury Types

It's not always clear what kind of injuries can happen from heat exposure—you need to look into all the different types. The way an injury takes place usually decides how it appears and how much recovery is needed which helps doctors and forensic experts understand what happened. Take car accidents, for example. By studying the injuries, you can notice how the impact and heat from a crash interact. Studies generally show that head injuries, for instance, tend to show up differently depending on factors like the kind of vehicle involved and how the crash happened, sometimes adding extra complications when settling claims for burns or heat damage (Paola et al., 2025). It's also worth noting that noticing how these elements mix—though it might seem a bit messy—can sharpen a forensic expert's insight, ultimately guiding how legal decisions are made in personal injury cases (Grukhovskiy et al., 2024). All in all, a wide and sometimes unpredictable way of looking at these injuries is key for both analyzing cases and handling the legal side.

11.1.9. Case Studies Illustrating Different Types

In forensic cases, thermal injuries can be very complex because the different factors often mix in ways that are hard to predict. For example, operating room fires have resulted from using monopolar diathermy which sometimes caused routine procedures to become risky and caused patients to suffer severe burns.

One review, for example, pointed out that such mishaps resulted in over 3,500 injuries and 178 deaths—mostly because of burns; clearly, getting a grip on the so-called fire triangle (ignition sources, fuels, oxidizers) is pretty crucial to stopping these disasters.

When they paid attention to accidents involving vehicles, experts found that the nature and location of injuries were not the same. Most of the time, head trauma was more severe in domestic vehicles than in those made overseas which suggests there might be other elements to think about. It seems that these differences, however subtle, push for more in-depth investigations to boost forensic evaluations (Grukhovskiy et al., 2024).

Test Your Knowledge

1. Define thermal injury.
2. State the main types of burns based on the agents that cause them.

11.2. Mechanisms of Injury

Learning Outcome

1. Identify heat transfer methods;
2. Explain the physiological response to thermal exposure;
3. Identify factors influencing burn severity;
4. Talk about how skin anatomy affects thermal injuries;
5. Study how the length and temperature of exposure can cause injury;
6. Focus on the pathophysiology of thermal injuries;
7. Describe healing processes and complications;
8. Understand the long-term effects of thermal injuries;
9. Discuss forensic implications of injury mechanisms.

Thermal injuries are difficult to understand and you should know what happens inside cells when heat is involved, as it plays a big role in many forensic cases. A variety of heat-related injuries can happen, including scalds and burns and these can disrupt the body's normal functions and sometimes cause severe harm.

In such cases, high heat can damage cell components like proteins and nucleic acids and the harm is usually irreversible, so the cells die. Understanding these changes is usually necessary to determine how the person died. Generally speaking, instances like cadaveric spasm—where muscles stiffen abruptly—can blur the picture during post-mortem checks, making things more complicated (Son et al., 2024). Similarly, animal cadaver studies highlight the complicated mix between physical injuries and heat damage, showing how both factors can shape the outcome of death investigations and affect the evidence gathered (Kazantsev and Yatsenko, 2024).

11.2.1. Heat Transfer Methods: Conduction, Convection, and Radiation

Heat transfer is very important when looking at burn injuries. In many forensic investigations, the way heat travels such as by conduction, convection or radiation, can show how serious the wounds are. When hot things come into contact with your skin, it can cause spot burns; convection which happens with air or water movement, may spread the damage to other parts. Radiation causes heat to be emitted by electromagnetic waves, so being in a fire can make a person feel intense heat even if there is no direct flame touch. Generally speaking, breaking down these heat-sharing methods is key for probing both thermal injuries and hypothermia, as studies in human physiology show how our bodies react under shifting temperatures, which underscores the need for fast intervention in hypothermic cases (Savioli et al., 2023) and for putting together safety plans in fire scenarios (Koromila et al., 2023) (Figure 11.8).

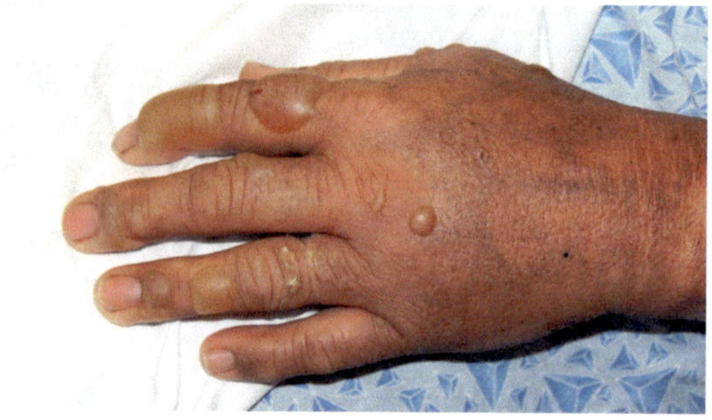

Figure 11.8. Heat transfer matters a lot when we're trying to understand burn injuries.

Source: https://burncenters.com/wp-content/uploads/2020/05/second-degree-scaled-e1588603811149.jpg.

11.2.2. Physiological Response to Thermal Exposure

When it gets hot, our bodies react differently

which gives us insights into how injuries happen in forensic cases. When it gets too warm, instead of just suffering silently, our blood vessels spread out (that's vasodilation) to let off extra heat and keep things steady inside. Usually, this small step can decide how severe a thermal injury becomes, mainly when the person is exposed to extreme conditions. Interestingly, research on Antarctic notothenioid fishes shows that sometimes these adaptations happen after the cell's instructions have already been laid out, hinting at a subtle, post-transcriptional tweak that might also occur in humans (Dowd et al., 2024). Also, studies with hypothermic rabbit models reveal that small, local shifts in temperature sensors can sway the entire body's response – a reminder that even tiny changes in heat regulation play a major role in injury outcomes (Wincoko et al., 2023). All in all, using all these observations helps us understand thermal injuries in detail.

11.2.3. Factors Influencing Burn Severity

Many things work together to determine how much damage a thermal injury causes. Considering just one element is not enough, since being close to the heat source and the condition of the environment often play a bigger role than anticipated. For instance, a study on the London bombings generally showed that crowd density, the layout of the enclosure, and the actual positioning of victims relative to the blast all combined to affect both injury patterns and mortality (Chukwu-Lobelu et al., 2017). Likewise, the atmosphere isn't just a background detail; research into vapor cloud explosions reveals that factors like wind conditions and the very makeup of the cloud tend to adjust the blast's force, which in turn tweaks the thermal damage observed (Atkinson et al., 2017). To summarize, keeping track of these various elements—even if it means accepting a bit of uncertainty here and there—is pretty crucial for accurately evaluating burn severity in forensic contexts (Figure 11.9).

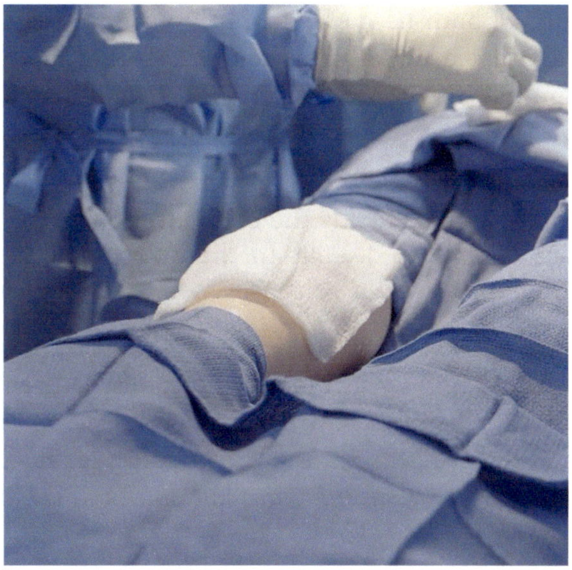

Figure 11.9. Thermal injuries aren't as straightforward as they might seem—many intertwined factors influence just how severe a burn can get.

Source: https://s3.amazonaws.com/lmg-drugdiscoverynews/assets/articleNo/15424/iImg/39217/stratagraft-epidermis-matte-side-l.jpeg.

11.2.4. Role of Skin Anatomy in Thermal Injuries

Skin is more than a layer—it actively protects us from many environmental dangers such as heat burns. Generally, the epidermis is the first to react to heat, while the dermis which contains nerves, blood vessels and support and the hypodermis, though less recognized, play important roles in a burn injury.

When these layers get hurt, complications such as infection or scarring can crop up, and these issues often become crucial details during forensic examinations (Egger et al., 2022). In many cases, a solid grasp of how the skin is built tends to guide decisions on both medical interventions and even legal aspects, as determining burn depth and extent isn't just about surface appearances (Armstrong et al., 2018). Basically, knowing how our skin is made helps us see why a small burn should get more attention, especially when putting all the forensic clues together.

11.2.5. Impact of Duration and Temperature on Injury

Forensic investigators rely on the length and intensity of a fire and these factors can affect what they observe. It has been noted by studies that variations in the time of exposure and the intensity of heat can result in different changes in human tissues which usually causes small shifts in the way injuries are understood. There's literature noting a standardized system for burn injury classification that seems to enhance the forensic community's ability to assess heat damage more straightforwardly (Williams et al., 2020).

Exploring the ways fractures can endure high temperatures teaches us a lot about the injuries that happen in fires. In several experiments comparing burned bones, researchers found a noticeable link between the degree of thermal alteration and distinct trauma patterns, which underscores the need for detailed examinations of both heat effects and blunt force injuries (Pendray et al., 2016). All in all, these results suggest that precise measurement of both temperature and exposure time is very important when examining the consequences of thermal events.

11.2.6. Pathophysiology of Thermal Injuries

Burns are only the start of what happens inside the body after a thermal injury and these reactions can make investigations more complicated. Cells in the body usually die from heat exposure by necrosis or apoptosis and their breakdown releases chemicals that can increase tissue damage and start a body-wide alert.

As a result, patients might develop hypovolemic shock, fail to breathe properly or experience problems with several organs which shows how severe the harm can be. In many explosion cases, for example, the heat doesn't only scar the skin and what's under it; it can reach internal organs too, thanks to a tangled mix of environmental factors and shifts in the body's hemodynamic status (Galante et al., 2021).

Plus, the way thermal injuries tweak gene expression—especially regarding low oxygen responses and inflammatory pathways—only adds to the need for careful forensic checks to figure out what went wrong and pin down the cause and manner of death (Gagliardi et al., 2021) (Figure 11.10).

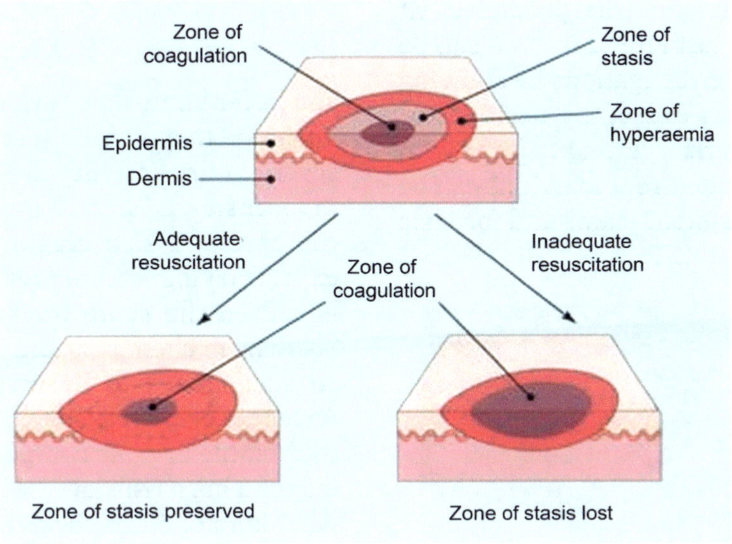

Figure 11.10. When someone is hit with high heat, cells usually die by necrosis or apoptosis, and as they break down, they leak inflammatory chemicals that can worsen tissue loss and start a body-wide alarm.

Source: By Shehan Hettiaratchy - Original publication: https://www.ncbi.nlm.nih.gov/pmc/articles/PMC421790/Immediate source: https://www.ncbi.nlm.nih.gov/pmc/articles/PMC421790/, Fair use, https://en.wikipedia.org/w/index.php?curid=54394246.

11.2.7. Healing Processes and Complications

Thermal injuries require close observation of how healing happens, as they often lead to many complications that can make recovery slow. It turns out that watching cells and chemicals interact is very important, especially for forensic cases where everything counts. It is usually found in research that burn recovery involves many different types of cells and chemical signals working together. For example, Single-cell ATAC sequencing has picked out several distinct cell subsets playing key roles in putting the skin back together, which underscores just how complex dermal healing can be (Wang et al., 2025). Then there's the issue of complications like healthcare-associated infections (HAIs) that tend to drag recovery along, making a thorough forensic investigation necessary to sort out causes and figure out who's responsible in medical settings. Sorting out claims tied to these problems typically calls for genuine forensic know-how that can navigate those tricky compensation systems effectively (Paola et al., 2025).

11.2.8. Long-term Effects of Thermal Injuries

Burn injuries usually mean more than just a hospital stay; they can cause lasting health and mental problems. Some people have to deal with pain that never really goes away and skin that is too sensitive which can interfere with their daily routine. Not all the damage is physical; many people also have to deal with mental problems which can lead to PTSD, anxiety or depression and change the way they see themselves or interact with others. Often, recovery requires using several pain relief methods, doing some physical therapy and getting mental support and these things usually work together in a way that can't be predicted. At times, the effects that last after a trauma can be important in forensic investigations by showing whether an injury was caused by accident or on purpose. To summarize, getting to grips with how deep and varied these repercussions can be is crucial for both treatment teams and forensic experts alike (Figure 11.11).

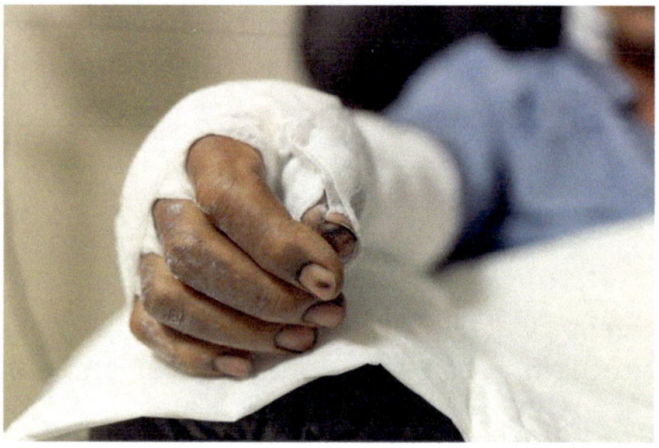

Figure 11.11. Burn injuries don't just end with a hospital stay—they often bring along a whole array of long-lasting body and mind troubles.

Source: https://www.rosnerlaw.net/images/blog/iStock-1400527321.2402091556550.jpg.

11.2.9. Forensic Implications of Injury Mechanisms

You never know how serious a thermal burn will be, since they can be just a minor scorch or a severe injury and they are not easy to figure out in forensic cases. Such injuries give hints about the case and also create many difficulties for experts trying to interpret them. Not every burn is caused the same way; some are from heat, some from chemicals and some from electricity, so each needs to be investigated differently. Recent work even suggests that checking out the volatile organic compounds (VOCs) released during a burn (Nńska et al., 2021) can help signal what kind of blaze occurred and where the heat came from. And in most cases, understanding how natural substances, like cannabinoids, play with tissues turns out to be pretty key in rounding out the overall forensic picture (Pellati et al., 2018).

Test Your Knowledge

1. What is meant by the mechanism of thermal injury?
2. How does dry heat (e.g., flame) cause tissue damage?

11.3. Forensic Analysis of Thermal Injuries

Learning Outcome

1. Learn identification of burn patterns;
2. Describe how forensic pathology helps with thermal injuries;
3. Identify techniques for documenting injuries;
4. Explain the use of photography and imaging;
5. Know the importance of witness statements;
6. Give correlation with other forensic evidence;
7. Identify challenges in assessing thermal injuries;
8. Know legal considerations in forensic analysis;
9. Focus on case studies of forensic investigations.

Investigating burns in forensic cases isn't always cut-and-dry. This often means looking at the obvious and then closely examining things under a microscope. Some veterinary studies, for instance, have shown that keeping an eye on carbon monoxide levels—by leaning on COHb checks alongside standard tissue exams—can point us in the right direction when determining fire-related deaths (Piegari et al., 2024). Sorting out if burns occurred while breathing or after death is important and recent studies indicate that oxidative stress markers can help a lot. One study even noted that higher malondialdehyde levels coupled with shifts in gene expression seem linked to heat damage, which in turn can help forensic experts figure out the timing of injuries (Habotta et al., 2023). Mixing these new methods, analysts are often able to build a clearer picture of what caused the thermal injuries which offers more information about the events.

11.3.1. Identification of Burn Patterns

Usually, investigators first examine the marks that are left from the burn. Burns may tell us about the intensity and duration of the heat exposure. An example is that water-like marks can show that an accelerant was used and burned spots may indicate where the person was when the fire started. Elemental tests on debris are conducted as usual and can usually discover small amounts of certain substances which adds more information to the investigation. Even with all the recent advances in forensic techniques, there's still a fair share of challenges; variability in how human skin reacts to heat and the ongoing search for standard protocols keep investigators on their toes (Armstrong et al., 2018; Rocchi et al., 2020) (Figure 11.12).

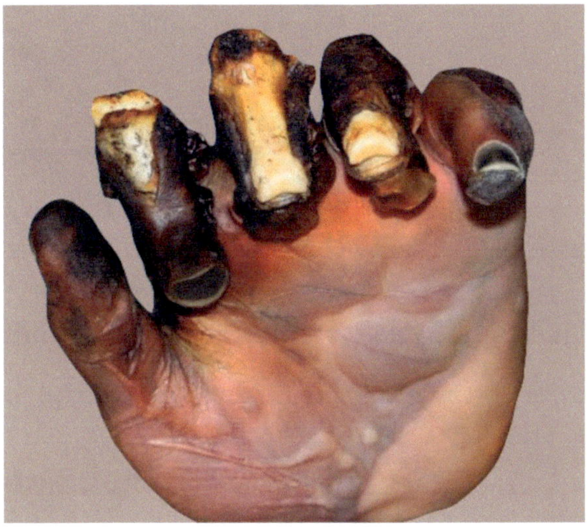

Figure 11.12. Identification of burn patterns.

Source: By goga312 at Russian Wikipedia, CC BY-SA 3.0, https://commons.wikimedia.org/w/index.php?curid=7771672.

11.3.2. Role of Forensic Pathology in Thermal Injuries

Thermal injuries are not handled using a single set of steps; instead, many approaches, some unexpected, are needed to help forensic pathology. For example, pathologists study the details of burns to tell if they happened before or after the person died. They investigate the effects of heat on the victim, check for repeated injuries and try to notice any health problems that may have changed the outcome. Usually, these investigations are not straightforward: details may appear again in different sections of the investigation. In many cases, post-mortem computed tomography (PMCT) turns out to be a pretty neat tool since it can expose skeletal injuries that aren't obvious by usual means (Lawler et al., 2023). Even though a carbon monoxide check is somewhat redundant, it adds more information to what happened. All of these pieces, when combined, help forensic experts offer insights that are key to nailing down causes of death; these conclusions not only support legal probes but also go a long way toward giving families a sense of closure (Beattie et al., 2018) (Figure 11.13).

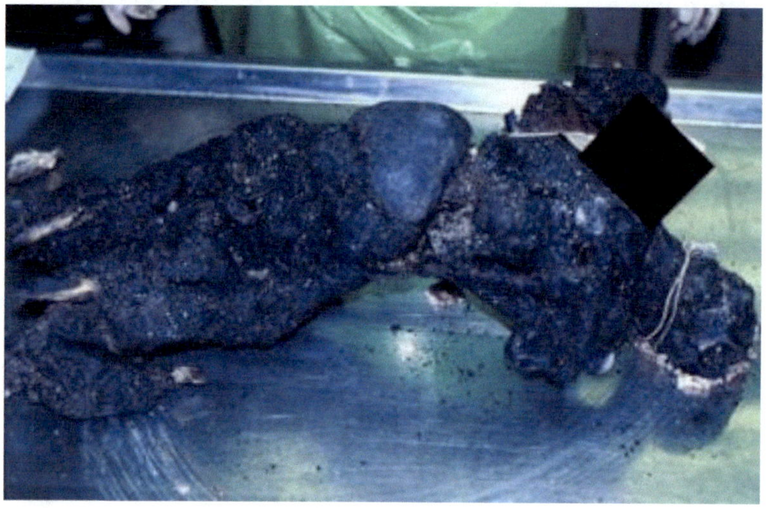

Figure 11.13. Role of forensic pathology in thermal injuries.

Source: https://img.medscapestatic.com/pi/meds/ckb/46/13146tn.jpg.

11.3.3. Techniques for Documenting Injuries

Heat injuries matter—a lot. Noticing reactions to heat is important in forensics because it affects the reading of evidence and the results of legal cases. Experts assess these injuries by looking at the overall scene and by closely examining all the details, using well-known methods to determine how much damage there is. Scientists often find cellular harm in tissues when they use a microscope, since heat-related changes are sometimes hard to notice without special tools. Engineers are also involved, offering explanations about how the injuries happen, mainly when explosions are involved. Generally, research reveals that blast injuries have certain characteristics such as internal bleeding and harmed muscles and so full documentation is necessary for proper forensic reporting. Together, these mixed approaches boost how reliable the conclusions are in cases of heat-related harm, keeping pace with the latest trends in forensic science and engineering (Fındık, 2024; Mykhaylenko et al., 2024).

11.3.4. Use of Photography and Imaging

Thermal injuries can cause forensic work and imaging technology to work in ways that are not always expected. Infrared (IR) photography, for example, lets experts pick up on subtle heat changes—tricky clues that help sort out different burn levels and other types of trauma. What stands out is that IR can reveal tiny temperature shifts on surfaces that generally match injury severity, making it a handy asset in an investigation (Asirdizer et al., 2016). If you use UV light in a different technique, it can help find hematomas that are not always visible. Research generally shows that UV-induced fluorescence brings out differences in tissue health even well past the initial incident, which in turn sharpens the accuracy of injury documentation (Glauche et al., 2017). To summarize, these imaging advances not only bolster evidentiary support but also deepen our overall grasp of trauma in forensic cases (Figure 11.14).

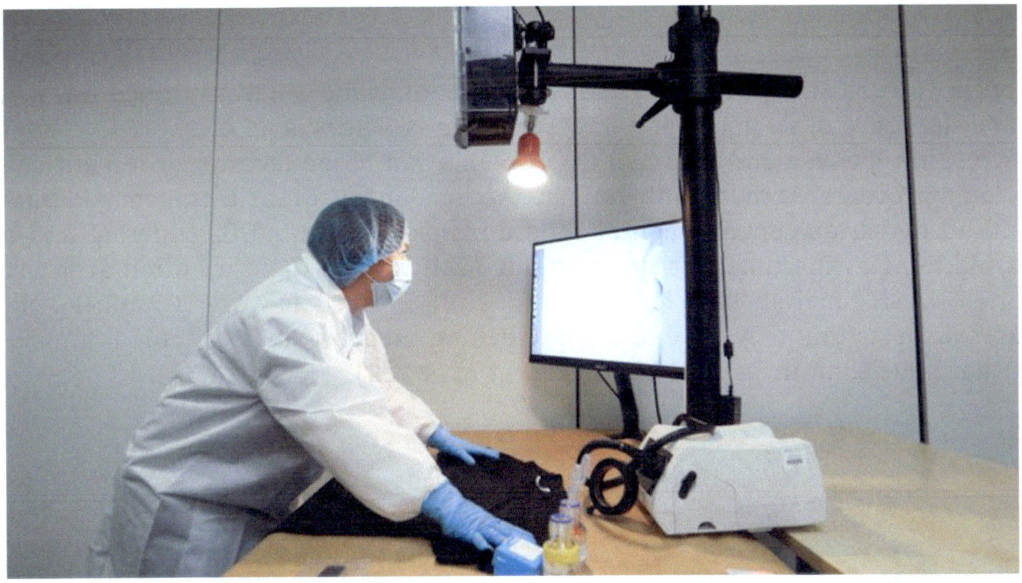

Figure 11.14. Forensic work and imaging tech often mix in unexpected ways when dealing with thermal injuries.

Source: https://e3.365dm.com/22/03/768x432/skynews-blood-forensics_5707919.jpg?20220316054701.

11.3.5. Importance of Witness Statements

What eyewitnesses say is very influential in burn investigations and it's not treated as minor information. In a lot of cases, people's personal stories help us understand the sequence of events as well as the important details that were repeated. A direct report could also mention how a victim came into contact with fire or heat which can be very important when deciding on the type and severity of the thermal injuries. Also, anyone present may mention if any safety steps were taken or describe what others were doing which can be very important when dealing with lawsuits.

11.3.6. Correlation with Other Forensic Evidence

Sometimes, investigators find that burns and other forensic signs become mixed in ways that are not expected. Checking for VOCs as well as heat injuries can help you notice things you may not have seen before. For example, Nńska et al. (2021) show us a broad spread of VOCs gathered from various bodily fluids, patterns that sometimes seem connected with conditions from heat exposure. It is fascinating —these bodily fluids and their markers are often signs of bigger stories. Then there's another twist: microRNAs (miRNAs), which, thanks to their stability and distinct patterns in fluids, add another layer to how we link heat injuries with biological evidence. In most cases, as Rocchi et al. (2020) point out, using these miRNAs as biomarkers helps in figuring out wound vitality and getting a rough time of death. All these bits of evidence are used together to explain what could have happened and to improve how thermal injury cases are understood in law. All in all, the mix of different kinds of forensic data proves that a detailed, occasionally messy process is necessary.

11.3.7. Challenges in Assessing Thermal Injuries

Assessing burns isn't as straightforward as it might seem. Many different things can make it hard to understand the cause of an injury and how serious it is. There is no one way for people to react to heat, since skin type, age and past health problems can all be factors, so it's difficult to know how much damage occurs. At that point, you need to look at the forensic aspects and burn patterns can be confused by various environmental conditions. Sometimes, VOCs show up and offer hints about the conditions at the time, yet the methods used to pick them up often aren't reliable for every material, which generally calls for extra validation in forensic work (Drabińska et al., 2021). In many cases, experts find they have to keep tweaking their methods to truly untangle the story behind thermal injuries in investigations (Lykou et al., 2020) (Figure 11.15).

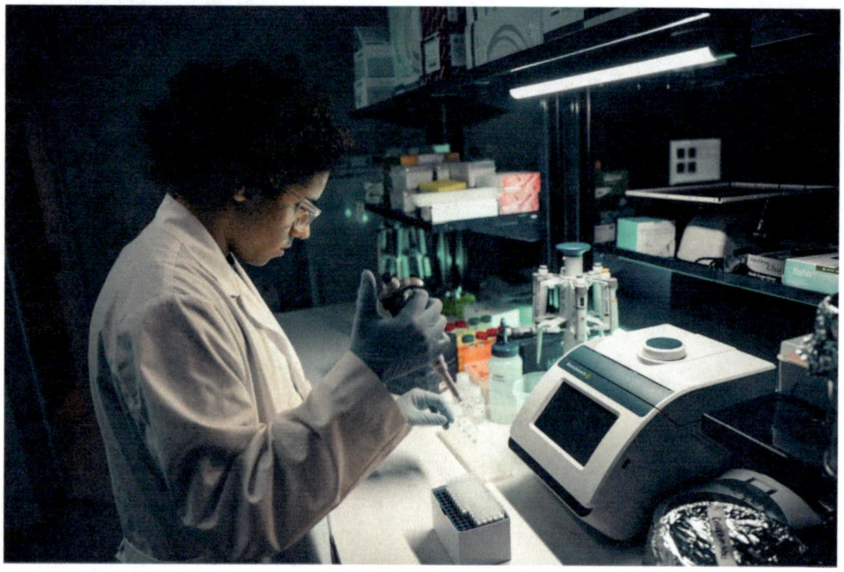

Figure 11.15. People respond to heat in wildly different ways—skin type, age, and even earlier health setbacks all play their part—making it tough to nail down a standard degree of damage.

Source: https://erau.edu/-/media/images/university/becoming-a-student/omics-2.jpg?as=0&hash =14A1D1961C22B31719F5D4C1C884EA9E.

11.3.8. Legal Considerations in Forensic Analysis

Heat-related injuries often bring together aspects of the law and the work of forensic experts in unpredictable ways. If the chain of custody for PMCT scans is strong, the evidence can be very influential in a court of law. In most cases, PMCT does a good job of flagging bone fractures linked to high temperatures, but it doesn't cover everything; that's why toxicological analyses are often brought along to fill in the gaps concerning a fire-related death (Lawler et al., 2023). Meticulous note-taking and a firm, albeit occasionally slightly off, commitment to forensic protocols go a long way to cushion against potential legal blows and keep findings trustworthy (Davis et al., 2025). In general, as laws and forensic science progress, experts have to be aware and ensure their work is scientifically sound and meets legal requirements so that justice for thermal trauma cases is served well.

11.3.9. Case Studies of Forensic Investigations

Forensic study of fatal burns often shows surprising facts about the well-being of the public and the state of society as a whole. Some case studies in places like St. Petersburg seem to show a drop in violent deaths, including burns, which might be linked, in most cases, to shifts in the local economy and health conditions (Bozhchenko et al., 2022). Research coming out of Johannesburg, on the other hand, points to a higher risk for fatal burns among young males and even hints at some seasonal ups and downs in these incidents (Keyes et al., 2021). It shows that we should always look at forensic information together with what is happening in society. Experts can use case studies to notice risks, develop better ways to prevent fires and influence safety policies and measures to prevent injuries. All in all, this flexible and slightly random way of working highlights the main role that forensic investigations have in helping to tackle thermal injuries in many communities.

Test Your Knowledge

1. What forensic features help distinguish antemortem from postmortem burns?
2. How can the appearance of blisters help show if a burn happened before the person died?

11.4. Psychological and Social Implications

Learning Outcome

1. Know the psychological impact on victims;
2. Explain societal perceptions of burn victims;
3. Identify the role of support systems in recovery;
4. Focus on stigmatization and discrimination;
5. Describe the legal ramifications for perpetrators;
6. Learn the public health implications of thermal injuries;
7. Identify education and prevention strategies;
8. Perform advocacy for burn victims;
9. Discuss case studies highlighting social issues.

Thermal injuries have effects on the skin and also on a person's emotions and place in society. Many survivors of severe burns or heat trauma experience PTSD, anxiety and depression which can affect their recovery. Since these situations usually come up unexpectedly, many people find themselves alone, dealing with changes in their self-image and facing old social labels. At the same time, family bonds are often weakened and people find that their relationships and support networks are under more pressure than usual. Experts in forensics usually point out that a person's emotions can change their statements and the accuracy of the evidence. Overall, getting a handle on these wider implications is key to building an environment that truly supports healing and rebuilding, thus helping forensic teams offer more rounded care and support to those affected (Galante et al., 2021).

11.4.1. Psychological Impact on Victims

Thermal burns leave scars on the body and also leave psychological wounds that are difficult to heal. Most survivors of these events often have to deal with mental health problems such as PTSD, anxiety and depression which may persist for a long time after their injuries heal. At times, this inner struggle appears without warning, making someone have frequent nightmares, sudden flashbacks and become more sensitive to daily stresses which affects their daily routines and relationships. Explosions, for example, stir up a particularly unique stress response, with the shock of the event triggering reactions that seem almost different in nature (Galante et al., 2021). Also, the continuous mental pressure may make it tougher for the patient to recover as planned. For these reasons, a solid support system—often including mental health counselling—is usually seen as essential to help individuals navigate both physical recoveries and the messy, lingering emotional aftereffects, easing their step back into society (Clarysse et al., 2019) (Figure 11.16).

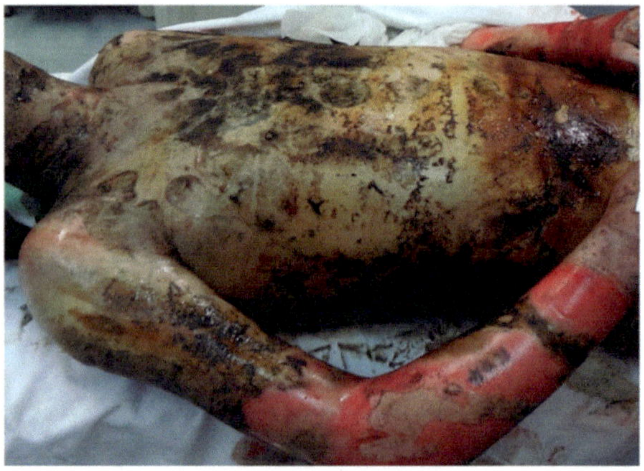

Figure 11.16. Thermal injuries don't just leave marks on the skin—they also etch deep, lasting wounds into a person's psyche.

Source: Żwierełło, Wojciech, Krzysztof Piorun, Marta Skórka-Majewicz, Agnieszka Maruszewska, Jacek Antoniewski, and Izabela Gutowska. 2023. "Burns: Classification, Pathophysiology, and Treatment: A Review" *International Journal of Molecular Sciences* 24, no. 4: 3749. https://doi.org/10.3390/ijms24043749.

11.4.2. Societal Perceptions of Burn Victims

The way society sees burn survivors covers up many layers of stigma and misunderstanding that are not easy to notice. Burn victims find that the problems they deal with are not only physical; how others view them can greatly affect their treatment. A lot of cultural stories present these individuals as people who suffer which usually leads to their feeling more isolated. Seeing the clear, often shocking marks from their injuries can make people uncomfortable or afraid which actually decreases understanding and increases loneliness. In discussions on international law targeting, it's often noted that a person's visual presence can strongly affect both legal processes and day-to-day social ties, hinting that burn visibility may indeed push them further to the margins (Parsa, 2023). Increased advocacy and education, generally speaking, are crucial for softening these harsh perceptions and building a more welcoming society, especially when the risks linked with these injuries reflect broader social attitudes (Duffey et al., 2020).

11.4.3. Role of Support Systems in Recovery

A burn injury is not easily treated with just medicine—usually, it requires a lot of medical help and emotional support. Actually, these injuries are handled by treating the physical issues and also planning for a long-term recovery so that daily life can be resumed slowly. Usually, a number of professionals—doctors, psychologists, social workers and sometimes others from the community—work on different aspects of recovery, each with their own ideas. With teamwork, many people can stick to their treatment plans and manage ongoing issues such as anxiety or PTSD that might appear after a trauma. Having family and community around often means the difference when recovery seems hard. As studies suggest , these supportive networks, by encouraging personal resilience, play an essential role in how well someone bounces back from thermal injuries—even when seen through the lens of forensic care (Lykou et al., 2020; Nńska et al., 2021) (Figure 11.17).

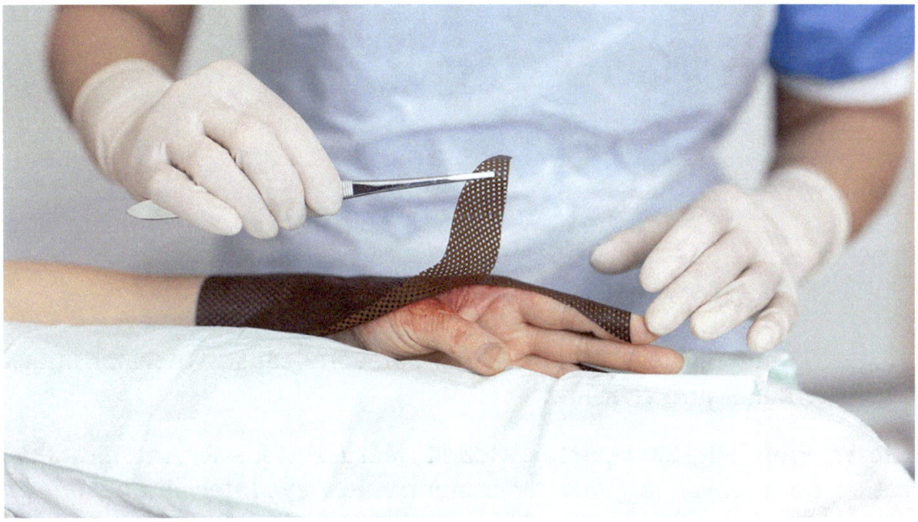

Figure 11.17. Recovering from a burn isn't as simple as just treating the wound—it usually means having many strong medical care and real emotional support.

Source: https://www.molnlycke.com/contentassets/935e8fa408f44c278fbb8b68ff2dfa3b/burns-8382-29_16-9_1200px.png.

11.4.4. Stigmatization and Discrimination

Having a thermal injury often brings social biases along with the pain which can seriously influence a person's life. A lot of the time, people who suffer from severe burns or other heat-related injuries must deal with the pain and also with being stigmatized which makes both their recovery and legal actions more difficult. Sometimes, the way media reports these injuries can make them seem more dramatic than they really are which only strengthens old, negative views of burn victims and forces them to stay on the margins of society. Being labeled in this way often affects a person's mental state and usually interferes with their ability to get proper legal attention. As noted in recent forensic writings, the ever-changing world of forensic science generally calls for fresh, innovative approaches to tackle these social issues, aiming to ease both the stigma and discrimination seen in medical and legal settings (Deo et al., 2022).

11.4.5. Legal Ramifications for Perpetrators

When there are thermal injuries, it is important to look at the rules of criminal and civil law. The court has to look at the facts and the reason for the act—was it just carelessness, a sudden outburst or deliberate cruelty?

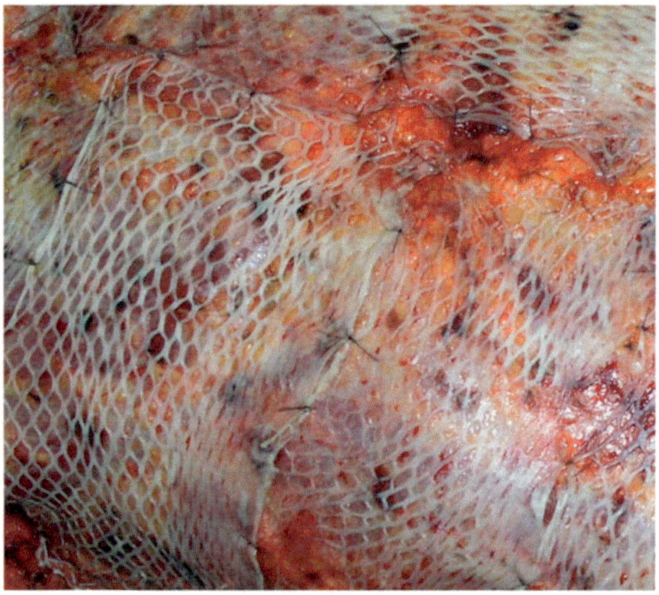

Figure 11.18. Figuring out the legal fallout when someone causes thermal injuries demands a careful look at both criminal and civil law.

Source: Żwierełło W, Piorun K, Skórka-Majewicz M, Maruszewska A, Antoniewski J, Gutowska I. Burns: Classification, Pathophysiology, and Treatment: A Review. *International Journal of Molecular Sciences*. 2023; 24(4):3749. https://doi.org/10.3390/ijms24043749.

Every case usually has its own penalties which may involve fines or time in prison. If a crime is civil in nature, the victim may try to recover compensation for their medical bills and pain which can create more problems for the offender in both money and emotions. Since cyber threats are always evolving, it's becoming obvious that laws need to be updated which means legislators have to balance safety with personal freedoms. Ultimately, these legal moves are meant to serve as a deterrent, encouraging potential wrongdoers to pause and reconsider actions that could lead to severe consequences, especially when cyber issues intersect with overall public safety (Singh et al., 2022) (Figure 11.18).

11.4.6. Public Health Implications of Thermal Injuries

Thermal injuries are increasing which is more than just about treating the wounds quickly. Because of environmental dangers, risks at work and even small accidents at home, we keep seeing a rise in accidents which requires us to update our prevention and care strategies. Fire safety education and proper training in handling hot substances should also be part of public health efforts, not only dealing with emergencies and rehabilitation. It's interesting how new tools, like 3D printing in forensic labs, help piece together the story behind these injuries—this added insight can lead to more precise reconstructions and even extend to improved predictive models for future cases (Carew et al., 2020). In many cases, these technological advances show that forensic science and public health are, in a way, wedded together, nudging us toward a more collaborative stance to ease the long-term impacts of thermal injuries on our communities (Jannetto et al., 2018).

11.4.7. Education and Prevention Strategies

Thermal injuries aren't as straightforward as they might appear. There are many challenges involved which require different educational and prevention measures. Local police and the community should also play a role, not just the doctors.

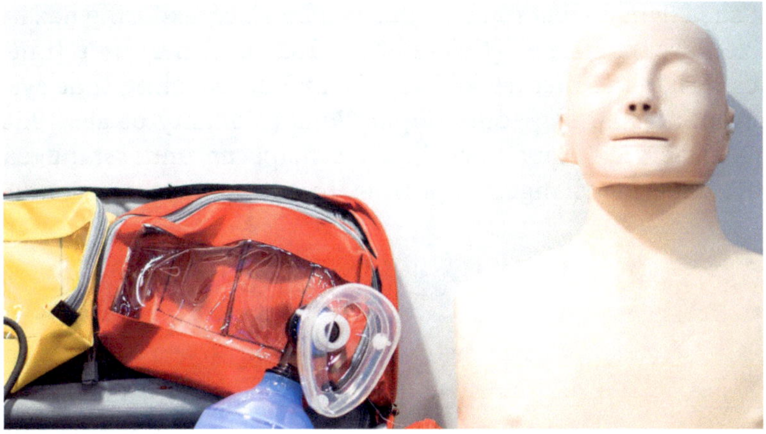

Figure 11.19. Understanding the warning signals and fallout of burns, along with getting a feel for the ins and outs of forensic checks, can change how emergencies are handled in most cases.

Source: https://www.cprclassesoakland.org/wp-content/uploads/2023/03/can-you-preform-cpr-on-a-burn-victim.jpg.

Being aware of the signs and consequences of burns, as well as knowing how to carry out forensic checks, can alter the way most emergencies are dealt with. Actually practicing how to spot burns can really help people act fast in any emergency. If public health campaigns target those who are most likely to suffer burns, they might stop burns before they happen. And if you bring your community into the learning process, it helps create a more alert, ready-to-react group, which fits in with broader trauma plans that lean on layered prevention efforts (Beck et al., 2019; Egger et al., 2022) (Figure 11.19).

11.4.8. Advocacy for Burn Victims

Burns can have a strong impact on a person's feelings and relationships which is often not recognized by others. Investigations often find that severe burns get tangled up with broader problems; for instance, dowry-related tragedies show how cultural and family pressures can intensify a victim's suffering (Kumar et al., 2024). It is obvious from these connections that burn victims are in a risky situation which usually means they need fair laws and strong support from the community. In many cases, burns account for a significant slice of injury-related deaths, signalling that focused efforts to raise awareness and prevention are essential (Verma, 2024). Advocacy efforts should, therefore, make sure communities know the risks of thermal injuries and work towards improving laws to safeguard those who might be hurt. Even if the changes happen slowly, society can make things better for burn victims and help them recover.

11.4.9. Case Studies Highlighting Social Issues

From studying many case studies, it becomes clear that the issues in society and forensic investigations can easily get mixed up when thermal injuries are part of the situation. A review of these examples often reveals that the way these injuries happen can be linked to a person's social and economic situation such as through unsafe housing and missing safety precautions in struggling areas. For instance, looking at measurements of VOCs—which serve as little clues about chemical presence in an environment—can shed light on where these burns take place, exposing hazardous conditions that tend to hit marginalized groups harder (Nńska et al., 2021). At the same time, when catastrophic events like pandemics strike, the picture seems to expand, revealing that systemic shortcomings further worsen vulnerabilities among some populations (Mohanty et al., 2020). All in all, joining social factors with forensic studies of burn injuries helps us understand each case better and strongly points out the need for changes in policies to address these essential problems.

Test Your Knowledge

1. What are the usual psychological reactions people have after getting severe burns?
2. What part does body image disturbance have in the recovery of burn survivors?

Summary

In a lot of forensic investigations, thermal injuries highlight the need for hospitals to re-examine their safety procedures. With over 3,500 incidents and some of them being fatal, we see that operating rooms are not safe and monopolar diathermy is often responsible for the problems. Because of these serious statistics, we must think of better ways to keep both patients and staff safe. It's also worth noting that insights from groups such as the General Directorate of National Security (Matadi et al., 2025) remind us that risks are wrapped up in broader social and cultural factors, too. All in all, a combination of tough training, creating clear guidelines and increasing awareness is important to decrease these accidents in hospitals.

Investigating thermal burns in crimes is not as simple as you might expect because there are many aspects to consider. Instead of just saying a burn is light or heavy, they can be anything from a mild scald to something serious and each type can bring its own set of problems to solve. They cause immediate medical harm, but they also give signs that might influence the outcome of the case as accidental or deliberate. You end up looking at everything: how hot the source was, how long someone was pushed into the heat, and even how each person's body seems to react, with these factors coming together (in most cases) to help experts put the puzzle together. New ways to read burn marks, albeit slowly, keep nudging the field forward, and when you throw in the way heat interacts with the surroundings, it becomes pretty clear that bringing together different kinds of expertise is key (Joseph et al., 2023; Stokes et al., 2023).

KEY TERMS FROM THIS CHAPTER

Age	Anxiety	Biological evidence
Bodily fluids	Caution	Conduction
Convection	Depression	Eyewitness
Hematomas	Radiation	Survivors
Validation	Volatile organic compounds (VOCs)	

Short Answer Questions

1. Differentiate between scalds and flame burns.
2. What is a contact burn and what are the signs that show it?
3. What do curling's ulcers involve and when are they seen in burn patients?
4. Name two cold-related injuries and briefly describe them.
5. Heat hematoma is a different condition from traumatic intracranial hemorrhage.
6. What are postmortem heat fractures and how can they be told apart from antemortem fractures?
7. What forensic clues help differentiate antemortem from postmortem burns?

Critical Thinking Questions

1. Which of these is a good sign of burns before death?

a. Charring of skin
b. Pugilistic attitude
c. Line of redness
d. Burned clothing

2. Which of the below is not a form of thermal injury?

a. Flame burn
b. Scald burn
c. Frostbite
d. Contusion

3. At what level of burn does the skin become completely damaged and nerve endings are destroyed?

a. First-degree
b. Second-degree
c. Third-degree
d. Fourth-degree

4. Soot in the trachea and bronchi means:

a. Death occurred before the fire
b. Inhalation of toxic gases postmortem
c. Inhalation while alive
d. Electrical burns

5. Heat rupture is most likely to be confused with:

a. Abrasion
b. Laceration

c. Incised wound

d. Gunshot wound

Answers to Critical Thinking Questions

1. (c); 2. (d); 3. (c); 4. (c); 5. (b)

References

1. Albaladejo, F. R., Soriano, B. J., & Gitto, L. (2024). Analysis of unique atypical screwdriver injuries. *Journal of Forensic Sciences*, *69*(6), 2302–2307. https://doi.org/10.1111/1556-4029.15610.
2. Alfsdotter, C. (2021). Forensic archaeology and forensic anthropology within Swedish law enforcement: Current state and suggestions for future developments. *Forensic Science International Reports*, *3*, 100178. https://doi.org/10.1016/j.fsir.2021.100178.
3. Armstrong, E. J., & Erskine, K. L. (2018). Investigation of drowning deaths: A practical review. *Academic Forensic Pathology*, *8*, 8–43. https://doi.org/10.23907/2018.002.
4. Asirdizer, M., Gumus, O., & Hekimoglu, Y. (2016). Usage of infrared-based technologies in forensic sciences. https://core.ac.uk/download/322426315.pdf (accessed on 29 May 2025).
5. Atkinson, G., Cowpe, E., Halliday, J., & Painter, D. (2017). A review of very large vapor cloud explosions: Cloud formation and explosion severity. *Journal of Loss Prevention in the Process Industries, 48*, 367–375. https://doi.org/10.1016/j.jlp.2017.03.021.
6. Baker, C., Nugent, B., Grainger, D., Hewis, J., & Malamateniou, C. (2024). Systematic review of MRI safety literature in relation to radiofrequency thermal injury prevention. *Journal of Medical Radiation Sciences*, *71*, 445–460. https://www.semanticscholar.org/paper/cab0e33de248a68c797a5f9fddf135019ffb178b (accessed on 29 May 2025).
7. Beattie, E., Fraser, J., MacPhee, N., Milne, et al. (2018). A comparison of penetration and damage caused by different types of arrowheads on loose and tight fit clothing. https://core.ac.uk/download/228178194.pdf (accessed on 29 May 2025).
8. Beck, B., Smith, K., Mercier, É., Gabbe, B. J., Bassed, R., Mitra, B., Teague, W. J., et al. (2019). Differences in the epidemiology of out-of-hospital and in-hospital trauma deaths. *PLoS ONE*, *14*, e0217158. https://doi.org/10.1371/journal.pone.0217158.
9. Bozhchenko, A. P., Isakov, V. D., Yagmurov, O. D., Yakovenko, O. O., & Nazarov, Y. V. (2022). Dynamics and structure of forensic medical investigations of violent death in St. Petersburg over the past 10 years. *Russian Journal of Forensic Medicine*, *8*, 37–46. https://doi.org/10.17816/fm694.
10. Broussard, J. R. (2016). Equipment for dying: A dramatistic critique of heroism and the crises assaulting returning soldiers [Doctoral dissertation, University Name]. https://doi.org/10.31390/gradschool_dissertations.103.
11. Carew, R. M., & Errickson, D. (2020). An overview of 3D printing in forensic science: The tangible third-dimension. *Journal of Forensic Sciences*, *65*, 1752–1760. https://doi.org/10.1111/1556-4029.14442.

12. Cattaneo, C., Tambuzzi, S., De Vecchi, S., Maggioni, L., & Costantino, G. (2023). Consequences of the lack of clinical forensic medicine in emergency departments. *International Journal of Legal Medicine, 138*, 139–150. https://doi.org/10.1007/s00414-023-02973-8.

13. Chukwu-Lobelu, R., Appukuttan, A., Edwards, D. S., & Patel, H. D. L. (2017). Burn injuries from the London suicide bombings: A new classification of blast-related thermal injuries. *Annals of Burns and Fire Disasters, 30*(4), 256–260.

14. Clarysse, K., Grosber, M., Ring, J., Gutermuth, J., & Kivlahan, C. (2019). Skin lesions, differential diagnosis and practical approach to potential survivors of torture. *Journal of the European Academy of Dermatology and Venereology, 33*, 1232–1240. https://doi.org/10.1111/jdv.15439.

15. Cláudia-Ferreira, A., Barbosa, D. J., Saegeman, V., Fernández-Rodríguez, A., Dinis-Oliveira, R. J., & Freitas, A. R. (2023). The future is now: Unraveling the expanding potential of human (necro) microbiome in forensic investigations. *Microorganisms, 11*, 2509. https://doi.org/10.3390/microorganisms11102509.

16. Das, N. G., Das, N., & Sil, A. (2025). Pattern and forensic significance of defense injuries in homicide cases: A cross-sectional study. *Cureus, 17*. https://www.semanticscholar.org/paper/b220d59af690d815386e317b288a0dd397b6051b (accessed on 29 May 2025).

17. Davis, J. R., Lane, H. W., & Stepaniak, P. C. (2025). Loss of signal: Aeromedical lessons learned from the STS-107 Columbia space shuttle mishap. https://core.ac.uk/download/pdf/42730063.pdf (accessed on 29 May 2025).

18. De Paola, L., Napoletano, G., Di Fazio, N., Marinelli, S., & Rinaldi, R. (2025). Healthcare associated infections: European comparative analysis and forensic expertise in compensation systems. *La Clinica Terapeutica, 176*(Suppl 1(2)), 59–65. https://www.semanticscholar.org/paper/e08e621ad4db54805441cd2126d50167eced0b3a (accessed on 29 May 2025).

19. Deo, N., & Singh, A. (2022). Cybersecurity and sustainable development. https://doi.org/10.55662/book.2022ccrs.009.

20. Doukas, D. (2022). Non-accidental injuries in dogs and cats: Review of post-mortem forensic evaluations and the social significance of small animal practice. *Journal of the Hellenic Veterinary Medical Society*, *73*, 3543–3552. https://doi.org/10.12681/jhvms.23296.

21. Dowd, W., & Kültz, D. (2024). Lost in translation? Evidence for a muted proteomic response to thermal stress in a stenothermal Antarctic fish and possible evolutionary mechanisms. *Physiological Genomics*. https://www.semanticscholar.org/paper/1535ed33100cd3f17d84a81a07e695934313763b (accessed on 29 May 2025).

22. Drabińska, N., Flynn, C., Ratcliffe, N., Belluomo, I., Myridakis, A., Gould, O., Fois, M., et al. (2021). A literature survey of all volatiles from healthy human breath and bodily fluids: The human volatilome. *Journal of Breath Research, 15*, 034001. https://doi.org/10.1088/1752-7163/abf1d0.

23. Duffey, R. B., & D'Auria, F. S. (2020). Nuclear energy and its history: Past consequences, present inadequacies and a perspective for success. *Energy and Power Engineering, 12*, 193–236. https://doi.org/10.4236/epe.2020.126014

24. Egger, J., Gsaxner, C., Pepe, A., Pomykala, K. L., Jonske, F., Kurz, M., Li, J., et al. (2022). Medical deep learning—A systematic meta-review. *Computer Methods and Programs in Biomedicine, 221*, 106874. https://doi.org/10.1016/j.cmpb.2022.106874.

25. Findik, F. (2024). Forensic materials and test methods. *Sustainable Engineering and Innovation, 6*(1), 103–118.
26. Fonollosa, J., Solórzano, A., & Marco, S. (2018). Chemical sensor systems and associated algorithms for fire detection: A review. *Sensors, 18*, 553. https://doi.org/10.3390/s18020553.
27. Gagliardi, S., Poloni, T. E., Pandini, C., Garofalo, M., Dragoni, F., Medici, V., Davin, A., et al. (2021). Detection of SARS-CoV-2 genome and whole transcriptome sequencing in frontal cortex of COVID-19 patients. *Brain, Behavior, and Immunity, 97*, 13–21. https://doi.org/10.1016/j.bbi.2021.05.012.
28. Galante, N., Franceschetti, L., Del Sordo, S., Casali, M. B., & Genovese, U. (2021). Explosion-related deaths: An overview on forensic evaluation and implications. *Forensic Science, Medicine, and Pathology, 17*, 437–448. https://doi.org/10.1007/s12024-021-00383-z.
29. Gardner, R. M., & Krouskup, D. R. (2018). *Practical Crime Scene Processing and Investigation*. CRC Press. https://doi.org/10.4324/9781315170596.
30. Glauche, J. (2017). Examination of invisible injuries: UV-induced fluorescence as a supplement to physical examination for blunt trauma injury. https://core.ac.uk/download/226126879.pdf (accessed on 29 May 2025).
31. Grukhovskiy, S. V., Velenko, P. S., Bychkov, A. A., Marchenkov, R. E., Globa, I. V., Berezovskiy, D. P., & Barinov, E. K. (2024). Forensic medical analysis of head injuries in drivers sustaining fatal in-vehicle trauma. *Russian Journal of Forensic Medicine, 10*(4), 509–516. https://doi.org/10.17816/fm16134.
32. Habotta, O. A., Ateya, A., Abdeen, A., Ibrahim, I., Badawy, M. M., & Zeina, A. M. (2023). Oxidative stress-related biomarkers as forensic biomarkers for burned skin vitality in rats. *Mansoura Veterinary Medical Journal, 24*(3), Article 10. https://doi.org/10.35943/2682-2512.1135.
33. Hunt, H. G. P., Blumenthal, R., Nixon, K., & Gomes, C. (2020). A multidisciplinary forensic analysis of two lightning deaths observed in South Africa. *International Journal of Disaster Risk Reduction, 51*, 101814. https://doi.org/10.1016/j.ijdrr.2020.101814.
34. Jannetto, P. J., Helander, A., Garg, U., Janis, G. C., Goldberger, B. A., & Ketha, H. (2018). The fentanyl epidemic and evolution of fentanyl analogs in the United States and the European Union. *Clinical Chemistry, 65*, 242–253. https://doi.org/10.1373/clinchem.2017.281626.
35. Joseph, D., Ahuja, P., Dockrell, M. E. C., Purchase, D., Price, R., Krishna, S., García-Muñoz, J., et al. (2023). *Trace Metals in the Environment*. IntechOpen eBooks. https://doi.org/10.5772/intechopen.1001530.
36. Kazantsev, R., & Yatsenko, I. (2024). Thanatognomonic substantiation of the forensic veterinary diagnosis in the death of dogs and cats due to hemodynamic disorders and hypoxemia. *Ukrainian Journal of Veterinary Sciences, 15*(2), 66–101. https://doi.org/10.31548/veterinary2.2024.66.
37. Keyes, C. A., & Liphoko, K. L. (2021). Five-year overview of fatal thermal and electrical burns in Johannesburg, South Africa. *South African Journal of Science, 117*. https://doi.org/10.17159/sajs.2021/8288.
38. Koromila, I., & Spyrou, K. J. (2023). Design fire methodology for vehicle spaces onboard ships. *Fire Technology, 59*, 1725–1759. https://doi.org/10.1007/s10694-023-01403-w.

39. Kumar, S., Prasad, K., & Aithal, P. S. (2023). Tech-business analytics in secondary industry sector. *International Journal of Applied Engineering and Management Letters*. https://doi.org/10.47992/ijaeml.2581.7000.0194.

40. Kumar, S., Shubhendu, K., Kumar, S., & Kumar, A. (2024). An insight into dowry deaths: The untold stigma and torment of a social evil. *Cureus*. https://doi.org/10.7759/cureus.76348.

41. Lawler, H., & Sanderson, S. (2023). Comparing the diagnostic accuracy of post-mortem CT with invasive autopsy in fire-related deaths: A systematic review. https://core.ac.uk/download/587835194.pdf (accessed on 29 May 2025).

42. Layden, J. E., Ghinai, I., Pray, I. W., Kimball, A., Layer, M., Tenforde, M. W., Navon, L., et al. (2019). Pulmonary illness related to e-cigarette use in Illinois and Wisconsin–Final report. *New England Journal of Medicine, 382*(10), 903–916. https://doi.org/10.1056/nejmoa1911614.

43. Lee, J., Sattar, I., Dodd, S., Schimmel, T., Manchikanti, S., Wong, J., & Armour, A. (2025). Assessing housing status of inpatient admissions for thermal injuries: Insights from a Canadian burn unit. *Journal of Burn Care & Research, 46*(Supplement 1), S218. https://www.semanticscholar.org/paper/cf625cedab5d31c52231c2b38fce32c176bcd6a2 (accessed on 29 May 2025).

44. Lu, G., & Fei, B. (2014). Medical hyperspectral imaging: A review. *Journal of Biomedical Optics, 19*, 010901. https://doi.org/10.1117/1.jbo.19.1.010901.

45. Lykou, G., Moustakas, D., & Gritzalis, D. (2020). Defending airports from UAS: A survey on cyber-attacks and counter-drone sensing technologies. *Sensors, 20*, 3537. https://doi.org/10.3390/s20123537.

46. Matadi, B. M., & Abouzahir, H. (2025). Retrospective study of work-related knee injuries: Analysis of 86 cases among the personnel of the General Directorate of National Security received by the Medico-Legal Institute of Casablanca. *Moroccan Forensic & Law*. https://www.semanticscholar.org/paper/35fd37cce0b8589014d9573cc35523c30bddedad (accessed on 29 May 2025).

47. May, T. R. (2010). Fire pattern analysis, junk science, old wives tales, and ipse dixit: Emerging forensic 3D imaging technologies to the rescue? https://core.ac.uk/download/232774036.pdf (accessed on 29 May 2025).

48. Mobayen, M., Ghaffari, M. E., Shahriari, F., Gholamrezaie, S., Haghani Dogahe, Z., & Chakari-Khiavi, A. (2021). The epidemiology and outcome of burn injuries in Iran: A ten-year systematic review and meta-analysis. *Research Square*. https://doi.org/10.21203/rs.3.rs-505860/v1.

49. Mohanty, S. K., Satapathy, A., Naidu, M. M., Mukhopadhyay, S., Sharma, S., Barton, L. M., Stroberg, E., et al. (2020). Severe acute respiratory syndrome coronavirus-2 (SARS-CoV-2) and coronavirus disease 19 (COVID-19)–anatomic pathology perspective on current knowledge. *Diagnostic Pathology, 15*. https://doi.org/10.1186/s13000-020-01017-8.

50. Mykhaylenko, O. V., Mishalov, V. D., Kozlov, S. V., & Varfolomeiev, Y. A. (2024). Forensic characteristics of injuries from thermo-baric explosive device. *Reports of Morphology, 30*(2), 24–30. https://doi.org/10.31393/morphology-journal-2024-30(2)-03.

51. Parsa, A. (2023). *Targeting in International Law* (184 pages, 7 B/W illustrations). Routledge. https://doi.org/10.4324/9781003121947.

52. Pellati, F., Borgonetti, V., Brighenti, V., Biagi, M., Benvenuti, S., & Corsi, L. (2018). *Cannabis sativa* L. and nonpsychoactive cannabinoids: Their chemistry and role against oxidative stress, inflammation, and cancer. *BioMed Research International, 2018*, 1–15. https://doi.

org/10.1155/2018/1691428.

53. Pendray, J. (2016). *The Identification of Blunt Force Trauma in Thermally Altered Remains Using Reconstruction and Computed Tomography* [Master's thesis, Boston University]. https://open.bu.edu/bitstream/2144/16171/1/Pendray_bu_0017N_11138.pdf (accessed on 29 May 2025).

54. Piegari, G., D'aquino, I., Salanti, G. V., Russo, V., De Biase, D., Caccia, G., Carfora, A., et al. (2024). Pathological alterations and COHb evaluations as tools for investigating fire-related deaths in veterinary forensic pathology. *Frontiers in Veterinary Science, 11.* https://www.semanticscholar.org/paper/d80038817779e52da8b577ef0b0f6503c0c0c88c (accessed on 29 May 2025).

55. Qayyum, K., Rehan, M., Arshad, Z., Iqbal, T., Sarwar, M. A., & Mahmood, R. (2024). Seasonal dynamics in burn profiles: A comprehensive analysis at the burn care center, Islamabad. *Journal of Burn Care & Research.* https://www.semanticscholar.org/paper/b2df551474b705a3159076fa28711cc624aece9f (accessed on 29 May 2025).

56. Rocchi, A., Chiti, E., Maiese, A., Turillazzi, E., & Spinetti, I. (2020). MicroRNAs: An update of applications in forensic science. *Diagnostics, 11*, 32. https://doi.org/10.3390/diagnostics11010032.

57. Rodríguez-Gonzálvez, P., Muñoz-Nieto, Á. L., Zancajo-Blázquez, S., et al. (2016). Geomatics and forensic: Progress and challenges. In *Forensic Analysis–From Death to Justice.* InTech. http://dx.doi.org/10.5772/63155.

58. Santos, R. M., Boyd, A. N., Walroth, T., Hall, A., King, J., Ahiskali, A., Walter, E., et al. (2024). A multicenter, retrospective outcome analysis of vancomycin area under the curve versus trough-based dosing strategies in patients with burn or inhalational injuries (MONITOR). *Journal of Burn Care & Research.* https://www.semanticscholar.org/paper/85e08d9a1edeb033e23ec6cc3da3dd88cc5f0e4a (accessed on 29 May 2025).

59. Savioli, G., Ceresa, I. F., Bavestrello Piccini, G., Gri, N., Nardone, A., La Russa, R., Saviano, A., et al. (2023). Hypothermia: Beyond the narrative review—The point of view of emergency physicians and medico-legal considerations. *Journal of Personalized Medicine, 13*, 1690. https://doi.org/10.3390/jpm13121690.

60. Sikora, J. P., Karawani, J., & Sobczak, J. (2023). Neutrophils and the systemic inflammatory response syndrome (SIRS). *International Journal of Molecular Sciences, 24*, 13469. https://doi.org/10.3390/ijms241713469.

61. Singh, V., & Gautam, R. (2022). Cybercrime, security and regulation in India. https://doi.org/10.55662/book.2022ccrs.005.

62. Son, I. G., Na, J. Y., Heo, J. H., & Ko, Y. S. (2024). Deceased male with a cigarette *in situ*: Is this a cadaveric spasm? *Korean Journal of Legal Medicine.* https://www.semanticscholar.org/paper/8de19a208f8e4877fdc0d3f6673c2eb4bec922f4 (accessed on 29 May 2025).

63. St Cloud State University. (2019). *2019 Huskies Showcase Abstracts.* https://core.ac.uk/download/232795819.pdf (accessed on 29 May 2025).

64. Stokes, K., Clark, K. R., Odetade, D., Hardy, M., & Goldberg Oppenheimer, P. (2023). Advances in lithographic techniques for precision nanostructure fabrication in biomedical applications. *Discover Nano, 18.* https://doi.org/10.1186/s11671-023-03938-x.

65. Verma, S. (2024). Profile of autopsy cases at Government Medical College Kanpur: A

retrospective study. *Medico-Legal Update*, *24*, 18–23. https://doi.org/10.37506/5adw7z05.

66. Wang, T., Zhu, B., Lu, J., Guo, X., Li, R., Yuan, Y., Chen, J., et al. (2025). Single-cell chromatin landscapes associated with the burnt skin healing process in rats. *Scientific Data*, *12*(1), 639. https://www.semanticscholar.org/paper/7c7a94966415b2dd5c395bc9e0545c89a87b2b11 (accessed on 29 May 2025).

67. Williams, A. N. (2020). A new classification system for analyzing burned human remains (Master's thesis). University of Montana. https://scholarworks.umt.edu/etd/11564 (accessed on 29 May 2025).

68. Wincoko, W., Yueniwati, Y., Sakti, S., & Ratnawati, R. (2023). The effect of thermal exposure to carbon fiber filament in the thermoreceptor area on the physiological response of hypothermic baby rabbits. *Acta Informatica Medica*, *31*, 92–95. https://www.semanticscholar.org/paper/cd9edc4fff3138ebd712bf1b931805acb016d6f2 (accessed on 29 May 2025).

69. Zissler, A., Stoiber, W., Steinbacher, P., Geißenberger, J., Monticelli, F., & Pittner, S. (2020). Postmortem protein degradation as a tool to estimate the PMI: A systematic review. *Diagnostics*, *10*, 1014. https://doi.org/10.3390/diagnostics10121014.

ASPHYXIAL DEATHS

12

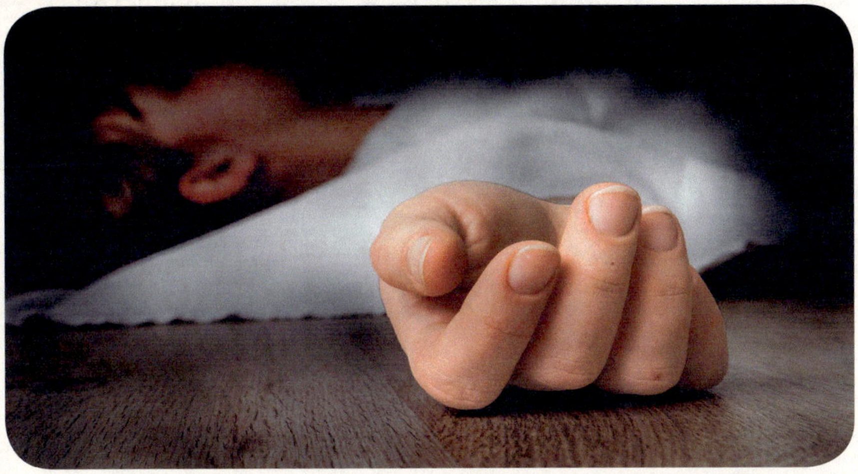

LEARNING OBJECTIVES

After studying this chapter, you will be able to:

1. Identify types of asphyxial deaths;
2. Explain the mechanisms of asphyxia;
3. Learn forensic investigation techniques;
4. Discuss challenges in asphyxial death cases.

Introduction

It is very important in forensics to realize that asphyxial deaths are often messy, so the key is to decide if a drowning was accidental or not. Drowning tragically takes about 362,000 lives each year around the globe, which pretty much shows that, in many cases, investigators need to mix insights from many different fields (Armstrong et al., 2018). Saying just one thing caused it is not enough, because being intoxicated, facing tough environmental conditions or having health issues often happen at the same time. Plus, when you watch how the body reacts during drowning—with immersion and submersion setting off complex heart and lung responses (Bierens et al., 2016)—you see the process is anything but straightforward. All in all, investigating asphyxial deaths closely and honestly helps find the real cause and encourages public health measures to prevent more such events, showing that teamwork is vital in forensic science.

Definition of Asphyxial Deaths

A loss of oxygen can cause a person to go from brain problems to unconsciousness and then death in a short time. Sometimes, something blocks the airway which prevents air from getting to the lungs. For instance, mechanical incidents like hanging (which squeezes the throat) or drowning—where the airway ends up submerged under water—illustrate just a couple of scenarios. A study reviewing 654 autopsies generally revealed that hanging was the most common method among those aged 21–30, while drowning tended to crop up more often in children under 10 (Ghadge et al., 2016). There's also a worrying trend among the youth: engaging in activities informally labeled as the choking game often leads to self-induced oxygen deprivation, and, in most cases, tragic outcomes (Busse et al., 2015). Clearly, understanding these varied ways of cutting off oxygen—crucial for forensic investigations—is key to accurately piecing together the cause and manner of death (Figure 12.1).

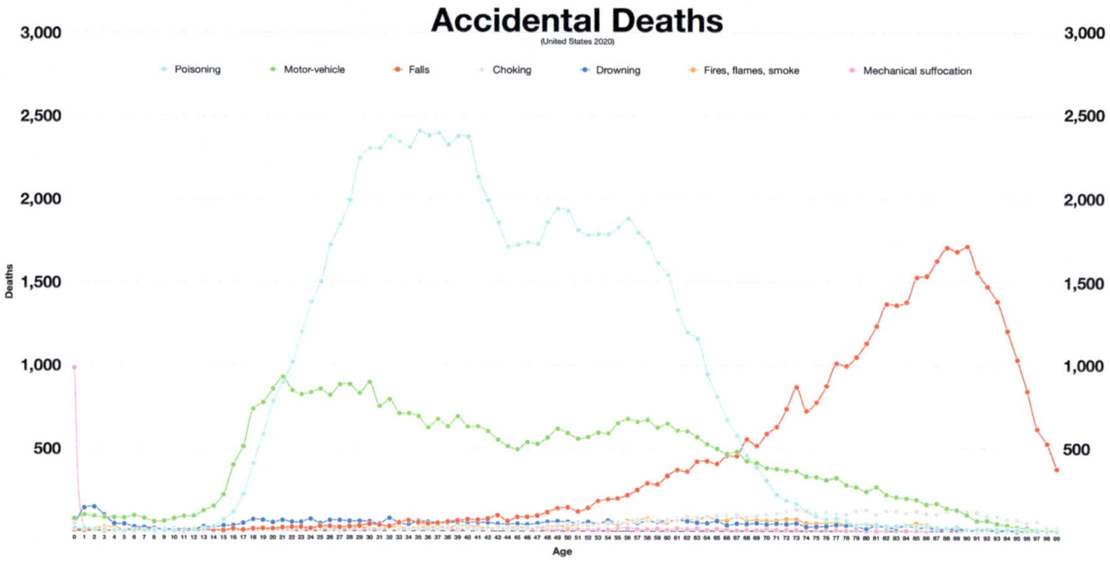

Figure 12.1. Asphyxial deaths.

Source: By Wikideas1 - Own work https://injuryfacts.nsc.org/all-injuries/deaths-by-demographics/deaths-by-age/data-details/, CC0, https://commons.wikimedia.org/w/index.php?curid=145191793.

Importance of Studying Asphyxial Deaths in Forensics

Examining asphyxial deaths can reveal interesting details about the cause of death which helps forensic experts find out exactly what happened. Forensic experts often notice particular changes in the tissues of people who died by hanging or ligature strangulation which often help guide criminal investigations. One study, for instance, examined the skin and the tissues right underneath and found subtle differences that allowed investigators to tell hanging apart from strangulation, boosting the reliability of their conclusions (Khanna et al., 2024). It's generally true that detailed tissue exams can't be overlooked; they play a crucial role in confirming both the cause and the manner of death, which is key in serving justice (Khanna et al., 2024). In the end, using modern analysis tools only strengthens this approach, giving a solid but flexible way to deal with the complexities of asphyxial deaths.

Overview of Common Causes of Asphyxial Deaths

Deaths due to asphyxia are not easy for forensic scientists to explain, so they have to look into many possible reasons for the loss of breath. Often, mechanical asphyxia—most notably hanging—shows up as the main culprit; in fact, recent findings suggest hanging makes up roughly 34.22% of these cases, especially among males in urban areas (Nadeem et al., 2024). Sometimes, drowning and strangulation cases appear and these require special attention and sometimes unforeseen examination during autopsies. Some studies generally note that checking both the visible and microscopic changes at ligature spots is key to reliably telling hanging apart from strangulation (Singh, 2023). Even though this approach might get a bit confusing now and then, it helps determine the cause of death and also reveals the background to these events. All in all, these points prove how important forensic science is for such complicated cases.

Historical Context of Asphyxial Death Investigations

Nowadays, forensic experts have a much different view of asphyxial deaths than they did before. Most people then assumed strange forces or simple mistakes caused these things which indicated they knew little about the body. It was around the late 1800s and early 1900s that studies using science showed that asphyxiation could be caused by the environment and different substances. Generally speaking, these insights led to the birth of forensic epidemiology, which uses ideas from public health to track death trends and tease out causes, thereby sharpening death investigations related to asphyxiation (Schumann et al., 2025). This broader approach even spilled over into the study of skeletal remains—hinting at deeper social and demographic connections in these cases (Rupa, 2024). All in all, these changes stress that combining various scientific areas is important for uncovering the small details in asphyxial deaths.

Relevance to Modern Forensic Science

Forensic science is always changing and new methods are always being introduced for examining asphyxial deaths. Death Investigators, for instance, now gather background details before the autopsy even kicks off; this extra step has been known to boost the quality of assessments (Villiers et al., 2020). It not only paints a fuller picture of what might have happened but also helps stop us from jumping into quick decisions—like leaning on the hotly debated Excited Delirium Syndrome, a diagnosis sometimes blamed on police violence (Fischer et al., 2024). Even minor changes in procedure can have a big impact which is why it's important to have good data and look over it carefully. To summarize, these evolving practices add a crucial layer of clarity and fairness, ensuring that each case of asphyxial death is handled with the right mix of scientific rigor and human judgment (Figure 12.2).

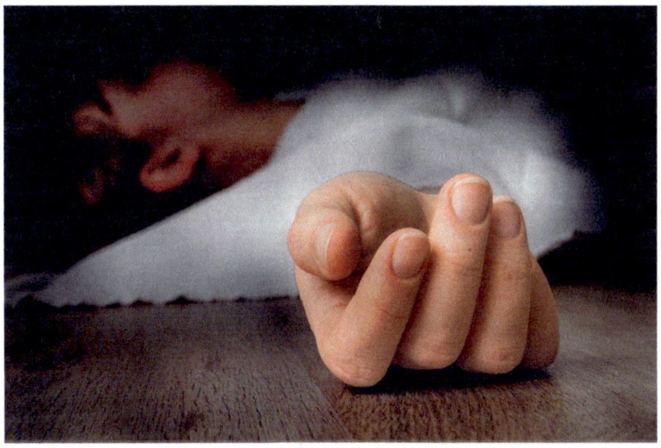

Figure 12.2. Forensic science isn't standing still—new methods keep cropping up that change how we dig into asphyxial deaths.

Source: https://www.verywellmind.com/what-is-asphyxiation-21972

12.1. Types of Asphyxial Deaths

Learning Outcome

1. Understand suffocation, strangulation, drowning, and choking;
2. Explain chemical asphyxia;
3. Focus on positional asphyxia;
4. Discuss traumatic asphyxia;
5. Know environmental asphyxia;
6. Describe neonatal asphyxia.

Forensic investigations rely on being able to tell apart the different types of asphyxial deaths. Another type is mechanical asphyxia which happens when the airway is blocked by something such as in strangulation or suffocation. Alternatively, drowning is a special type of asphyxial death that requires a more detailed and involved investigation to tell it apart from others. Recent studies indicate that mechanical asphyxia is pretty prevalent, with data showing that hanging happens more often than either drowning or strangulation (Iqbal et al., 2024). Another useful tool is the Drowning Index (DI); by analyzing organ weights, it gives forensic experts a way to compare drowning incidents with other asphyxial cases (Dhakar et al., 2024). All in all, making sure classifications are precise helps autopsy results and increases our knowledge about mortality related to asphyxia.

12.1.1. Suffocation

Investigating suffocation deaths can be very complicated because there are many confusing aspects. Examples like plastic bag asphyxiation prove that things are not always simple—the mix of our bodies and the environment can make it hard to understand what happened. A lack of oxygen and high carbon dioxide levels can cause the heart and lungs to stop working very quickly and this can happen without anyone noticing. Studies lately suggest that these incidents are increasing which is concerning since more young people may be using helium inhalation instead of other methods. It is interesting that using inert gases such as helium seems to be making the numbers of suffocation-related suicides higher. In many situations, the findings from autopsies come off as rather vague, meaning forensic professionals have to be extra alert to catch the subtle cues that reveal the full story behind these deaths (Dhakar et al., 2024; Saulė Kaubrytė et al., 2024) (Figure 12.3).

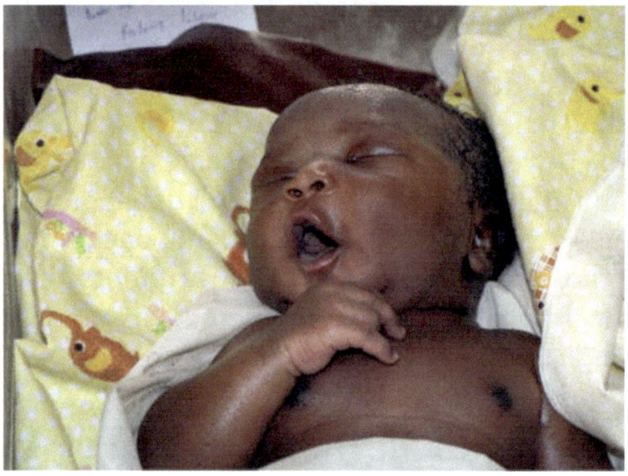

Figure 12.3. Suffocation deaths.

Source: https://img.etimg.com/thumb/msid-68989520,width-480,height-360,imgsize-749851,resizemode-75/bed-sharing.jpg.

12.1.2. Strangulation

Deaths caused by asphyxia and strangulation in particular, can be very difficult to investigate because they bring a lot of hidden challenges. Micro computed tomography has stepped in these days, catching injuries that might have been missed, especially in fragile sites like the larynx (Baier et al., 2019). It highlights the details of trauma and also adds more support to important forensic assessments used in court. In many homicide cases, nailing down the weapon used turns out to be a key clue for steering investigations in the right direction (Fletcher et al., 2022). Experts are able to find patterns of injury on the body by using clear images and carefully examining them which often links the suspect to the crime. Overall, these fresh innovations are slowly reshaping forensic work, making the whole process a bit clearer and, frankly, a lot more objective (Figure 12.4).

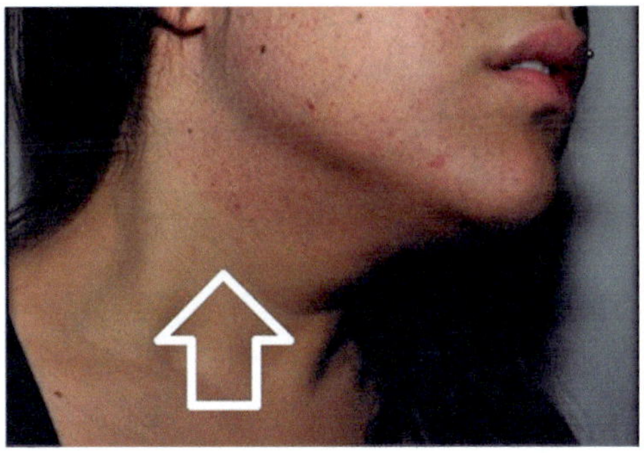

Figure 12.4. Strangulation.

Source: https://godoymedical.net/wp-content/uploads/2014/05/methods.jpg.

12.1.3. Drowning

Nowadays, forensic science is more advanced and a main issue is telling whether a person died from drowning or some other kind of asphyxia. Drowning is hard to diagnose, as the signs at autopsy are usually the same as those seen in hanging or strangulation. At present, scientists are examining the DI; it is useful for forensic pathologists by comparing the weights of organs and the ratios of fluids in a body. In a lot of cases, weighing the lungs and spleen provides more details which increases the accuracy of medicolegal conclusions. Even looking closely at ligature marks can show important differences between hanging and strangulation which may aid further investigation. To summarize, mixing these approaches not only deepens our understanding of asphyxial deaths but also reinforces the trustworthiness of forensic conclusions, which is pretty important in the quest for justice (Dhakar et al., 2024; Khanna et al., 2024) (Figure 12.5).

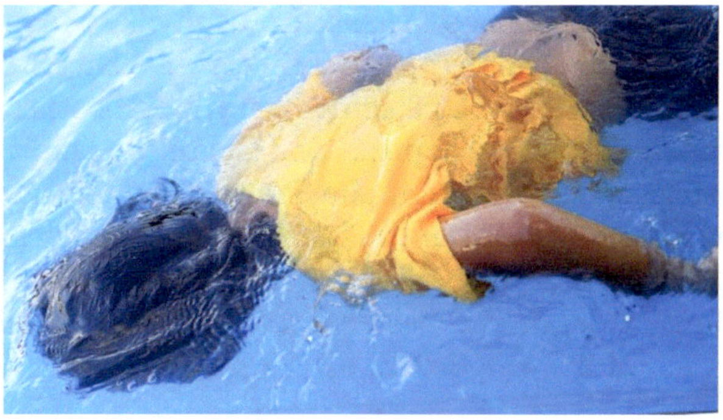

Figure 12.5. Drowning.

Source: https://s.rfi.fr/media/display/9bd13958-dbc0-11ea-adfd-005056a98db9/w:980/p:16x9/SAMU%20Vendee%20Twitter%20image%20to%20warn%20of%20drowning_July%202020.jpg.

12.1.4. Choking

Many people, mainly kids and at-risk adults, still experience choking accidents because they often can't look after themselves. Small toys, coins and even small pieces of food can quickly get stuck in the airway and stop a child from breathing. In many cases involving adults, the food that gets stuck is often a hard piece like a bone which is another reason to watch your eating. The risk ramps up for those with cognitive challenges too—there are several reports (Biradar et al., 2015) where folks ended up eating without taking enough care, which only makes things worse. Being aware of how choking occurs helps us find better ways to prevent it and also helps in both emergency care and forensic investigations. Improved public education about these choking hazards and the proper first-aid steps might, quite frankly, help cut down on these tragic accidents that sometimes end in asphyxia and even death (Biradar et al., 2015).

12.1.5. Chemical Asphyxia

Knowing the signs of asphyxia, especially those caused by chemicals, is very important for forensic investigators. Chemical asphyxia is not the same as mechanical asphyxia which involves something blocking the airways; it occurs when chemicals stop the body from using oxygen properly. In a lot of cases, carbon monoxide, various cyanides and some heavy metals stick to hemoglobin or interfere with the cell's breathing which results in hypoxia and death. Spotting these substances during an autopsy can show the cause of asphyxiation and support the creation of a toxicological profile. Recently, studies have been taking a closer look at things like pericardial fluids—this sometimes sheds light on how the body's metabolism shifts after chemical exposure, thereby helping forensic experts estimate the time of death and better understand what happened in asphyxial cases (Book et al., 1993; Locci et al., 2023) (Figure 12.6).

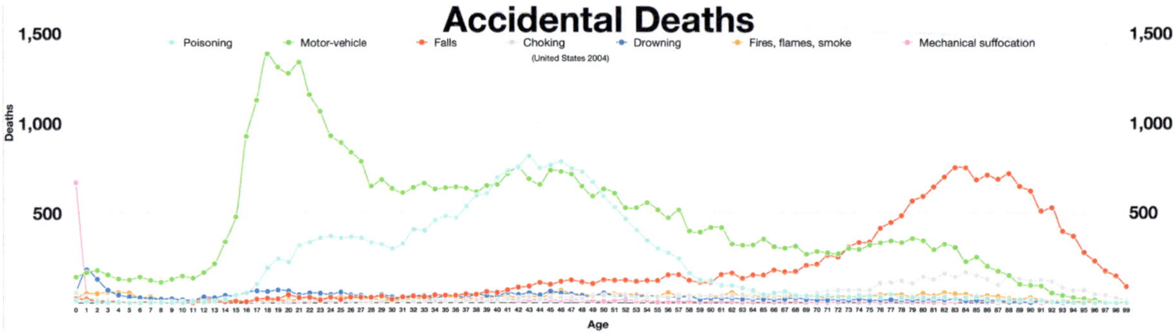

Figure 12.6. Finding chemical compounds during an autopsy can directly point to the cause of asphyxiation and help build a toxicological profile.

Source: By Wikideas1 - Own work https://injuryfacts.nsc.org/all-injuries/deaths-by-demographics/deaths-by-age/data-details/, CC0, https://commons.wikimedia.org/w/index.php?curid=145191792.

12.1.6. Positional Asphyxia

Positional asphyxia is a difficult matter in forensic pathology – it happens when the way someone lies down blocks enough oxygen to cause suffocation. A lot of the time, it's not easy to determine the cause of death, so experts turn to small pieces of evidence, mainly when nothing else stands out as the reason. I recall one particularly sad case involving a woman who was extremely undernourished and found in an unstable sitting position; her lungs were congested and her circulation just wasn't getting enough going, which ultimately led to her demise (Ishigami et al., 2020). Sometimes, this breathing trouble even shows up alongside neck trauma, nudging examiners to be extra careful during autopsies (Akhlaghi et al., 2013). Usually, putting together the puzzle and guiding legal and medical decisions depends on how these factors interact.

12.1.7. Traumatic Asphyxia

Deaths caused by asphyxia aren't always easy to understand – many different things can happen and traumatic asphyxia is often the most important for forensic experts. It is common for this type to occur when blunt trauma presses the chest and neck which quickly stops normal breathing. You might find bruises or contusions on the outside, but the serious injuries inside are often not clear during an autopsy which makes it hard to put the pieces together. Detecting broken bones in the throat area, like fractures in the hyoid or laryngeal region, is key since that damage is pretty tightly linked with asphyxia and may offer vital clues into what actually occurred (Vashist et al.,

2025). Also, knowing whether a death was caused by traumatic asphyxia or something else, like drowning, means relying on specific methods – for example, the Drowning Index, which generally helps nail down the particular circumstances behind the death (Dhakar et al., 2024) (Figure 12.7).

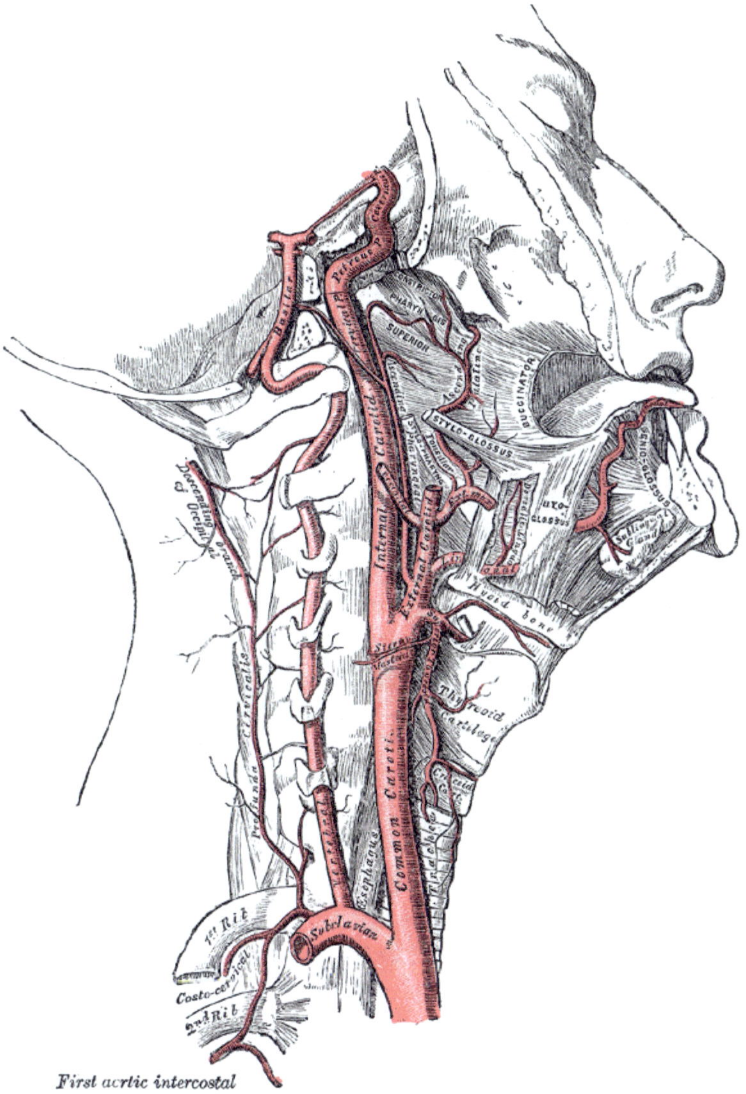

Figure 12.7. Traumatic asphyxia.

Source: By Henry Vandyke Carter - Henry Gray (1918) Anatomy of the Human Body (See "Book" section below)Bartleby.com: Gray's Anatomy, Plate 513, Public Domain, https://commons.wikimedia.org/w/index.php?curid=559527.

12.1.8. Environmental Asphyxia

It's not only a blocked airway that can kill – often, other environmental problems are the reason there is less oxygen. Many times, this happens when someone is in an air-poor or toxic gas-filled room which is what we usually call environmental asphyxia. People often realize these dangerous places are a problem when it's almost too late which makes it harder for investigators. These days, forensic science has found that it's important to examine the area around the body, as well as the body itself, because new developments in forensic biology point to this approach. Research, for example, has repeatedly hinted that the environment can have a huge effect on medico-legal outcomes—this puts a real urgency on spotting and addressing risks where asphyxial dangers might be lurking (Al-Kandari, 2012). Thus, knowing about environmental asphyxia is important for correct death analysis and developing effective prevention methods.

12.1.9. Neonatal Asphyxia

Neonatal asphyxia is a major problem when we examine deaths caused by suffocation in the forensic setting. Many times, a newborn does not breathe for the first time which can soon result in serious health problems or death. Some factors such as problems in the womb or during delivery, are linked; if the breathing issue is not addressed quickly, it could result in permanent damage to the brain. Forensic experts, when examining such tragic cases, need to dig deep into what exactly went wrong—whether it's related to drowning, mechanical blockage of the airways, or something else—so that they can draw accurate conclusions (Dhakar et al., 2024). Generally speaking, the stats show that asphyxia still ranks high among causes of newborn death, which keeps both doctors and forensic investigators extra vigilant (Iqbal et al., 2024) (Figure 12.8).

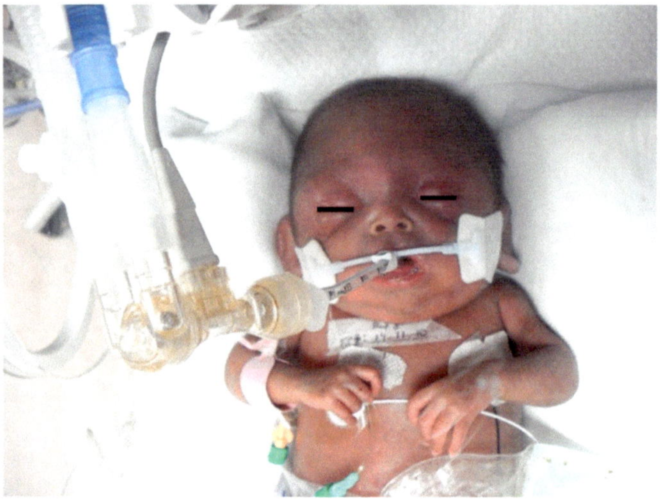

Figure 12.8. Neonatal asphyxia.

Source: Mota-Rojas D, Villanueva-García D, Solimano A, Muns R, Ibarra-Ríos D, Mota-Reyes A. Pathophysiology of Perinatal Asphyxia in Humans and Animal Models. *Biomedicines*. 2022; 10(2):347. https://doi.org/10.3390/biomedicines10020347

Test Your Knowledge

1. What are the main types of asphyxial deaths encountered in forensic medicine?
2. Explain the mechanism of strangulation and how it leads to death.

12.2. Mechanisms of Asphyxia

Learning Outcome

1. Understand oxygen deprivation;
2. Explain carbon dioxide retention;
3. Focus on airway obstruction;
4. Identify neurological effects;
5. Learn physiological responses to asphyxia;
6. Know the pathophysiology of asphyxial deaths;
7. Describe the role of the cardiovascular system;
8. Discuss the impact on brain function;
9. Know the long-term effects of asphyxia.

If the body doesn't get enough oxygen, it can lead to asphyxia which allows carbon dioxide to build up. There are actually several methods by which this problem can take place. Sometimes, when there is external pressure on the body such as during strangulation or suffocation, it stops normal breathing and we call this mechanical asphyxia. Another case is drowning which leads to water in the lungs and interrupts gas exchange; strangely, this can still result in oxygen loss even if there is plenty of oxygen nearby. Chemicals are used as well and carbon monoxide can prevent hemoglobin from using oxygen which can be deadly even if there is no visible obstruction. Forensic experts usually rely on spotting these various paths since each one leaves its own clues during the autopsy to help explain the situation. Recent studies have generally grouped these dynamics into distinct categories (Dhakar et al., 2024; Iqbal et al., 2024).

12.2.1. Oxygen Deprivation

Asphyxia goes beyond a lack of oxygen; it causes many other problems in the body. If there is not enough oxygen, the cells misbehave which can cause organs to fail. You might notice that a fair number of these fatal events pop up especially among young people in city settings, often tied to mechanical issues or hanging incidents (Iqbal et al., 2024). At the same time, there's been some interesting work showing that nature might have a little trick up its sleeve; studies on Amburana cearensis suggest it could help ease damage from both oxygen and glucose shortages—and even calm the surge of glutamate that sometimes harms neurons (Sanches et al., 2025). To summarize, these insights point to a delicate tug-of-war between bodily responses and forensic clues, underlining that there's still a lot we need to figure out about asphyxia's tragic impact (Figure 12.9).

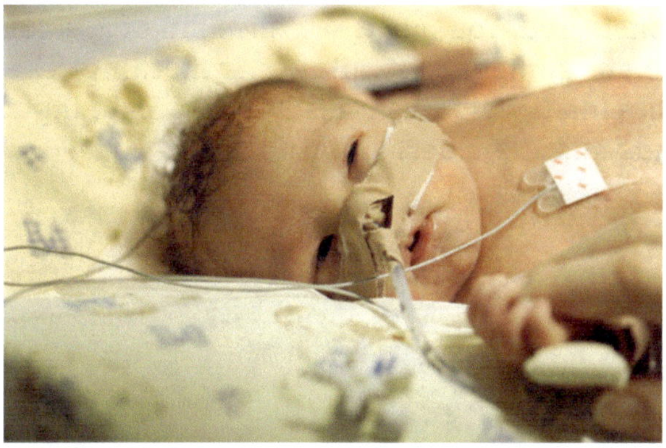

Figure 12.9. Oxygen deprivation.

Source: https://s22948.pcdn.co/wp-content/uploads/2017/06/asphyxia-oxygen-deprivation.jpg.

12.2.2. Carbon Dioxide Retention

Asphyxia sets off a series of events in the body mostly because carbon dioxide stays in the system for too long. If oxygen levels are low, CO_2 increases and usually leads to hypercapnia which is too much CO_2 in the blood. An accumulation of carbon dioxide can disrupt the balance between acids and bases which can cause respiratory acidosis and harm important organs. In examining asphyxial deaths, you find that the amount of CO_2 in the air is closely connected to the type of death and this is especially clear in mechanical asphyxia, where external pressure increases the CO_2. Research generally shows that male victims, particularly in urban areas, are hit harder by this issue (Iqbal et al., 2024). And, curiously enough, understanding how CO_2 retention works is super important for forensic work—not only does it help determine the cause of death, but it also sheds light on the manner of death in complicated cases with multiple asphyxial factors at play (Gerstel et al., 2021).

12.2.3. Airway Obstruction

Airway obstruction can cause a forensic investigation to go in a completely different direction, mainly when asphyxia is being considered. You might see this kind of accident when someone swallows something they shouldn't which can easily cause choking in kids and the elderly.

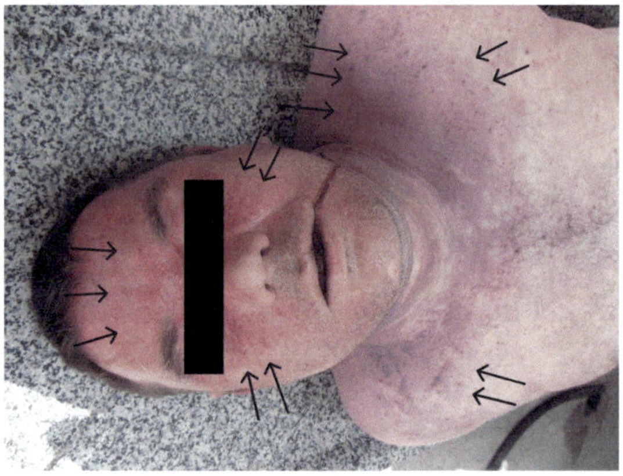

Figure 12.10. Airway blockage can turn a forensic investigation on its head—especially when asphyxial deaths are on the table.

Source: Kiryakova T, Yovchevska I, Tihchev V, et al. (October 22, 2024) A Rare Case of Sudden Fatal Airway Obstruction Caused by an Undiagnosed Laryngeal Lesion. Cureus 16(10): e72103. doi:10.7759/cureus.72103.

In many adult cases, though, it tends to be that a piece of food gets lodged smack-dab in the airway, and if not eased out quickly, it can end up being fatal (Biradar et al., 2015). Usually, forensic experts think it's important to look closely since a basic autopsy could miss certain signs of the cause of death. In one instance, for example, a post-mortem computed tomography (PMCT) scan revealed some surprising details—finding small fractures in the hyoid bone and signs of bleeding that, though subtle, turned out to be key in understanding the full picture behind an asphyxial death (Arcangeli et al., 2020) (Figure 12.10).

12.2.4. Neurological Effects

Forensic experts usually start by studying how a lack of oxygen affects the brain which is not as simple as it looks. A lack of oxygen in the brain which happens gradually, usually leads to a drop in brain function that can become very serious and permanent. Histological examinations have been the main way to diagnose asphyxia deaths, but researchers now think these tests might not always catch all the details. Although examining tissues after a death can show many kinds of damage, it is not always possible to tell if the heart stopped because of asphyxia or some other reason. Recent investigations, in most cases, show that looking at metabolomics—tracking unique metabolic changes during different stages of oxygen loss—adds a richer layer of detail to what forensic pathologists can work with (Locciet al., 2021). Also, with the rise in risky behaviors like self-asphyxia among young people, it's becoming increasingly obvious that we need more, well-rounded strategies to ease the neurological impacts of these incidents (Busse et al., 2015).

12.2.5. Physiological Responses to Asphyxia

The physical reactions during asphyxia can determine the outcome of a serious event. Low oxygen in the blood makes the body breathe faster and sends blood to the most important organs. If the shortage goes on for a long time, cells soon become stressed and may begin to change in ways that cannot be reversed. In many cases, forensic teams search for particular biomarkers that hint at these internal shifts—since standard autopsy findings are sometimes too vague (Sacco et al., 2024). Checking out local signs, like ligature marks on the neck, often helps experts decide if injuries happened while the person was still alive—a point that modern immunohistochemical techniques have made clearer (Varfolomeiev et al., 2024). Overall, these methods have boosted our ability to pinpoint asphyxial deaths, giving us valuable clues about what went down (Figure 12.11).

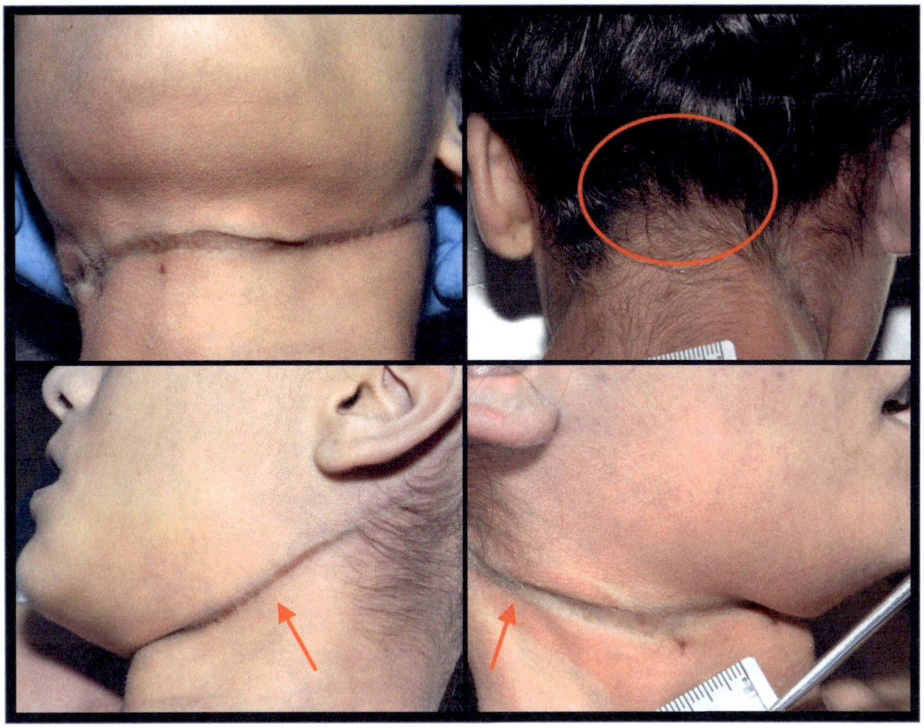

Figure 12.11. Physiological responses under asphyxia can tip the outcome of a critical situation.

Source: https://www.pathologyoutlines.com/imgau/forensicsasphyxia_Various01.jpg.

12.2.6. Pathophysiology of Asphyxial Deaths

Asphyxial deaths involve many problems in the body that gradually cause death. Drowning is an example; the water inside the lungs stops the usual airflow and also disrupts how oxygen is delivered to the body's organs. When the lungs fill with water, the normal breathing process is interrupted and usually makes the body suffer from hypoxia which leaves the cells in distress. In many forensic checks, tiny traces of diatoms appear as subtle markers that hint at exactly when and how these tragic events took place (Pal et al., 2017). Interestingly, studies generally show that men seem to fall victim to asphyxial incidents more often—probably because many personal habits and the environments they spend time in makes them more vulnerable (Beltrán Aroca et al., 2021). All these points mean that, while drowning at first appears straightforward, it is important to explore the real processes involved to prevent such tragedies and to improve the quality of forensic investigations.

12.2.7. Role of the Cardiovascular System

The way the heart helps with asphyxial deaths is sometimes overlooked—it's about the blood system delivering oxygen and removing carbon dioxide. When a person struggles to breathe, their oxygen level drops and their body tries to help by making the heart beat faster and blood pressure change, to keep the important organs working. For the most part, these quick fixes work for a little while, but if the low oxygen persists, the whole situation can end in cardiac arrest. Experts in forensics often look at these moments since they tend to leave hints about the person's metabolism which can suggest asphyxia was involved in the death. Researchers are now exploring these changes using techniques like NMR metabolomics, which is steadily deepening our grasp on how asphyxia affects the system (Cecchetto et al., 2022; Locci et al., 2020) (Figure 12.12).

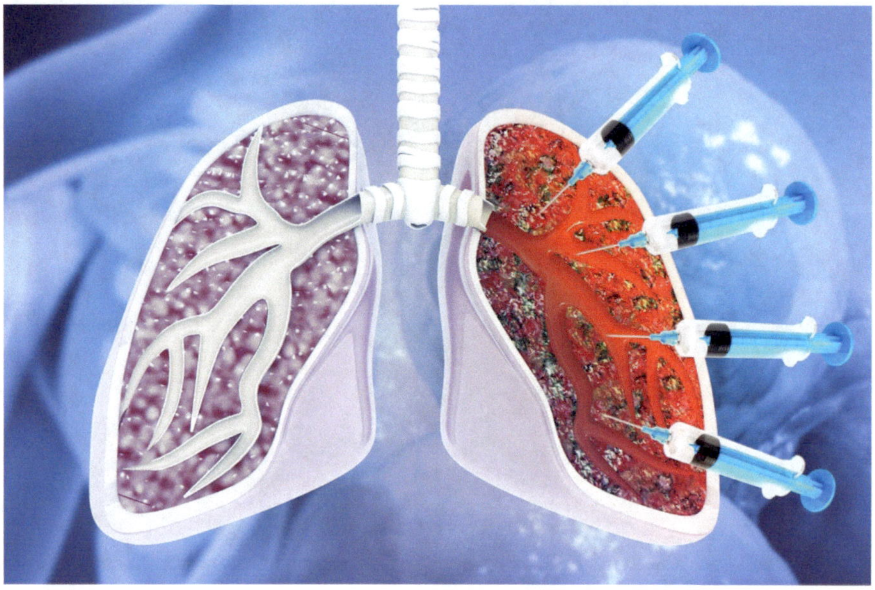

Figure 12.12. The heart's role in asphyxial deaths isn't given the simple attention it deserves—it's about how our blood system keeps oxygen flowing while getting rid of carbon dioxide.

Source: https://www.princeea.com/wp-content/uploads/2025/03/shutterstock_2233366207.jpg.

12.2.8. Impact on Brain Function

There is a strong connection between asphyxia and how the brain functions which helps explain asphyxial deaths. If oxygen is removed from the brain, it quickly becomes distressed and suffers damage that can't be fixed in a few minutes. Sometimes, nerve cells start to die just because they are not getting enough oxygen. Recent studies generally suggest that metabolomics can help sort out different triggers behind a cardiac arrest, providing an objective way to gauge the injury the brain takes when oxygen is scarce (Locciet al., 2021). Older tissue checks tend to miss the actual reason for arrest, but new metabolic profiling can catch the changes that happen just before it happens. Because forensic resources are stretched in South Africa, it is even harder to fully solve asphyxial cases. In most cases, it appears that fresh, innovative methods in death investigations are needed to untangle how asphyxia messes with brain function (Villiers et al., 2020).

12.2.9. Long-term Effects of Asphyxia

The brain may be affected in ways that last after asphyxia and this is something experts in forensics look for. In lots of cases, when oxygen is scarce for too long, zinc ends up accumulating in the mitochondria, and that buildup tends to mess with nerve cells, especially in sensitive spots like the CA1 area of the hippocampus (Medvedeva et al., 2022). A problem in mitochondrial function may trigger events that eventually cause cognitive problems in those who survive. At the same time, inflammation gets in on the action; for example, the activation of mast cell tryptase appears to drive inflammatory responses further after asphyxia-triggered cardiac arrest (Ocak et al., 2020). All in all, knowing about these effects is important for forensic professionals because it explains how people's actions and mental abilities may be affected which helps with both legal and clinical decisions.

Test Your Knowledge

1. How does hypoxia contribute to the mechanism of asphyxia?
2. What role do toxic gases (such as carbon monoxide) play in the mechanism of asphyxial death?

12.3. Forensic Investigation Techniques

Learning Outcome

1. Explain scene investigation protocols;
2. Know autopsy procedures for asphyxial deaths;
3. Describe toxicology testing;
4. Discuss the use of imaging techniques;
5. Describe the collection of evidence;
6. Know the role of forensic pathologists;
7. Perform documentation and reporting;
8. Learn legal considerations in asphyxial death cases;
9. Discuss case studies and their implications.

Asphyxial deaths are difficult to solve—it often takes many different forensic methods to find out what really happened. They often put together what witnesses say with the results from the autopsy which can make the process seem unpredictable. In cases involving newborns and tiny children, Batalis et al. (2017) show that a suspect's confession can sometimes tip the balance, and a careful look at tissue can bring forward clues about asphyxia. In drowning deaths, figuring out the cause is very important and diatom testing is now one of the main ways to do this. As Pal et al. (2017) point out, spotting diatoms can clearly back up drowning as the culprit, offering crucial biological evidence that not only helps tag the case but also strengthens the overall investigative process.

12.3.1. Scene Investigation Protocols

The first thing done in an asphyxial death case is to secure the scene which launches the entire investigation. Without protocols, this process would be much more difficult and the details of the case might be compromised. The first thing to do is secure the scene which prevents anything from being contaminated and keeps the raw evidence safe. Next, taking lots of photos, sketches and even some notes helps investigators put together the events that led to the tragedy. Those who investigate also need to be flexible and collect samples that might reveal metabolic signs of what led to death. General speaking, emerging techniques such as NMR metabolomics have started to shed more light on conditions before and after death, which in most cases sharpens our grasp of asphyxial deaths and their legal angles—as noted in the evolving trends in forensic medicine (Locci et al., 2020) (Figure 12.13).

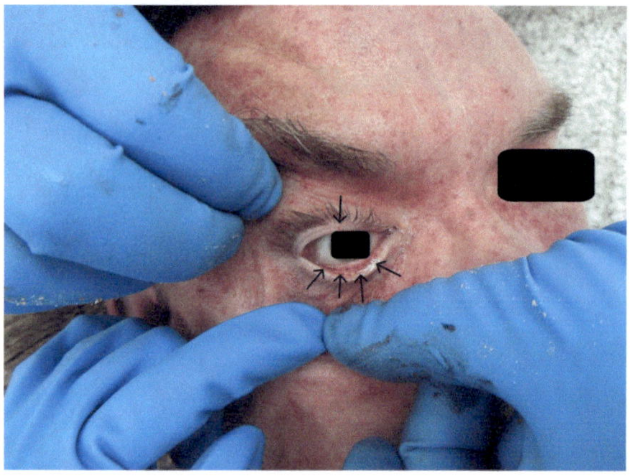

Figure 12.13. Forensic work on asphyxial deaths begins with getting the scene locked down—it's what sets the entire investigation in motion.

Source: Kiryakova T, Yovchevska I, Tihchev V, et al. (October 22, 2024) A Rare Case of Sudden Fatal Airway Obstruction Caused by an Undiagnosed Laryngeal Lesion. Cureus 16(10): e72103. doi:10.7759/cureus.72103.

12.3.2. Autopsy Procedures for Asphyxial Deaths

The first step in looking at deaths by asphyxiation is to study the autopsy which aims to find the cause of suffocation. In situations where someone's been exposed to problematic gases (like in low-oxygen environments or cramped areas with irrespirable air), the focus naturally shifts to closely checking the lungs and nearby tissues for any signs that point to asphyxia (Rangu et al., 2016). Sometimes the case is even more difficult such as when someone is strangled or has a foreign object in their body which requires investigators to use knowledge from both forensics and psychology. I remember one particular case where the death was eventually ruled accidental, caused by a weird combo of suffocation and a vagal response triggered by an errant object, underscoring just how important it is to factor in the broader crime scene picture (Atanasijević et al., 2009). To summarize, these careful steps help piece together a fuller, if sometimes muddled, understanding of what led to these fatal outcomes (Figure 12.14).

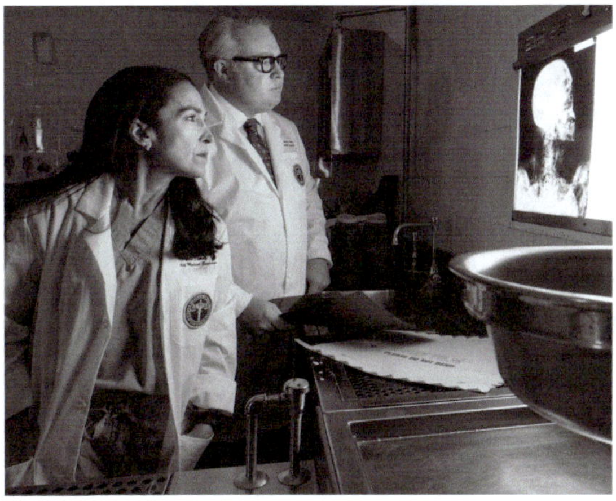

Figure 12.14. Examining deaths by asphyxiation starts with a deep dive into the autopsy process—one that tries to uncover exactly how suffocation happened.

Source: https://news.emory.edu/features/2023/03/em_speakers_for_the_dead_profile_of_new_york_city_chief_medical_examiners_16-03-2023/assets/CO6mCc4fIL/02-900-900x727.jpg.

12.3.3. Toxicology Testing

To discover the cause of asphyxia deaths, toxicology tests are very useful. It tries to find out which substances could be affecting the body, whether they were present before or after the asphyxiation, in general. Sometimes, the cause of drowning is not obvious, but a laboratory analysis could point out drugs or other intoxicants which a traditional autopsy might not notice. Some research even suggests that a notable chunk of these cases involves toxic substances, with signs of intoxication echoing many environmental and situational influences across various groups (Nadeem et al., 2024). Tools like the Drowning Index, for example, help experts sort through the messy difference between drowning and other asphyxial deaths by highlighting subtle toxic markers (Dhakar et al., 2024). All in all, toxicology testing helps a lot in figuring out how these deaths take place.

12.3.4. Use of Imaging Techniques

Modern imaging is being used in investigations of asphyxial deaths, helping to notice things that older methods might have missed. A CT scan done after death—or postmortem CT—allows experts to see inside the body and notice even the smallest changes that could go unnoticed otherwise. For instance, one study showed that generally speaking, AI-assisted CT analysis managed to nail drowning case classifications at around 92% accuracy for victims who weren't resuscitated (Ogawara et al., 2022). It helps investigators see those small, barely visible changes as well as giving them an advantage when the case gets complicated. Granted, while many of these techniques are still polishing up, the mix of advanced imaging with a push for common diagnostic cues is steadily reshaping the whole process and might even lead to better safeguards against these unfortunate deaths (Albano et al., 2024).

12.3.5. Collection of Evidence

Forensic science depends on collecting all the evidence which is especially clear in cases of asphyxial deaths. Everyday clues start to add up when techniques like NMR metabolomics help unravel the body's own chemical signals –

almost like a snapshot of what changed before and after death (Locci et al., 2020). Micro-computed tomography (or micro-CT, as many call it) pops in next, offering a fresh take on examining tiny details in biological samples; this method can sometimes point to how long someone's been gone or even suggest a possible cause (Cecchetto et al., 2022). In most cases, mixing these newer approaches with older methods shows that solving tough forensic puzzles usually benefits from a mix of ideas and expertise (Figure 12.15).

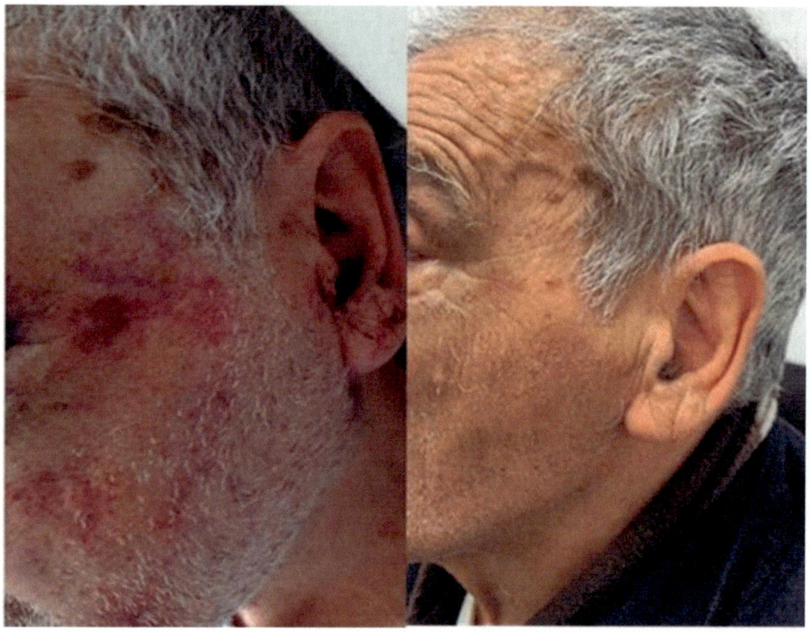

Figure 12.15. Forensic science often hinges on gathering every bit of evidence, a point that comes home in cases involving asphyxial deaths.

Source: De Paola L, Piersanti V, Tripi D, Marinelli E, Zaami S, Napoletano G. Clinical, Psychiatric, and Medicolegal Issues in Non-Fatal Strangulation: A Case Report. *Forensic Sciences*. 2024; 4(4):475-486. https://doi.org/10.3390/forensicsci4040031.

12.3.6. Role of Forensic Pathologists

Forensic pathologists are called in right away when someone's breathing suddenly stops under unclear circumstances. They examine each detail during an autopsy to see if the death was caused by drowning, suicide or something worse, mainly when water is involved. It can be messy; they have to gather evidence from the scene, check for signs of intoxication and also consider if any medical problems contributed to the accident. By investigating, their work helps police understand the events and, most of the time, also supports public health plans to avoid similar tragedies in the future. Science keeps nudging them to rethink their approach—COVID-19, for instance, has pushed them to adjust autopsy methods so things stay both precise and safe (Aquila et al., 2020). In a way, their findings stretch out past the immediate case, slowly reshaping how society understands asphyxial deaths overall (Armstrong et al., 2018).

12.3.7. Documentation and Reporting

The results of an asphyxial death investigation depend greatly on the documentation which also affects the legal outcome. Investigators often write down every detail they see; they consider where the body is found, what the surroundings look like and anything said by witnesses which together might explain the death.

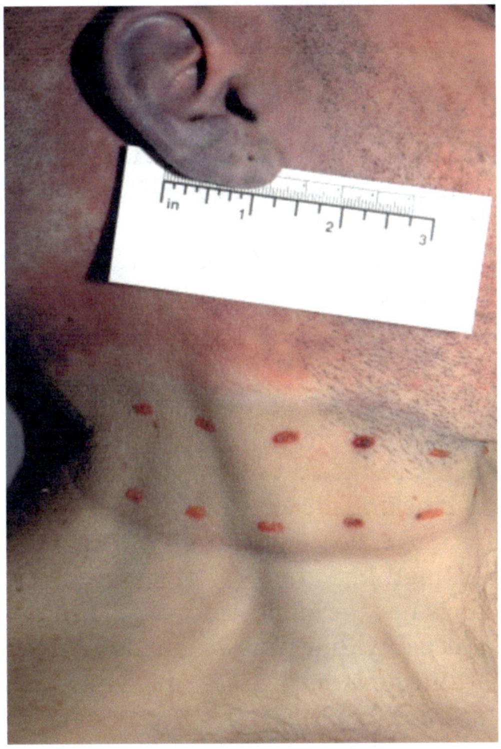

Figure 12.16. Documentation in asphyxial death investigations.

Source: https://ars.els-cdn.com/content/image/3-s2.0-B9780323917964000118-f11-06-9780323917964.jpg.

This process isn't merely for immediate use, it also turns into an essential resource in court where every tiny detail matters (Armstrong et al., 2018). At the same time, combining autopsy results, toxicology data and other tests takes the same level of care, so that all information is recorded correctly, even if it repeats a little. Ultimately, such thorough and sometimes a bit messy documentation reinforces forensic standards and boosts the odds of achieving genuine justice in cases where tangled details often obscure the real truth (Figure 12.16).

12.3.8. Legal Considerations in Asphyxial Death Cases

Deaths caused by asphyxia can be very difficult to analyze in forensic pathology. Asphyxia often presents special difficulties for autopsies and post-death examinations which are key to understanding what took place. Sometimes, the push for clarity leans on fresh biomarker research; take postmortem protein analysis, which shows promise in flagging specific changes at death (Robinson, 2022). Legal rules are also very important—since any small mistake can cause big issues in court. Observing how the body cools and shifts after death—its temperature changes and other subtle transformations—is key not only for guessing the post-mortem interval but also for meeting legal standards (Hamilton et al., 2017). All in all, the combination of scientific research and legal needs proves that all details matter when putting together the picture of asphyxial deaths.

12.3.9. Case Studies and Their Implications

Looking into asphyxial deaths is not an easy task – it's almost like trying to put together a jigsaw puzzle with pieces spread in many places. Many times, forensic experts look into specific cases to spot the details that can be easily missed and these situations sometimes make investigators reconsider their postmortem analysis techniques. Take COVID-19 fatalities, for example; in most cases, these situations have pushed professionals to tweak their usual autopsy protocols to deal with a range of unique risks, which, in turn, shifts how forensic practices operate during widespread health emergencies (Aquila et al., 2020). When it comes to drowning, not all water-related deaths are cut and dry – occasionally, factors like pre-existing conditions or unforeseen external influences blur the picture, making the diagnosis more complicated than expected (Armstrong et al., 2018). Looking at a range of case studies improves the way diseases are diagnosed and also helps create better public health strategies. All in all, combining insights from different cases is very important for growing our understanding and the tools applied in the field.

Test Your Knowledge

1. How do forensic investigators use different techniques to find out that asphyxia led to the person's death?
2. How are ligature marks around the neck useful for investigating strangulation cases?

12.4. Challenges in Asphyxial Death Cases

Learning Outcome

1. Explain the differentiating between types of asphyxia;
2. Be aware of the wrong ways evidence is understood;
3. Understand cultural and social implications;
4. Know the limitations of forensic technology;
5. Discuss ethical considerations in investigations;
6. Know the impact of witness testimonies;
7. Identify legal challenges in prosecution;
8. Focus on the need for interdisciplinary Collaboration.

Forensic experts find asphyxial deaths difficult because the usual signs present in other deaths are not always found. Instead, examiners end up piecing together the events from circumstantial clues and scene details—a process that, in many heartbreaking cases involving infants and young children, sometimes leans heavily on a suspect's own confession rather than just physical evidence (Batalis et al., 2017). Diatom analysis, for instance, can at times offer a link in drowning cases by associating the presence of diatoms with the diagnosis; however, this method isn't always a fit for every asphyxial situation (Pal et al., 2017). All these aspects show that using both traditional and modern forensic methods is necessary to solve these complicated cases.

12.4.1. Differentiating between Types of Asphyxia

It is soon clear to forensic teams that different ways of blocking the airways can cause asphyxia in different ways. Suffocation which happens when something blocks the airway from the outside, is not the same as strangulation which can be done with a rope or hands and usually leaves different marks. Yet, drowning usually adds more difficulties since it can cause water inhalation and other injuries.

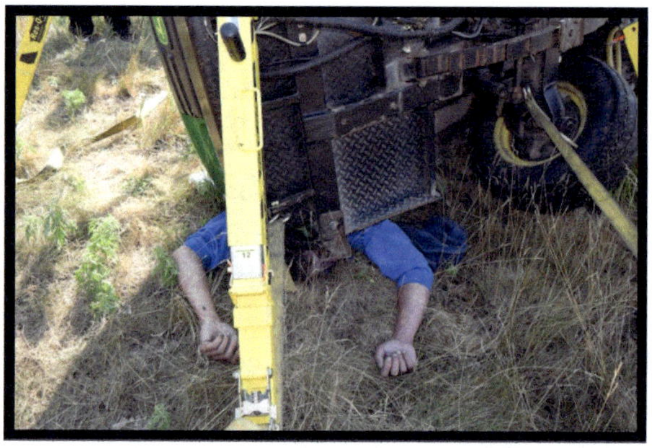

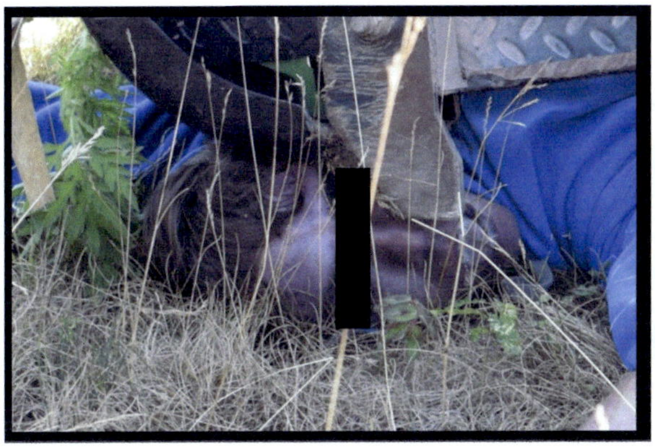

Figure 12.17. Forensic teams investigating asphyxial fatalities soon notice that not every way of cutting off breathing is the same.

Source: https://www.pathologyoutlines.com/imgau/forensicsasphyxiaVarious08.jpg.

Most of the time, these differences are very important for legal investigations because they can decide if the death is a homicide or just an accident. It's also important to note that the variation in injuries, depending on which tool or method is used during an asphyxial act, adds another layer to the investigation, reminding us why a meticulous inquiry is so essential (Fletcher et al., 2022) (Figure 12.17).

12.4.2. Misinterpretation of Evidence

It is important to understand evidence well when investigating asphyxial deaths in forensics. Small differences in anatomy can easily trip up a pathologist during an autopsy – sometimes a tiny crack in the hyoid area, which many link to asphyxia, might be so subtle it gets overlooked, leading to conclusions that aren't quite right (Vashist et al., 2025). Diagnosing drowning isn't any simpler; signs found in an autopsy can be nearly identical whether or not drowning was involved, so things can get messy (Dhakar et al., 2024). Small mistakes in this area can result in major legal and safety issues, generally. It proves that being aware of these subtle points makes forensic methods become stronger, although the world is not always perfect.

12.4.3. Influence of Environmental Factors

Your environment, economic status and ability to get help seem to affect asphyxial deaths more than we might think. Urban places, for example, tend to report more cases of such deaths, with mechanical asphyxia (think hanging) showing up more often, according to recent studies (Nadeem et al., 2024). Rural areas are not the same as urban ones, mainly because of things like lower income and fewer mental health resources.

It's also important to note that pressures like job loss and family fights, which often worsen mental health problems, can lead to a noticeable rise in suicidal asphyxiation (Balaji et al., 2024). In most cases, grasping these influences is a key step in crafting interventions that can better target the risks across different groups (Figure 12.18).

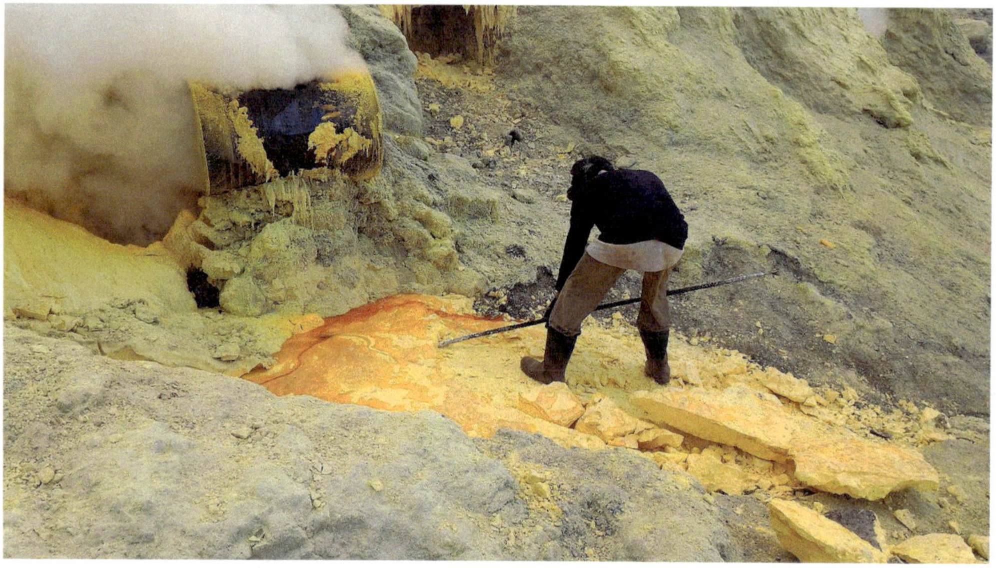

Figure 12.18. Environmental surroundings seem to shape asphyxial deaths in a way that isn't entirely random—where you live, your economic situation, and even how easily you can get help play a part.

Source: https://upload.wikimedia.org/wikipedia/commons/thumb/4/43/Sulphur_Mining_at_Kawah_Ijen_3.jpg/1200px-Sulphur_Mining_at_Kawah_Ijen_3.jpg.

12.4.4. Cultural and Social Implications

Deaths caused by asphyxiation raise problems that go beyond the experiments—they also change the way we view our culture. The use of forensic tools, for example micro Computed Tomography, is not only about having the latest technology; it changes the way courts and communities look at these cases. Take strangulation, for example—when we nail down its signs with extra clarity, it kind of changes the way folks talk about domestic violence (Baier et al., 2019). Digging into older cases, our science points out the cultural settings of these tragedies which may suggest that inequality and systemic violence played a role. In various ways, combining forensic science and cultural knowledge allows for solving cases and influencing how society looks at its laws and policies.

12.4.5. Limitations of Forensic Technology

Forensic experts are always challenged by asphyxial deaths, because our current methods may not always detect every detail. Rather than clearly separating hanging, drowning or suffocation, the Drowning Index gives helpful tips for spotting drowning, but it fails when there are autopsy details mix together; conditions such as hanging or suffocation can look surprisingly similar (Dhakar et al., 2024). Even if the Index looks useful, it is still possible for doctors to make a mistake since many asphyxiation paths have similar symptoms. Examining tissue samples does help to tell hanging apart from ligature strangulation, but even these tests can fall short due to similar tissue reactions (Khanna et al., 2024). All this shows that we need to push for better forensic techniques, ensuring more accurate results and fairer legal outcomes when unraveling these tricky cases (Figure 12.19).

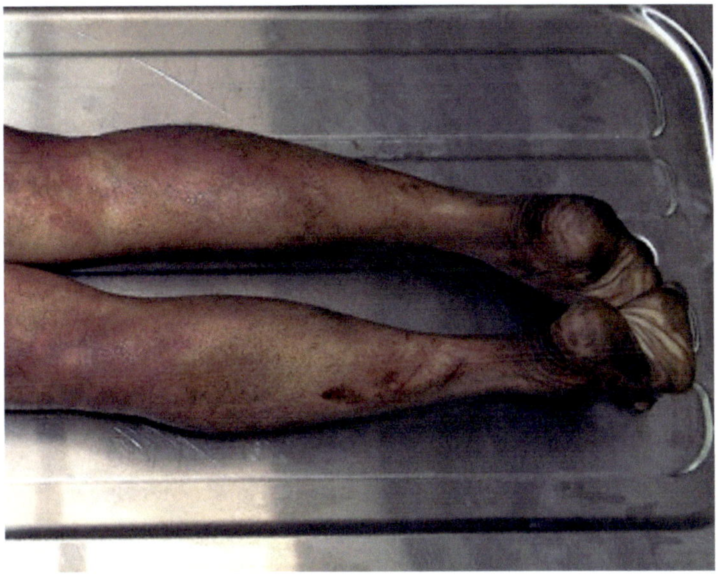

Figure 12.19. Asphyxial deaths keep forensic work on its toes – our current tools just don't always catch every nuance.

Source: https://ars.els-cdn.com/content/image/1-s2.0-S1752928X10000910-gr7.jpg.

12.4.6. Ethical Considerations in Investigations

It is challenging to solve asphyxial death cases and getting justice means making sure to find important evidence while still respecting the privacy of the deceased and their family. Investigators must balance their need for clues with the risk of mishandling sensitive information which could cause people to lose trust in the investigation. Most of the time, obeying the law matters, because it ensures the results will hold up in a court of law. At the same time, as technology keeps advancing, our ethical rules should also adjust to handle matters such as managing digital records and the privacy problems they bring. In short, it seems that we still need to keep having open discussions. about these ethical issues, helping build trust and keep everyone accountable in the quest to uncover the truth in asphyxial death investigations (Mandayam, 2024; Rashmi, 2025).

12.4.7. Impact of Witness Testimonies

A witness statement can change the direction of an investigation, mainly in cases where asphyxia is involved. The details in what people say are often what guide the whole legal investigation and decide whether an incident is an accident, a suicide or a homicide. In several forensic studies, researchers have noticed that even minor mismatches between what witnesses recall and what autopsy reports show can sometimes expose hidden layers of criminal intent (Mittal et al., 2023). Folks at the scene may add details that either back up or even call into question the physical evidence, which generally highlights why a deep, careful look is needed (Knight et al., 2014). To summarize, witnesses help bridge the gap between scattered clues and a fuller grasp of asphyxial incidents; this underscores, in most instances, why a broad and sometimes beautifully imperfect approach is so crucial in forensics (Figure 12.20).

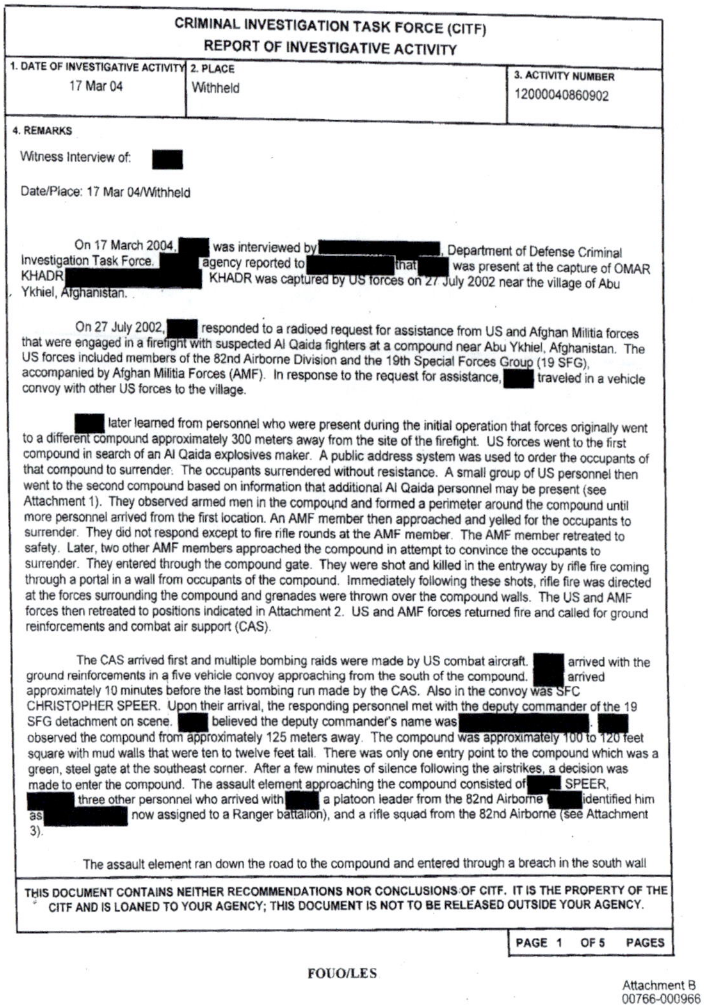

CRIMINAL INVESTIGATION TASK FORCE (CITF)
REPORT OF INVESTIGATIVE ACTIVITY

1. DATE OF INVESTIGATIVE ACTIVITY	2. PLACE	3. ACTIVITY NUMBER
17 Mar 04	Withheld	12000040860902

4. REMARKS

Witness Interview of: [redacted]

Date/Place: 17 Mar 04/Withheld

On 17 March 2004, [redacted] was interviewed by [redacted], Department of Defense Criminal Investigation Task Force. [redacted] agency reported to [redacted] that [redacted] was present at the capture of OMAR KHADR [redacted] KHADR was captured by US forces on 27 July 2002 near the village of Abu Ykhiel, Afghanistan.

On 27 July 2002, [redacted] responded to a radioed request for assistance from US and Afghan Militia forces that were engaged in a firefight with suspected Al Qaida fighters at a compound near Abu Ykhiel, Afghanistan. The US forces included members of the 82nd Airborne Division and the 19th Special Forces Group (19 SFG), accompanied by Afghan Militia Forces (AMF). In response to the request for assistance, [redacted] traveled in a vehicle convoy with other US forces to the village.

[redacted] later learned from personnel who were present during the initial operation that forces originally went to a different compound approximately 300 meters away from the site of the firefight. US forces went to the first compound in search of an Al Qaida explosives maker. A public address system was used to order the occupants of that compound to surrender. The occupants surrendered without resistance. A small group of US personnel then went to the second compound based on information that additional Al Qaida personnel may be present (see Attachment 1). They observed armed men in the compound and formed a perimeter around the compound until more personnel arrived from the first location. An AMF member then approached and yelled for the occupants to surrender. They did not respond except to fire rifle rounds at the AMF member. The AMF member retreated to safety. Later, two other AMF members approached the compound in attempt to convince the occupants to surrender. They entered through the compound gate. They were shot and killed in the entryway by rifle fire coming through a portal in a wall from occupants of the compound. Immediately following these shots, rifle fire was directed at the forces surrounding the compound and grenades were thrown over the compound walls. The US and AMF forces then retreated to positions indicated in Attachment 2. US and AMF forces returned fire and called for ground reinforcements and combat air support (CAS).

The CAS arrived first and multiple bombing raids were made by US combat aircraft. [redacted] arrived with the ground reinforcements in a five vehicle convoy approaching from the south of the compound. [redacted] arrived approximately 10 minutes before the last bombing run made by the CAS. Also in the convoy was SFC CHRISTOPHER SPEER. Upon their arrival, the responding personnel met with the deputy commander of the 19 SFG detachment on scene. [redacted] believed the deputy commander's name was [redacted]. [redacted] observed the compound from approximately 125 meters away. The compound was approximately 100 to 120 feet square with mud walls that were ten to twelve feet tall. There was only one entry point to the compound which was a green, steel gate at the southeast corner. After a few minutes of silence following the airstrikes, a decision was made to enter the compound. The assault element approaching the compound consisted of [redacted] SPEER, [redacted] three other personnel who arrived with [redacted] a platoon leader from the 82nd Airborne [redacted] identified him as [redacted] now assigned to a Ranger battalion), and a rifle squad from the 82nd Airborne (see Attachment 3).

The assault element ran down the road to the compound and entered through a breach in the south wall

THIS DOCUMENT CONTAINS NEITHER RECOMMENDATIONS NOR CONCLUSIONS OF CITF. IT IS THE PROPERTY OF THE CITF AND IS LOANED TO YOUR AGENCY; THIS DOCUMENT IS NOT TO BE RELEASED OUTSIDE YOUR AGENCY.

PAGE 1 OF 5 PAGES

FOUO/LES

Attachment B
00766-000966

Figure 12.20. Witness statements can flip an investigation, especially when dealing with those tricky asphyxial cases.

Source: https://en.wikipedia.org/wiki/File:OC-1_Witness_Statement_on_Omar_Khadr.pdf.

12.4.8. Legal Challenges in Prosecution

Forensic investigations of asphyxial deaths are complicated by many legal obstacles, so prosecuting them is far from simple. The exact reason behind a death is found by using forensic tools and making sure technology and the law are closely connected. A good example is micro Computed Tomography which has revealed many injuries without such evidence, these crimes might never be uncovered, proving how important it is to have strong proof in court. In most cases, recent studies suggest that the clarity and fairness offered by these technologies can sway legal outcomes (Baier et al., 2019). When laws and forensic methods change, the judicial system must keep learning and updating. All in all, being careful yet flexible helps to protect justice and the integrity of the investigations.

12.4.9. Need for Interdisciplinary Collaboration

It's not possible to understand asphyxial deaths by thinking about them in only one way. They bring together the team of investigators, doctors and lawyers to work closely, mainly when the case shows signs of homicide or accidental drowning. It can be necessary to mix the practical knowledge of forensic pathology with legal understanding to figure out asphyxia. Diana (2018) points out that putting together a crime scene—where forensic anthropology might toss out a clue about, say, the circumstances around a newborn's death—can be a game changer. Then, as Boussaid et al. (2017) show figuring out if injuries stem directly from drowning or from something else entirely isn't always cut-and-dry. In short, this teamwork between different areas of expertise improves the reliability and accuracy of investigating these kinds of deaths.

Test Your Knowledge

1. What are the biggest problems when trying to find out the cause of death in asphyxial cases?
2. How does the absence of outside trauma make it harder to investigate asphyxial deaths?

Summary

Handling asphyxial cases is not simple, because they are often full of detailed forensic information. I have looked into several types of asphyxia and it turns out that telling if a death was caused by drowning instead of other forms of asphyxia isn't always simple. Interestingly, the DI seems to offer a fresh way to sharpen diagnostic accuracy in these investigations (Dhakar et al., 2024). Studies often show that asphyxial deaths occur way more frequently among males and in urban spots, hinting at deeper societal trends that, in most cases, deserve a closer look—especially when you start considering ties with socio-economic factors and mental health issues (Nadeem et al., 2024). In short, better forensic methods and more awareness among the public could affect both legal results and the community responses, stressing how vital it is (albeit a bit messily) to have experts from various fields work together to cut down these tragic incidents.

Uncovering the details of asphyxial deaths in forensics often brings up many surprises and the process is usually messy. It is sometimes the case that small, but important, injuries are missed during a regular autopsy. For example, postmortem X-rays can capture tiny fractures in the hyoid-larynx area—little breaks that might hint at asphyxia but slip by during standard examinations (Vashist et al., 2025). They reveal hidden injuries and also point out that the neck is full of unique features that can make things more complicated. Then there's the numerical side of things. Studies using the DI have shown that comparing organ weights can offer a practical if not always straightforward, way to tell drowning apart from other asphyxial cases (Dhakar et al., 2024). Usually, using both imaging techniques and quantitative results strengthens forensic investigations when the evidence is not very clear.

KEY TERMS FROM THIS CHAPTER

Bruising	Chemical asphyxia	chemical exposure
Choking	Contusions	Drowning
hemoglobin	Lungs	metabolism
Positional asphyxia	Spleen	Strangulation
Suffocation	toxicological profile	Ventilation

Short Answer Questions

1. What is meant by asphyxial death?
2. Name the common causes of asphyxial deaths.
3. What is usually seen in the autopsy of a strangulation case?
4. How does drowning lead to asphyxial death?
5. What does postural asphyxia mean and in what circumstances is it usually found?
6. How can carbon monoxide poisoning cause asphyxial death?
7. Why is frothy blood important in cases of drowning?
8. How is suffocation different from strangulation and what is each of these terms?
9. How does smothering cause asphyxial death?
10. What problems are there when trying to diagnose positional asphyxia in infants and elderly people?

Critical Thinking Questions

1. **The primary mechanism of death in strangulation is:**
   a. Respiratory arrest due to airway blockage
   b. Hypoxia due to blood supply obstruction
   c. Cardiac arrhythmia
   d. Drowning
2. **Which of the following signs is commonly seen in drowning deaths?**
   a. Cyanosis of the lips
   b. Ligature marks on the neck
   c. Frothy fluid in the mouth and nose
   d. Petechial hemorrhages in the eyes
3. **The presence of ligature marks around the neck suggests:**
   a. Hanging
   b. Strangulation
   c. Smothering
   d. Drowning
4. **Smothering is typically characterized by:**
   a. Obstruction of the airway by a foreign object
   b. Compression of the chest and neck
   c. Complete obstruction of the nose and mouth
   d. Submersion in liquid
5. **Suffocation due to a closed space (e.g., confined area) usually leads to death by:**
   a. Cardiac arrest due to hypoxia

b. Progressive carbon dioxide poisoning
c. Airway obstruction
d. Thermal shock

Answers to Critical Thinking Questions

1. (b); 2. (c); 3. (b); (c); 5. (b)

References

1. Akhlaghi, M., Okazi, A., Ghorbani, M., Taghaddosi-Nejad, F., Mazinani, R., Mehdizadeh, F., & Sanjari, K. (2013). Causes of death accompanying soft tissue neck hemorrhage. *International Journal of Medical Toxicology and Forensic Medicine, 3*(1, Winter), 10–19. https://doi.org/10.22037/ijmtfm.v3i1(Winter).3982.
2. Albano, G., La Spina, C., Buscemi, R., Palmeri, M., Malandrino, G., Licciardello, F., Midiri, M., et al. (2024). Systematic review of fatal sodium nitrite ingestion cases: Toxicological and forensic implications. *Toxics, 12*(2), 124. https://doi.org/10.3390/toxics12020124.
3. Al-Kandari, N. M. J. (2012). *A Forensic Study of Unnatural Deaths in Kuwait: Epidemiological, Virtual Autopsy and DNA Investigations* (Doctoral thesis). University of Central Lancashire.
4. Amit Kumar, & Harmanjeet Singh. (2023). Histopathological changes in neck structures in cases of asphyxial deaths. *International Journal of Science and Research (IJSR)*. https://www.semanticscholar.org/paper/14849c373e1b8844251b236fd8f37db8aedd7f28 (accessed on 29 May 2025).
5. Aquila, I., Sacco, M. A., Abenavoli, L., Malara, N., Arena, V., Grassi, S., Ausania, F., et al. (2020). Severe acute respiratory syndrome coronavirus 2 pandemic. *Archives of Pathology & Laboratory Medicine, 144*, 1048–1056. https://doi.org/10.5858/arpa.2020-0165-sa.
6. Arcangeli, M., De Matteis, A., Del Fante, Z., Di Fazio, N., Fazio, V., La Russa, R., & Quattrocchi, A. (2020). The importance of post-mortem computed tomography (PMCT) as a complementary diagnostic technique to traditional autopsy in a case of asphyxia related-death. https://core.ac.uk/download/326235075.pdf (accessed on 29 May 2025).
7. Armstrong, E. J., & Erskine, K. L. (2018). Investigation of drowning deaths: A practical review. *Academic Forensic Pathology, 8*, 8–43. https://doi.org/10.23907/2018.002.
8. Atanasijević, T., Jovanović, A. A., Nikolić, S., Popović, V., & Jasović-Gasić, M. (2009). Accidental death due to complete autoerotic asphyxia associated with transvestic fetishism and anal self-stimulation - case report. *Psychiatria Danubina, 21*(2), 246–251.
9. Baier, W. (2019). Applications of micro-CT in the criminal justice system of England and Wales: An impact assessment. https://core.ac.uk/download/337784712.pdf (accessed on 29 May 2025).
10. Balaji, N., Ahamed, B. T., Kumar, P. P., Balaji, R. V., & Balasubramanian, S. (2024). Mechanical asphyxial deaths: An autopsy based cross sectional study in a tertiary care hospital. *Indian Journal of Forensic Medicine & Toxicology, 18*(2), 168–173. https://doi.org/10.37506/mg87wh78.

11. Banerjee, S. (2024). Importance of food forensics and its mandatory implications in health safety and compliance. *IP International Journal of Forensic Medicine and Toxicological Sciences*. https://www.semanticscholar.org/paper/943142dbc4a1fb9a7335940f721e2ab6d232ca78 (accessed on 29 May 2025).

12. Batalis, N. I., Brown, T. T., Collins, K. A., Corey, et al. (2017). A retrospective study of the investigation of homicidal childhood asphyxial deaths. http://deepblue.lib.umich.edu/bitstream/2027.42/144651/1/jfo13666_am.pdf (accessed on 29 May 2025).

13. Beltrán Aroca, C. M., Dye, A., Gill, J. R., et al. (2021). Epidemiology and autopsy findings of 500 drowning deaths. https://core.ac.uk/download/614632649.pdf (accessed on 29 May 2025).

14. Bierens, J. J. L. M., Lunetta, P., Tipton, M., & Warner, D. S. (2016). Physiology of drowning: A review. *Physiology, 31*, 147–166. https://doi.org/10.1152/physiol.00002.2015.

15. Biradar, G., Bakkannavar, M., Shankar, P. K. G., et al. (2015). Choking in a psychiatric patient–a case report. https://core.ac.uk/download/327998830.pdf.

16. Book, R. G. (1993). Autoerotic and assisted sexual asphyxias. https://core.ac.uk/download/427731168.pdf (accessed on 29 May 2025).

17. Boussaid, M., Mesrati, M. A., Belhadj, M., Salem, N. H., Chadly, A., & Aissaoui, A. (2017). Cervical injuries in drowning cases. https://orbi.uliege.be/bitstream/2268/214107/1/1-s2.0-S0379073817302773-main.pdf (accessed on 29 May 2025).

18. Busse, H., Harrop, T., Gunnell, D., & Kipping, R. (2015). Prevalence and associated harm of engagement in self-asphyxial behaviors ('choking game') in young people: A systematic review. *Archives of Disease in Childhood, 100*(12), 1106–1114. https://doi.org/10.1136/archdischild-2015-308187.

19. Cecchetto, G., Cecchin, D., Fais, P., Fichera, G., Franchetti, G., Giraudo, C., & Viel, G. (2022). Forensic applications of micro-computed tomography: A systematic review. https://core.ac.uk/download/590239484.pdf (accessed on 29 May 2025).

20. Chighine, A., Conte, C., De-Giorgio, F., d'Aloja, et al. (2023). Metabolomics investigation of post-mortem human pericardial fluid. https://core.ac.uk/download/614058577.pdf (accessed on 29 May 2025).

21. Dani, R. (2024). Comparative study of femur bone in human and non-human species. *International Journal of Forensic Sciences*. https://www.semanticscholar.org/paper/11428549a286d7a0315c52ed1e085da60fdfa826 (accessed on 29 May 2025).

22. De Villiers, K. (2020). Assessing the functionality and value of introducing death investigators into forensic pathology service in South Africa. https://core.ac.uk/download/528261014.pdf.

23. Dhakar, R. K., Baraw, R., Tomar, M. S., & Singh, S. (2024). Comparative analysis of drowning index: Relevance in drowning deaths versus non-drowning asphyxia deaths. *Indian Journal of Forensic Medicine & Toxicology*. https://www.semanticscholar.org/paper/38091e428f70f42b27bd4e7920264e9324700e8e (accessed on 29 May 2025).

24. Ferariu Petronela Diana. (2018). Forensic investigation of homicide or bodily injury of a newborn by his mother. *RAIS Conference Proceedings*. https://rais.education/wp-content/uploads/2018/11/024FP.pdf (accessed on 29 May 2025).

25. Fischer, E., & Jukola, S. (2024). Bodies of evidence: The 'Excited Delirium Syndrome' and

the epistemology of cause-of-death inquiry. *Studies in History and Philosophy of Science, 104*, 38–47. https://doi.org/10.1016/j.shpsa.2023.12.009.

26. Fletcher, E. (2022). *Weapons of Choice: A Statistical Comparison Between Different Weapons And Resulting Injuries, Opportunist Weapon Selection and Forensic Awareness* [Doctoral thesis, Murdoch University]. https://researchportal.murdoch.edu.au/esploro/outputs/graduate/Weapons-of-choice-A-statistical-comparison/991005541193807891#file-0 (accessed on 29 May 2025).
27. Gerstel, W., McCormick, M., McKenney, K. H., & Kitsap. (2021). The Association for Women Geoscientists. *Scientia*. https://www.semanticscholar.org/paper/c3e4955becf2e8244c960de276e48e51afdf1f61 (accessed on 29 May 2025).
28. Ghadge, M. R., Samel, D. R., Kulkarni, D. V., & Pate, R. (2016). Socio-demographic factors in mechanical asphyxial deaths in Thane region, Maharashtra, India. *International Journal of Research in Medical Sciences, 4*(9), 4078–4083. https://doi.org/10.18203/2320-6012.ijrms20162937.
29. Hamilton, S., & Green, M. (2017). Gross post-mortem changes in the human body: Forensic analysis of the dead and the depositional environment. In *Forensic Science Handbook* (Chapter 1). https://doi.org/10.1002/9781118953358.ch1.
30. Iqbal, F., Ullah, F., Ahmed, I., Samad, A., Tanoli, A. A., & Aziz, I. (2024). An autopsy-based retrospective analysis of asphyxia-related deaths. *BMC Journal of Medical Sciences, 5*(1), 92–95. https://doi.org/10.70905/bmcj.05.01.0286.
31. Ishigami, A., Kubo, S. I., Hara, K., Waters, B., Tokunaga, I., & Nishimura, A. (2019). Fatal accidental asphyxia in the reverse jack-knife position on a chair with wheels. *Legal Medicine (Tokyo, Japan), 36*, 81–84. https://doi.org/10.1016/j.legalmed.2018.11.001.
32. Kaubrytė, S. S., Chmieliauskas, S., Kažukauskė, G., Laima, S., Vasiljevaitė, D., & Stasiūnienė, J. (2024). Investigating confined space asphyxias: Plastic bag involvement and gas inhalation–A case series and literature review. *Acta Medica Lituanica, 31*, 217–230. https://www.semanticscholar.org/paper/6e544af60f6e91d0d07ed0e52e75c8b3d924d269 (accessed on 29 May 2025).
33. Khanna, K., Jakhar, J., Dagar, T., Titiksha, Gill, M., Pal, V., & Yadav, G. (2024). Histopathological examination findings in ligature mark in post-mortem cases of asphyxial deaths: A prospective study. *International Journal of Innovative Research in Medical Science*. https://www.semanticscholar.org/paper/a31fd4004902598c4ad799dfb4eb946c9163f01e (accessed on 29 May 2025).
34. Knight, L. D., & Stoppacher, R. (2014). Investigation of deaths and injury of prison inmates. *Academic Forensic Pathology, 4*, 351–365. https://doi.org/10.23907/2014.047.
35. Locci, E., Bazzano, G., Chighine, A., Locco, F., Ferraro, E., Demontis, R., & d'Aloja, E. (2020). Forensic NMR metabolomics: One more arrow in the quiver. *Metabolomics, 16*(11), 118. https://doi.org/10.1007/s11306-020-01743-6.
36. Locci, E., Chighine, A., Noto, A., et al. (2021). Metabolomics improves the histopathological diagnosis of asphyxial deaths: An animal proof-of-concept model. *Scientific Reports, 11*, 10102. https://doi.org/10.1038/s41598-021-89570-0.
37. Medvedeva, Y. V., Yin, H., Bazrafkan, A., Yeromin, A. V., Ji, S. G., Weiss-Hung, E. J., Sharman, E.,

et al. (2022). Blocking mitochondrial Zn2+ accumulation after ischemia reduces mitochondrial dysfunction and neuronal injury. *The Journal of Neuroscience, 42*, 5281–5292. https://www.semanticscholar.org/paper/bbc067adb1d080da78b079e20e71e44117abc084 (accessed on 29 May 2025).

38. Mittal, P., Sharma, B., & Mittal, N. (2023). Fall or homicide...? The imbroglio answered at autopsy...! *IP International Journal of Forensic Medicine and Toxicological Sciences, 8*, 35–43. https://doi.org/10.18231/j.ijfmts.2023.007.

39. Nadeem, F., Ahmad, I., Ali, A., Khan, M. A., Wasif, M., & Afridi, H. K. (2024). Trends of asphyxial deaths and its association with various demographic factors reported to Forensic Medicine Department Peshawar; an autopsy-based retrospective study. *Journal of Medical Sciences*. https://www.semanticscholar.org/paper/7831715fdc882d136c55e74fd530578f75f33ada (accessed on 29 May 2025).

40. Ocak, U., Ocak, P. E., Huang, L., Xu, W., Zuo, Y., Li, P., Gamdzyk, M., et al. (2020). Inhibition of mast cell tryptase attenuates neuroinflammation via PAR-2/p38/NFκB pathway following asphyxia cardiac arrest in rats. *Journal of Neuroinflammation, 17*. https://www.semanticscholar.org/paper/00c8641760fe61fc056edd2bdac2aeefc79fd81b (accessed on 29 May 2025).

41. Ogawara, T., Usui, A., Homma, N., & Funayama, M. (2022). Diagnosing drowning in postmortem CT images using artificial intelligence. *The Tohoku Journal of Experimental Medicine, 259*, 65–75. https://doi.org/10.1620/tjem.2022.j097.

42. Pal, S. K., Sharma, A., Sehgal, A., & Rana, A. (2017). Diagnosing death with diatoms: A retrospective study of forensic cases in Himachal Pradesh, India. *International Journal of Medical Toxicology and Forensic Medicine, 7*(2), 124–137. https://doi.org/10.22037/ijmtfm.v7i2(Spring).16373.

43. Rangu, S. C., Sundaragiri, S., & Rangu, S. (2016). Suffocation due to irrespirable gases in confined spaces: Accidental deaths of rescuers. *International Journal of Research in Medical Sciences, 4*(5), 1775–1777. https://doi.org/10.18203/2320-6012.ijrms20161271.

44. Rashmi. (2025). Ethical considerations in digital forensics. *International Journal of Innovative Research in Engineering & Multidisciplinary Physical Sciences*. https://www.semanticscholar.org/paper/0f91a82b2f57774a8aef15f76351eac462e5e983 (accessed on 29 May 2025).

45. Robinson, Z. (2022). Evaluation of postmortem protein expression in determining cause of death (University Honors Thesis, Paper 1189). https://doi.org/10.15760/honors.1218.

46. Sacco, M. A., & Aquila, I. (2024). Post mortem molecular biomarkers of asphyxia: A literature review. *International Journal of Molecular Sciences, 25*. https://www.semanticscholar.org/paper/b002348eed38556bfd4fa7d97b8fe8577cbe6a17 (accessed on 29 May 2025).

47. Sanches, F. S., Ramos, F. D. S., Costa, C. C. O. S., Nascimento, R. P. D., Souza, B. S. F., Costa, M. F. D., Costa, S. L., Ribeiro, P. R., Ferreira, R. S., & Silva, V. D. A. D. (2025). Dichloromethane extract from *Amburana cearensis* (Allemão) A.C. Sm. seeds and its coumarin reduce ROS production and protect PC12 cells against glutamate excitotoxicity and oxygen-glucose deprivation. *Antioxidants, 14*(4), 440. https://doi.org/10.3390/antiox14040440.

48. Schumann, J., Hlela, M. B. K. M., Oliverio, S., & Bugeja, L. (2025). Forensic epidemiology: Bridging public health and legal investigations to address modern challenges. *WIREs Forensic Science*. https://www.semanticscholar.org/paper/8d42e639b2fd95ebac486b2022a91acf9e43384a (accessed on 29 May 2025).

49. Varfolomeiev, Y., Pletenetska, A., & Bondar, S. (2024). Detection of the vital origin of the strangulation mark in mechanical asphyxia as an indicator of the development of forensic medicine. *Forensic-Medical Examination*, Higher State Educational Establishment of Ukraine Bukovina State Medical University. https://doi.org/10.24061/2707-8728.1.2024.2.

50. Vashist, Y., Malik, Y., Kundu, P., Sharma, S., Rajindran, R., & Sharma, G. (2025). Hyoid bone imaging—boon in asphyxia deaths autopsy—A retrospective study. *Journal of Indian Academy of Forensic Medicine*. https://doi.org/10.1177/09710973251327657.

51. World Health Organization, Council for International Organizations of Medical Sciences (CIOMS). (2001). *Current Challenges in Pharmacovigilance: Report of CIOMS Working Group V*. https://doi.org/ISBN 92 9036 074 7.

INDEX

B

C

Q

R

S

T

U

V

W

X